The Johns Hopkins Hospital

SCHOOL OF NURSING

1889-1949

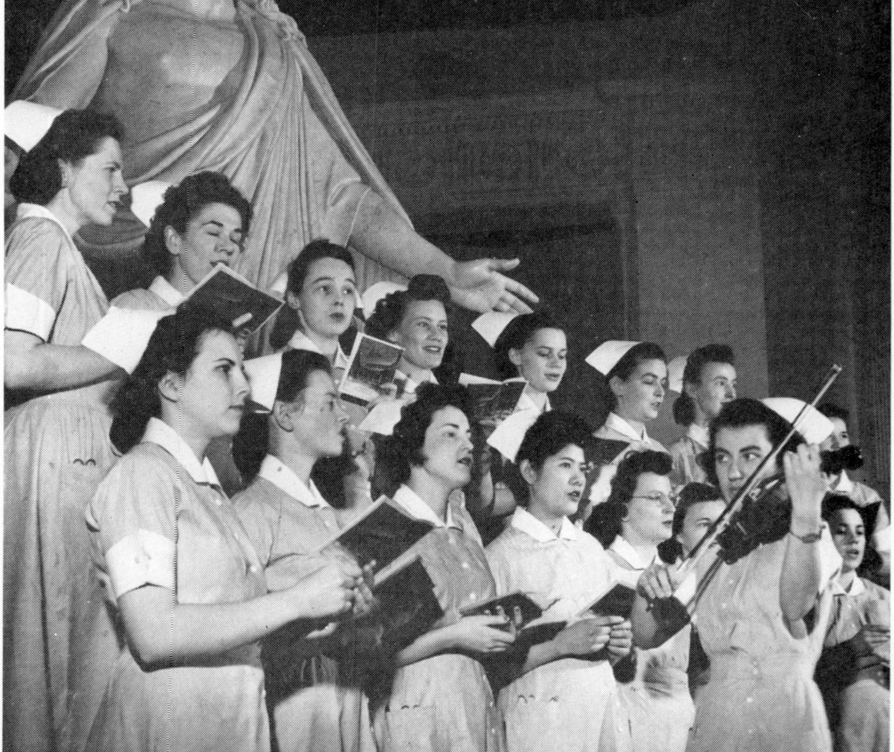

The Johns Hopkins Hospital SCHOOL OF NURSING

1889-1949

by

ETHEL JOHNS

and

BLANCHE PFEFFERKORN

Baltimore: 1954

THE JOHNS HOPKINS PRESS

Distributed in Great Britain, India, and Pakistan by Geoffrey Cumberlege: Oxford University Press, London, Bombay, and Karachi. Printed in the U.S.A. by Vail-Ballou Press. Library of Congress Catalog Card Number: 54-8006

Foreword

In 1946 the Alumnae Association of the Johns Hopkins Hospital School of Nursing decided to sponsor the writing of the history of the school, feeling that the story of its founding and development would be a valuable contribution to the history of nursing.

A committee was appointed:

- Jessie Black McVicar, '30, Chairman 1946–48; member 1948–54
- Annabelle Gleason Brack, '29, member 1946–48; Chairman 1948–54
- Mary Cloud Bean, '95
- Helen Wilber Athey, '05
- Effie J. Taylor, '07
- Elizabeth Thomas Kent, '08
- Claire Ridgely Craigen, '12
- Hester K. Frederick, '12
- Alta Elizabeth Dines, '14
- Anna D. Wolf, '15
- Virginia M. Dunbar, '23

Cecilia A. McMahon, '28
K. Virginia Betzold, '33

That this difficult project, often overwhelming in its many aspects, has come to a successful conclusion is due in no small measure to the enthusiasm and untiring efforts of the members of this committee. They were fortunate in the choice of Ethel Johns and Blanche Pfefferkorn as authors. Both have had distinguished careers in nursing, and have written books and numerous articles on nursing and nursing education.

Ethel Johns was born and educated in England. She graduated from the Winnipeg General Hospital School of Nursing in Canada and later did postgraduate work as a special student at Teachers College, Columbia University. While serving as the director of the Vancouver General Hospital School of Nursing, Miss Johns took part in the organization of the Department of Nursing and Health in the University of British Columbia and subsequently became its first director. Miss Johns attained international recognition as field director attached to the Paris office of the Rockefeller Foundation, assisting in the organization of schools of nursing in Hungary and Roumania.

Later she returned to Canada as editor of *The Canadian Nurse*, the official organ of the Canadian Nurses Association. Upon her retirement, Miss Johns was named by the Association to receive on behalf of all its members the honorary degree of Doctor of Laws, conferred by Mount Allison University as a mark of recognition of the services rendered by the nurses of Canada to their country.

Because of her close tie with the Johns Hopkins Hospital School of Nursing through the writing of this history, Miss Johns was elected to honorary membership in the Johns Hopkins Hospital Nurses Alumnae Association in 1953.

Blanche Pfefferkorn, a native Baltimorean, graduated from the Johns Hopkins Hospital Training School for Nurses in 1911. She received the Bachelor of Science degree from Columbia University in 1916, and later was awarded the Isabel Hampton Robb Fellowship for graduate study in Teachers College, Columbia University.

For many years Miss Pfefferkorn was engaged in the field of nursing education and research. She was instructor and assistant professor of nursing at the University of Cincinnati School of Nursing and Health; executive secretary of the National League of Nursing Education; research worker at the Bellevue School of Nursing; and for seventeen years prior to her retirement in 1949 director of studies of the National League of Nursing Education. We are proud to claim her as one of our most distinguished alumnae.

The Johns Hopkins Hospital Nurses Alumnae Association presents this history with pride in the accomplishments of the School of Nursing and faith in its future.

HELEN GROSE FALLON, '30, *President*
Johns Hopkins Hospital Nurses Alumnae Association, Inc.

Baltimore, Maryland
September 30, 1953

Johns Hopkins Hospital

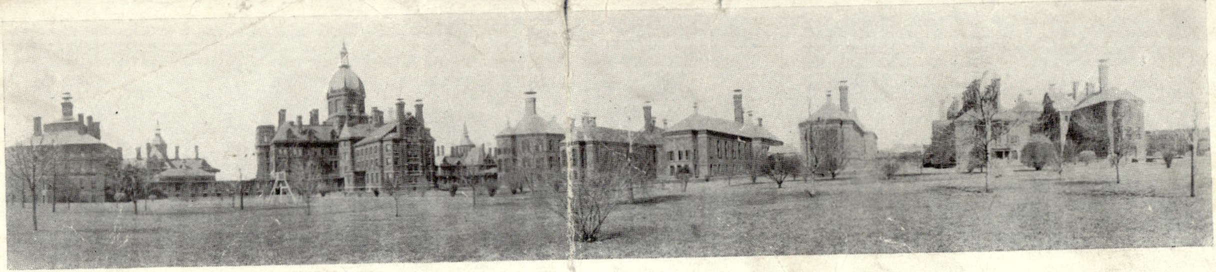

1899

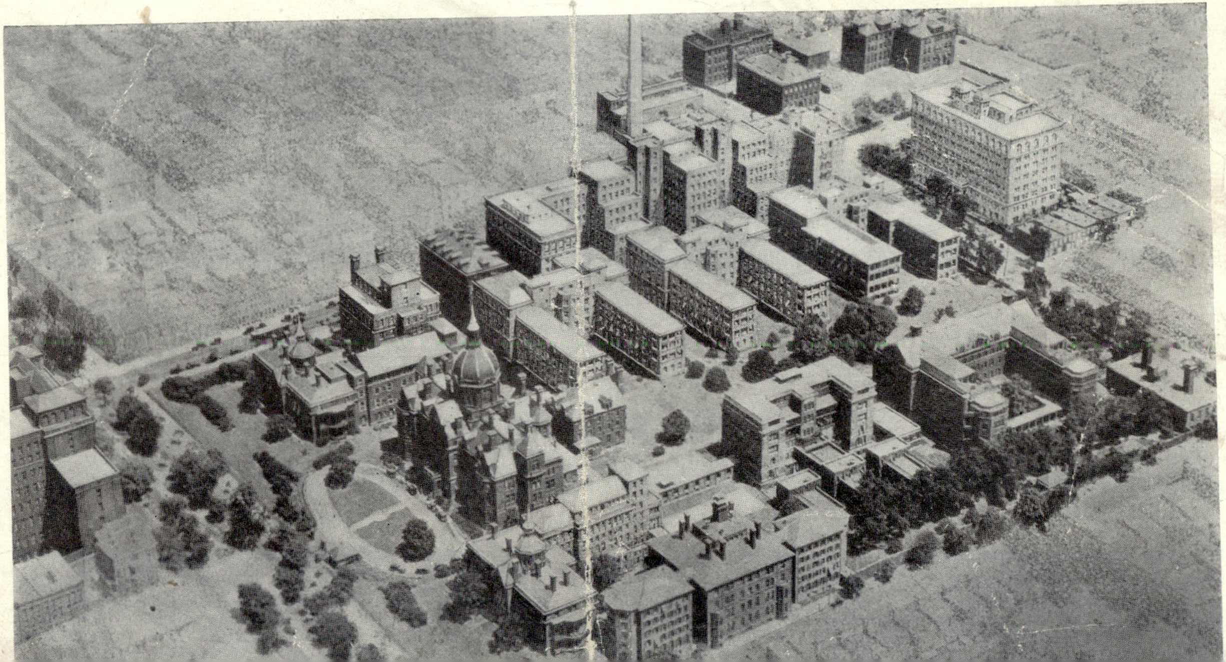

Acknowledgments

THIS story of the founding and early development of the Johns Hopkins Hospital School of Nursing extends over a period of forty years, that is to say from 1867 to 1907, and is based almost entirely on original documents preserved in the archives of the Hospital, the School of Nursing and the Alumnae Association. Free access to these sources was generously accorded me by the Director of the School of Nursing, Miss Anna D. Wolf, and by other authorities, a privilege for which I am most grateful. My thanks are also due to Dr. Alan M. Chesney, Dean of the Medical Faculty, the Johns Hopkins University School of Medicine, for his courtesy in permitting me to read an unpublished historical sketch, written by Dr. Henry Mills Hurd, which was not only valuable in itself but also proved to be indispensable in interpreting documentation derived from other sources.

Permission to quote from personal correspondence was granted by members of the family of Isabel Hampton Robb and a similar privilege was accorded by the family of Mary Adelaide Nutting. Some very interesting biographical material, bearing on the early life of Isabel Hampton Robb, previously prepared by Dr. Edith Ware on behalf of the Johns Hopkins Hospital Nurses Alumnae Association, was freely drawn upon, and access to an unique collection of historical items was generously afforded by Ruth Brewster Sherman. Little, Brown and Company, and Harper and Brothers both allowed certain excerpts to be quoted from books respectively published by them.

During the earlier stages of the project, the Alumnae Association (with the kind permission of the Director of the School of Nursing) arranged for me to reside in the Main Nurses Home and I was thus near enough to the School and to the Hospital to observe the distinctive qualities of both. There were also opportunities to talk with nurses who had been associated with the School from the beginning. To listen to Lavinia Dock as she told the thrilling tale of the first few years was an unforgettable experience and the pungent comments of Elsie Lawler shed new light on many a complicated situation. Although space will not permit individual mention of the nurses who so patiently submitted to questioning, I should like to assure all of them that it was they who made it possible to reflect in some measure, the dignity, the devotion and the serenity of those early days.

A special tribute is due to Mrs. C. Bernard Brack, chairman of the History Committee, for her unfailing support and encouragement and for the stimulus afforded by her keen sense of literary values. I am most grateful to Mrs. Guthrie J. McVicar, chairman of the Committee on Review, for arranging personal contacts that were very helpful from an historical point of view, and for her sympathetic interpretation of situations that might otherwise have been baffling to anyone not a member of the School. Sincere appreciation is also tendered to Mrs. Trevor New who gave expert assistance in the preparation of the manuscript.

It is freely admitted that, for the sake of brevity, some of the documents quoted in full might have been summarized. Yet any departure from the original text always seemed to detract from its true significance. These men and women not only made history —they also wrote it. On the evening before I began my task, I listened to an address given at the Johns Hopkins University by the eminent American historian, Douglas Southall Freeman. His stern admonition still rings in my ears: "As they wrote it, so let it stand."

E. J.

* * *

To write the history of a great institution is a privilege. To write the history of one's own school is a special privilege; it also imposes a special obligation—to write as unbiasedly as possible and to convey to the reader an awareness of the aspirations, the struggles, the disappointments, and the accomplishments that gave the institution its stature. It is the duty of the historian to weigh and to select from the available evidence, to present unfavorable as well as favorable events, and to interpret according to his best judgment the facts as they were—not as he would like them to have been.

To fulfill this duty the writer of contemporary history needs the help and counsel of many people. To the many individuals who aided in the making of the second part of this history, I wish to acknowledge my indebtedness and to express my appreciation. If I do not mention all by name I am none the less grateful for their assistance.

I think first of the librarians. Mrs. Zola Riches, librarian in the School of Nursing, always had time to find a particular reference. Ellen F. Watson, assistant in the General Reference Department of the Enoch Pratt Free Library, rendered unfailing help in solving special problems and in locating special sources of information. Ruth L. Tyler, in charge of the Reading Room of the William H. Welch Medical Library, introduced me to the stacks in Welch. Clement G. Vitek, librarian in the offices of the *Sunpapers* of Baltimore, permitted me access to the clipping files of those papers, a privilege I valued highly.

I am especially indebted to Mrs. Lorana A. Smart. Mrs. Smart expertly typed and retyped the manuscript, assisted with the editing, and shared the author's concern that details of the copy should be correct.

Two people without whom I would have been at a loss to uncover the School archives were Grace Davis, registrar, and Esther Murray, assistant registrar, in the School of Nursing. They are veritable mines of information. For more than two years I interrupted their day and infringed upon their time, and if occasionally I tried their patience they never once showed it. To them I owe particular thanks.

Still others to whom I owe thanks are Dr. Edwin L. Crosby, director of the Johns Hopkins Hospital, and Anna D. Wolf, director of the School of Nursing, who allowed a bound set of the *Johns Hopkins Nurses Alumnae Magazine* to accompany me to California and to remain there during the sixteen months I was working on the history in Sierra Madre; to Dr. Alan M. Chesney who permitted me to read an unpublished manuscript, entitled *History of the First-Quarter of the Johns Hopkins Hospital, 1889–1914*, by the late Dr. Henry M. Hurd, first superintendent of the Johns Hopkins Hospital, which was later edited and extended by the late Dr. Lewellys F. Barker, onetime professor of medicine in the School of Medicine and physician-in-chief in the Hospital; to Dr. Winford H. Smith, former director of the Hospital for more than thirty years, who has a remarkable memory and who untangled some perplexing questions; to Loula E. Kennedy who gave valuable assistance in developing the library study; to Miriam Ames who read the first manuscript of "Nursing the Community"; to Dorothy Plum, bibliographer in the library of Vassar College, for an indefinite loan of the *Announcement of the Training Camp for Nurses at Vassar College;* to Mrs. May Ermer McNeill, executive secretary of the Johns Hopkins Hospital Nurses Alumnae Association, who saw to it that I had the necessary supplies and otherwise gave assistance; to Mrs. Ann G. Krauk, secretary to the director of the Hospital, for making available Hospital records.

Most of all I wish to record my gratitude to the members of the Committee on the History of the School of Nursing who had the laborious responsibility of reading my several manuscripts. Their criticisms and suggestions helped greatly in the revision. To have been associated with the committee members, individually and as a group, for more than three years has been a satisfying experience.

Finally I must not forget the men and women of Johns Hopkins who were prodigal with their pens and who left to posterity a storehouse of priceless records.

B.P.

Table of Contents

PART TWO: 1907–1949

SPECIAL STUDIES

APPENDIX

List of Illustrations

TABLES

DIAGRAMS

Part One: 1869-1907

The Founder

ALTHOUGH much has been written about the famous University and Hospital which bear his name, comparatively little light seems so far to have been shed on Johns Hopkins himself. He remains a shadowy and enigmatic figure, never quite emerging either from his rather forbidding portraits or from the conventional biographical sketches which somehow seem to hide more than they reveal. And yet there can be no doubt that he was a remarkable man—able and imaginative, ruthless and compassionate.

Born in the last decade of the eighteenth century, he came of a Quaker family who had come to the new colony of Maryland in search of the religious tolerance and equality of civil rights denied to them elsewhere and who must have found the serenity of landscape and climate almost as refreshing as did Captain John Smith of Virginia who in 1607 thus set down his first impressions of it:

"There is but one entrance by Sea into this Country, and that is a very goodly Bay, 18 or 20 myles broad. . . . Within is a country of fruitful and delightsome land. . . . Not mountainous nor yet low . . . but pleasant plaine hills and fertile valleyes, one prettily crossing another and watered so conveniently with fresh brookes and springs. . . . Heaven and earth never agreed better to frame a place for man's habitation. . . . The chiefe of winter is halfe December, January, February, and halfe March. . . . The cold is extreame sharpe, but here the Proverbe is true, that no extreame long continueth."

In spite of this tranquil setting, the social and political conditions under which Maryland came into being can hardly be described as liberal. The Royal Charter granted by King Charles the first to Cecil Calvert, second Lord Baltimore, appointed him to be "Lord Proprietor of all land and water within its boundaries with full authority, imperial, aristocratic and feudal." Furthermore, Calvert and his principal associates, like their Royal Master, were staunch Roman Catholics and admission to the colony might well have been confined to persons of that faith. It is recorded, however, that among the hundred and twenty-eight souls who sailed for the New World in "The Ark and the Dove" there were "some Protestants and even a few Anglicans" who had been promised that they might worship as they pleased.

After a long and stormy voyage, "The Ark and the Dove" cast anchor on the fifth day of March in the year 1635 in Chesapeake Bay and the ship's company took peaceful possession of the "fruitful and delightsome land" that had gladdened the heart of Captain John Smith of Virginia. Some thirty-five years later, a Quaker gentleman, Wenlock Christison by name, came to Maryland from Massachusetts in order to escape religious persecution and built a family mansion which he hopefully named "The End of Controversie." Then, as time went on, other members of the Society of Friends sought a similar haven and among them were the great-grandparents of Johns Hopkins.

His father and mother, Samuel Hopkins and Sarah Janney, were the proprietors of "Whitehall," a thriving tobacco plantation in Anne Arundel County, and it was here that in 1795 their second son was born and was given the name of his paternal great-grandmother, Margaret Johns. Until the boy was twelve years old, the family were in comfortable circumstances but in 1807 the Society of Friends declared the ownership of slaves to be morally unjustifiable and Samuel Hopkins not only granted his able-bodied slaves their freedom but also assumed the support of those no longer fit to work. Deprived of slave labor, the plantation ceased to flourish and the family fortunes dwindled accordingly. The education of a growing family of children at last became so heavy a burden that Samuel Hopkins decided to send Johns to Baltimore to live with and work for his uncle, Gerard Hopkins, a prosperous merchant who had established himself in what George Washington described as "the risingest town in America except the Federal City." Helen Hopkins Thom,[1] a grand-niece of Johns Hopkins, has given a vivid picture of how it must have looked to the eager lad when he saw it for the first time:

"A few stately mansions dotted the surrounding hills while the town itself, built close to the land-locked harbor, was only a few years old, having been given its charter as a city in 1796. There were no tall structures and few public buildings of any sort and the streets were paved with cobble-stones. . . . The tall masts of the clipper ships towered above the wharves and the straggling streets, lined with low houses, mostly of frame, seemed centered at the foot of the hills and close to the water. . . . A giant flag floated from Fort McHenry, its stars and stripes, new-born and self-conscious, a flaunting defiance in the face of the English vessels at anchor, loading their cargoes of tobacco. Covered Conestoga wagons, spattered with mud, crowded in from the West, forming lines down the main streets, their blue-shirted teamsters gathering for refreshments at the numerous inns."

Other and gentler aspects were observed by Frances Trollope [2] when a few years later she paid a brief visit to Baltimore: "It is one of the handsomest cities to approach in the Union. The noble column erected to the memory of Washington, and the Catholic Cathedral with its beautiful dome are seen at a great distance. . . . Even the private dwellings had an air of magnificence from the abundance of white marble with which many of them were adorned." Mrs. Trollope was equally impressed by "the vast number of churches and chapels in the city in proportion to its extent" and by such evidences of culture as "the handsome museum super-

[1] Helen Hopkins Thom, *Johns Hopkins, A Silhouette*. Baltimore, The Johns Hopkins Press, 1929

[2] Frances Milton Trollope, *Domestic Manners of the Americans*. New York, Knopf, 1949

intended by one of the Peale family, well known for their devotion to natural science and works of art."

As for the ladies of Baltimore, they quite enchanted her: "I never saw anywhere so many beautiful women at one glance, all dressed with that attention to taste and smartness which seems to be the distinguishing characteristic of the Baltimore females of all ranks." Elsewhere in the United States, it had seemed to Mrs. Trollope that "women, even the very highest, occupy themselves with their household concerns in a manner that precludes the possibility of their becoming elegant and enlightened companions. In Baltimore, Philadelphia and New York, I met with some exceptions." Any Quaker lady whom Mrs. Trollope may have encountered in Baltimore must surely have been included in this select company, for she would be regarded by the male members of the Society of Friends as a mental and spiritual equal who might even be "moved to speak in Meeting" if she so desired. She would look well to the ways of her household and while her "plain dress" might be sober in hue it would be made of rich material that fell in graceful lines as she went her stately way.

It was in a setting such as this that Johns Hopkins first met his cousin Elizabeth and that they fell in love with one another. From the beginning, he had been happy in his uncle's home and when he was only nineteen had shown such an amazing talent for business that he was sometimes left in charge: "I want thee to put an old head on young shoulders" said Gerard Hopkins when he set off on a long journey and, upon his return, found that his confidence in his nephew had been justified. Yet when it came to accepting him as a son-in-law, Gerard Hopkins hesitated to run counter to the Quaker belief that marriage between cousins was neither seemly nor desirable and flatly refused to give his consent to an engagement. Johns was ready to defy this display of parental authority while Elizabeth felt constrained to obey her father. Neither of them ever married but they remained close friends all their lives.

After the break with his uncle, Johns Hopkins struck out for himself. Henceforth he devoted his energies to various commercial enterprises and especially to the development of the Baltimore and Ohio Railroads, which he later regarded as the most productive of his many holdings. In business dealings he was bold and self-reliant but often high-handed. Swift and even generous in large undertakings, he was inclined to be niggardly about small expenditures. Certainly no ascetic, he lived comfortably in the lavish style of the time, kept a good table, and offered his friends the best wine that money could buy. Although he never travelled widely, he sought the company of those who had and took a lively interest in the artistic adornment of the house and gardens at Clifton, a summer home which he had built on a wooded ridge overlooking the waters of the Patapsco. The stately mansion still stands, surrounded by some fine old trees, in what is now a public park.

Somehow or other, the getting and spending of money never quite satisfied Johns Hopkins and all through the dull fabric of his outer life there ran a bright thread of idealism that was to lead him to the fulfillment of a dream. It is possible that the public benefactions of his friend George Peabody may have touched his imagination and set him thinking, but it is not easy to trace the source of his interest in higher education for he himself was not a highly educated man and it is remarkable that he should have conceived so comprehensive a plan for the establishment of a university, associated with a medical school. Nevertheless, Dr. Henry Mills Hurd, the first superintendent of the Johns Hopkins Hospital, was firmly convinced that although several persons claimed to have influenced him, these bold and original ideas were essentially his own. His interest in hospitals and in nursing obviously stemmed from his personal experience during a terrible epidemic of cholera that broke out in Baltimore in 1832 when he contracted the disease and nearly died of it. Appalled by the utter lack of either hospital accommodation or nursing service, he subsequently became a member of the governing boards of several charitable institutions, among them the Maryland Hospital for the Insane which at that time occupied part of what was later to become the site of the Johns Hopkins Hospital.

In 1867, while Johns Hopkins, Francis T. King and Judge George Dobbin were all serving as members of the Board of Visitors of the Maryland Hospital, an investigation of the nursing service disclosed that "the nurses did not possess either method, order, invention or energy, or are sufficient in number or intelligence to discharge their duties." In that same year, Johns Hopkins caused two Bills to be introduced into the General Assembly of the State of Maryland authorizing the formation of two corporations to be known as the Johns Hopkins Hospital and the Johns Hopkins University. The Hospital was not to open its doors for twenty-two years, but as early as 1867 its founder named Francis T. King as the president of its Board of Trustees and Judge George Dobbin as a charter member of that body. The insight into the problems of nursing service that all three acquired as members of the Board of Visitors at the Maryland Hospital may have prompted Johns Hopkins to make sure that the Hospital which was to bear his name should also serve as a center for the education of nurses.

Early in 1873, Johns Hopkins began to feel the full weight of his seventy-eight years. The ultimate disposition of his large estate had long been decided upon and he had given specific directions in his will regarding its use for the establishment and maintenance of the Johns Hopkins University and the Johns Hopkins Hospital. So far, he had been unwilling either to relinquish control of his business affairs or to part with any of his wealth, but now he realized that his strength was slowly ebbing and that the reins were slipping out of his hands. On the tenth day of March he summoned his lawyer, Charles J. M. Gwinn, and directed him to draft a letter to his Trustees in which certain instructions concerning the Johns Hopkins Hospital were embodied. An excerpt from that letter clearly shows what he had in mind with respect to nursing service and the education of nurses:

"I desire you to establish, in connection with the hospital, a training school for female nurses. This provision will secure the services of women competent to care for the sick in the hospital wards, and will enable you to benefit the whole community by supplying it with a class of trained and experienced nurses."

This letter was presented to the Board of Trustees at a meeting held on March 11, 1873, and was duly incorporated in the Minutes. It is evident, therefore, that the School of Nursing actually had its origin during the lifetime of the Founder even though its doors were not to open until sixteen years after his death. To quote Dr.

Hurd: "As far as can be ascertained, this is the first instance in which before a Hospital was built, directions were given by the founder for the establishment of a training school through which the services of competent women might be secured to nurse the patients and to supply the community with trained and experienced nurses."

All through the long hot summer and the cool autumn days, Johns Hopkins looked out from the wide windows of Clifton toward the hill on which his Hospital would stand. It was still his dream that the University would be built at Clifton and that the intervening ridge of high land between it and the Hospital would become a great educational center. None of this would he live to see but somehow it was comforting to remember that Elizabeth Hopkins still lived on a pleasant street in Baltimore in the dignified home that he had given to her. If only she could have been persuaded to free herself from the authority of her father and the Society of Friends, she would have married him and there might have been children to inherit the wealth he had striven so hard to win. As the shadows deepened into winter, Clifton seemed strangely desolate and forlorn. On Christmas Eve, the turbulent lonely life came to an end and the restless spirit entered into peace.

Doctor Billings

and the School of Nursing

GREAT deliberation was exercised by the Trustees in dealing with the provisions of Johns Hopkins' bequest. They were compelled to move slowly since the terms of the will did not permit the use of capital funds for building purposes and it was therefore necessary to restrict expenditures to the income available from interest. Furthermore, Johns Hopkins had requested that the best possible advice be obtained from experts in the hospital field before building operations began at all and it was to this task that the Trustees first addressed themselves.

At a meeting held on November 13, 1874, it was decided that "five distinguished physicians" each of whom was regarded as an authority should be requested to prepare essays concerning the best methods of construction and general organization. They were also asked to submit recommendations with respect to "the accommodations needed for the training school for nurses and whether they should be within the Hospital building or separated from it." The consultants thus chosen included Dr. John S. Billings, Assistant Surgeon in the United States Army; Dr. Norton Folsom, Superintendent of the Massachusetts General Hospital; Dr. Joseph Jones, professor of chemistry and clinical medicine in the University of Louisiana and surgeon in the Confederate Army during the Civil War; Dr. Caspar Morris, of Philadelphia; and Dr. Stephen Smith, of New York. By the end of 1875, all five essays had been received by the Board of Trustees and though all were utilized to some extent in subsequent planning, the essay presented by Dr. Billings was considered the best and led to his appointment in July, 1876, as supervisor of the construction of the Hospital.

As might have been expected, there was considerable difference of opinion among the consultants as to the best method of organizing the training school for nurses. Dr. Joseph Jones, doubtless influenced by his military background, made some rather drastic recommendations: "Each of the twenty female head nurses and the forty assistant female nurses should be appointed by the president of the Hospital, and each head nurse and her assistants should be permanently attached to one ward and limited rigidly to the discharge of duty therein." He also contended that the proper place for the instruction of nurses was in the ward itself and that no separate school for nurses was needed: "If, however, the President and the Board of Trustees should deem special instruction necessary, the resident surgeon and one or more attending physicians of the hospital might instruct the nurses by lectures and practical demonstrations." Dr. Jones further recommended that nurses should not be less than twenty-five years of age nor more than sixty, and that no assistant nurse should be kept on duty for longer than twelve hours "for if the health and strength of the nurses be not carefully husbanded their efficiency will sooner or later be impaired."

The recommendations of both Dr. Morris and Dr. Smith were somewhat vague and inconclusive but Dr. Folsom suggested that the school should be "a separate organization under the charge of the Hospital." Dr. Billings held strong convictions with respect to the training of nurses and, as the official supervisor of the construction of the Hospital, he was in a position to influence the thinking of the Trustees. During the Civil War he had served with distinction as an army surgeon, an experience which was to color his attitude toward nursing service and education for some time to come. In 1864 he had been transferred from active duty to the War Department in Washington where he played an important part in the reorganization of military hospitals on a peacetime basis and in the improvement of the Marine Hospital Service. His outstanding ability as a pioneer in the field of public health soon became manifest as did his keen interest in medical education. From the outset, he fully realized the educational implications of his new task and a letter to the Trustees of the Johns Hopkins Hospital indicates his approach:

"It should be remembered that our buildings and machinery are simply tools and instruments, and that the real Hospital, the moving and animating soul of the institution, which is to do its work and determine its character, consists of the brains to be put in it. Whether it shall be a truly great Hospital and a charity such as was intended by its founder, is not a matter solely of arrangement and plan of buildings, it depends upon not more than half-a-dozen men and one or two women. . . . The most difficult thing in forming this Hospital is to find the proper and suitable persons to be the soul and motive power of the institution."

Dr. Billings' first step was to seek advice abroad and he made a three-months tour of observation during which he visited hospitals in Holland, Germany, Austria, Italy, France and Great Britain. He seldom mentioned the names of persons with whom he conferred and there is, therefore, no record of any meeting with Florence Nightingale although he must certainly have heard of her current activities as a sanitarian and as a participant in the organization of the Army Medical School. However, he did visit St. Thomas's Hospital in London and it seems probable that he talked with Mrs. Wardroper, its Matron. If so, he must have gotten a first-hand impression of "the Nightingale system" since, at that time, Miss Nightingale maintained a closer contact with the School than ever before.

Early in January 1877 Dr. Billings addressed a letter to Mr. Francis T. King, president of the Board of Trustees, in which he gave his impressions of what he had seen in Europe. For the most part, his recommendations bore directly upon various aspects of hospital construction, especially upon those which had to do with sanitation and the prevention of the spread of infection. Finally, and with visible reluctance, he tackled the vexing question of nursing service:

"In previous reports, I have refrained from alluding to the subject of female nurses, to the organization of the training school or to the relation which it should have to the Hospital, because I had not sufficient information to feel authorized to advise on this subject. I have inquired carefully as to the working of the nursing system in the several hospitals which I visited, and in addition to what has been published on the subject, which is almost exclusively by those favourable to what is known as the Nightingale system. I have also consulted the opinions of those most experienced in hospital management, which opinions are by no means as favourable as I had anticipated, and are unanimous in the statement that one of the most difficult problems in connection with this Hospital will be the organization of its system of nurses if anything like the Nightingale plan is to be adopted.

"As the time has now come when some decision must be made as to the scope and character of the training school, and the kind of nurses we should endeavor to obtain and to provide for, I will briefly state the opinions I have formed.

"As I understand the intention of the Founder and the opinions of the Trustees, this training school is not to be put in the hands of any religious order, and I therefore exclude all such from consideration.

"Miss Nightingale's views as to female nurses and their amplification and exposition by Mrs. Wardroper and Miss Lees—and by publications of the Bellevue Hospital training school—are well known. By this school it is held that female nurses should be as far as possible, refined, educated women, fitted to move in good society—who should be thoroughly trained in everything pertaining to the management of the sick—from the washing of bedpans to the regulation of temperature and ventilation and the noting of symptoms for the physician—who should be good cooks and seamstresses—gentlewomen also, thoroughly kind-hearted, yet with firmness and decision, and power of control of unruly patients. They should know as much as the surgeon about the dressing of wounds and as much as the physician about the meaning of symptoms—yet they must have no tendency to become medical women, or to set up their own opinions in practice. They must, of course, be of unspotted morals and chastity.

"It is acknowledged that to secure and retain such women is difficult—and that to do it, the accommodations and arrangements must be of a special kind. It is insisted that women of this kind must not be subordinate to any man—and that it is only a woman who can understand and manage them—that the Superintendent of the female nurses should be the sole head of all the women employed in the hospital—and that she should not herself be subordinate to the Superintendent of the hospital but should report only to the Board of Trustees, nay, logically, the conclusion is that the Board of Trustees should be composed partly of women in order to carry out the principle that no woman shall be subordinate to a man.

"Upon these views, I would remark that I do not believe it is possible to obtain such women for nurses, except from religious motives, that the great majority of the nurses in the St. Thomas's Hospital are not of this character, but are of the class from which the better kind of English domestic servants are obtained, that the denunciations of attempts to govern women by men are not worth considering except as indicating that those who utter them are not desirable persons to be associated with in an institution of this kind, and that I think that the experiences as to female nurses of European hospitals or training schools are not of much value to us here in Baltimore since the circumstances are so different, and the class of women whom we may expect to induce to enter and remain as nurses is so unlike the class from which European hospitals are supplied that failure will be the result of attempting to transplant their methods here.

"The opinions of those connected with the training school for nurses at New Haven appear to me much more worthy of consideration. Instead of attempting to establish an independent female hierarchy, which will consider from the commencement that one of its main objects is to endeavor to be independent of all males, who are to be considered as the natural enemies of the organization, I find in the New Haven Hospital a superintendent of the female nurses who devotes her time and attention to teaching the women how to nurse—and a matron who is the housekeeper of the establishment, each of these attending to her own department, and reporting to the authorities of the Hospital.

The establishment in New Haven is a small one but the same principle will apply in this Hospital. The superintendent of the training school will have plenty to do to attend to that, if she does it properly, and I can see no possible good in having her also attempt to supervise the kitchen, the laundry, etc.

"As a rule, I agree with the general opinion that women are better nurses than men but two or three of the best nurses I ever saw were males, and for some cases all physicians would strongly prefer such to any woman. A really well trained first-class male nurse can always find employment but there are very few such, and in this country there is no place where they can be trained. If the right sort of material presents itself I think it would be worth while for the authorities of this Hospital to try the experiment of training a few, say half-a-dozen male nurses, for whom I am sure there will be no lack of employment. One great difficulty with both male and female nurses is that if of a superior class, they wish to become doctors and doctoresses.

"As I understand the duties of a female nurse, they lie chiefly in the ward itself, that is her room, the absence of which is sometimes complained of, and her place of rest while on duty is in the middle of it.

"If a female nurse is a properly organized and healthy woman, she will certainly at times be subject to strong temptation under which occasionally one will fall, and this occurs in all hospitals where women are employed, without any exception whatever. Something may be done, however, to remove opportunities—and I believe the construction proposed effects this as far as it is worthwhile to attempt it."

These forthright opinions were an integral part of a closely reasoned formal report and therefore reflect the attitude of Dr. Billings, at that particular time, to women in general and nurses in particular. According to his biographer,[1] "His severe regard for the truth, his austere feeling for duty were such that he could not be fascinated by beauty nor dazzled by brilliancy. . . . Dr. Billings' feeling for the fair sex was that of a sincere friend or a kindly mentor." Dr. Garrison once asked General

[1] Fielding H. Garrison, *John Shaw Billings, A Memoir*. New York, G. P. Putnam's Sons, 1915

Alfred Woodhull about the attitude of women towards Dr. Billings and received a curt and enigmatic reply: "I think that women would have liked him if he had given them a chance—he didn't."

Yet it is evident that some women, a few of whom happened to be nurses, did like him. As a young man, he had served as an intern at St. John's Hospital in Cincinnati and here came under the gentle influence of Sister Anthony and the nuns who worked with her. "His grave serious ways, his austere life, the look of mild melancholy in his blue eyes, won their regard in such wise that he became known among these ladies as 'St. John of the Hospital.' " A few years later, during the campaign before Richmond, Sisters of Charity helped him to care for the wounded and this and kindred experiences may have led to the conviction that only the religious motive could induce women of character and refinement to become nurses.

At the Johns Hopkins Hospital he was confronted with the stubborn fact that the founder had not wished the direction of the School of Nursing to be placed in the hands of any religious order and this alternative was consequently ruled out. Johns Hopkins had also made it clear that the purpose of the School was to prepare women, rather than men, to become trained nurses and, as a result, Dr. Billings' plaintive appeal to the Trustees for "the training of a few, say half-a-dozen male nurses" had fallen on deaf ears. Did all this mean that he might be compelled to accept "the Nightingale system" with its bold defiance of masculine authority and its audacious demand that nurses be allowed to manage their own affairs?

So far as the employment of male nurses was concerned, it happened that in one instance things did go his way. On July 15, 1879, while the Hospital was still under construction, the builder's records contained the following entry:

"An Accident. About one o'clock this afternoon Mr. John K. Bruff, foreman of the bricklayers at work on the kitchen building, while going up a ladder to where his men were at work fell to the cellar below, a distance of 30 feet, breaking his right leg between the ankle and the knee. He was removed to the basement floor of the Octagon Ward. Dr. Alan P. Smith was

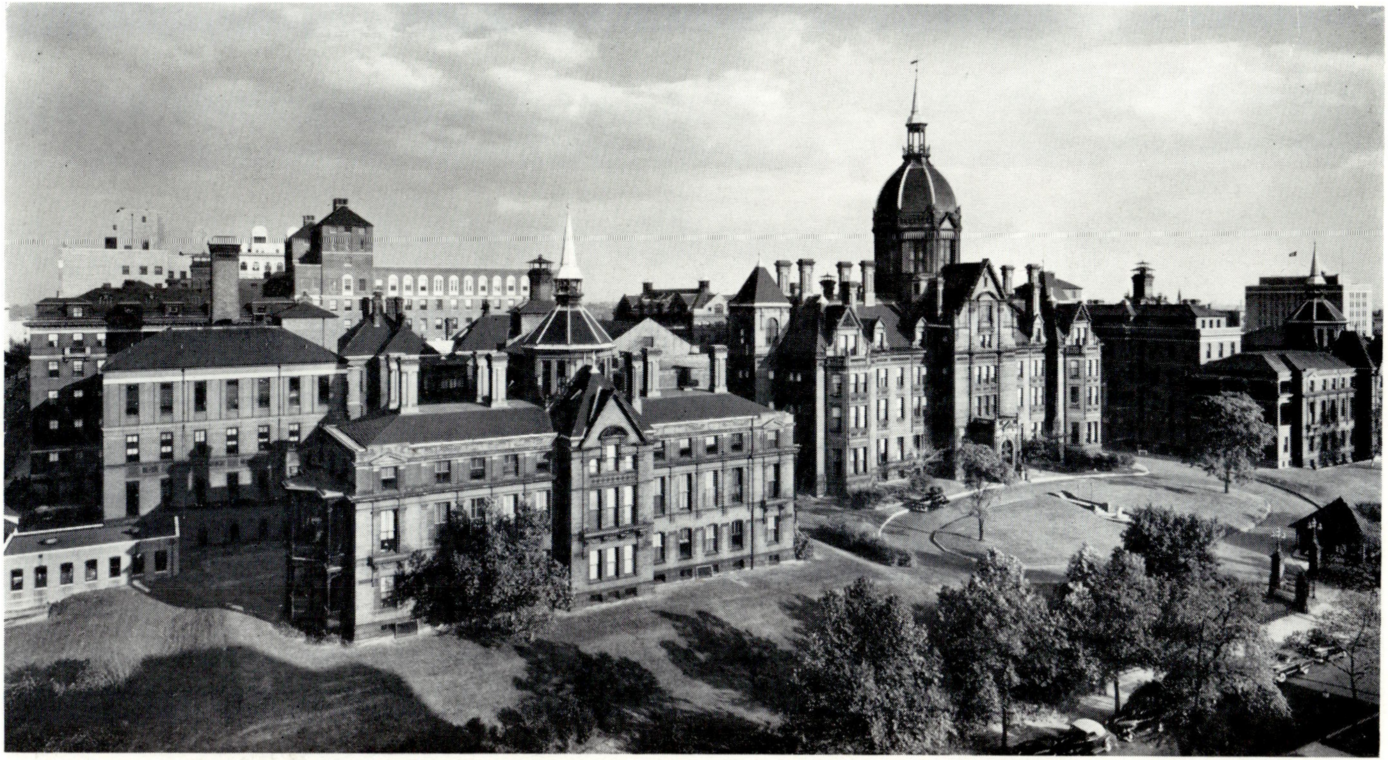

The Johns Hopkins Hospital

HOLMES I. METTEE

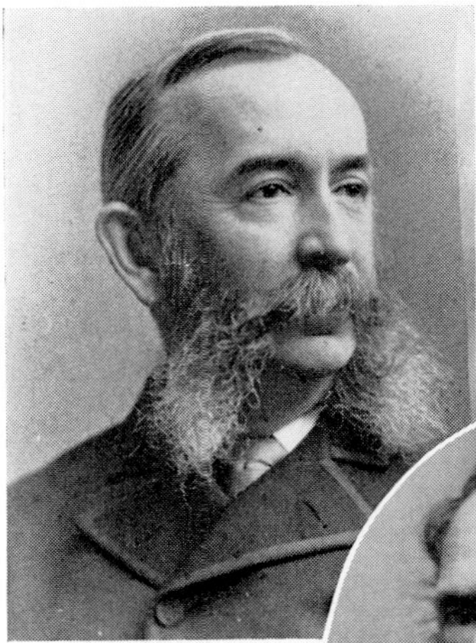
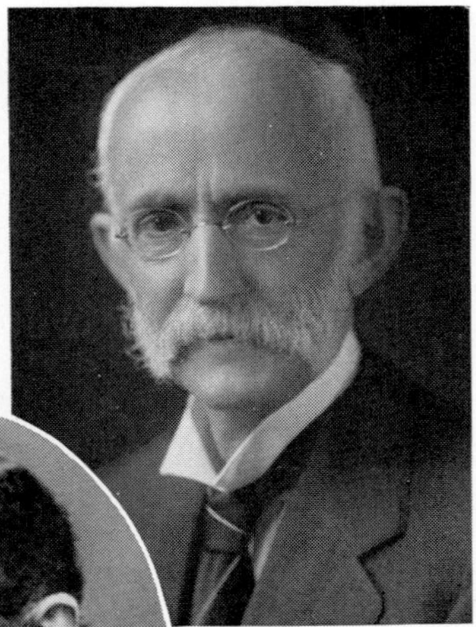
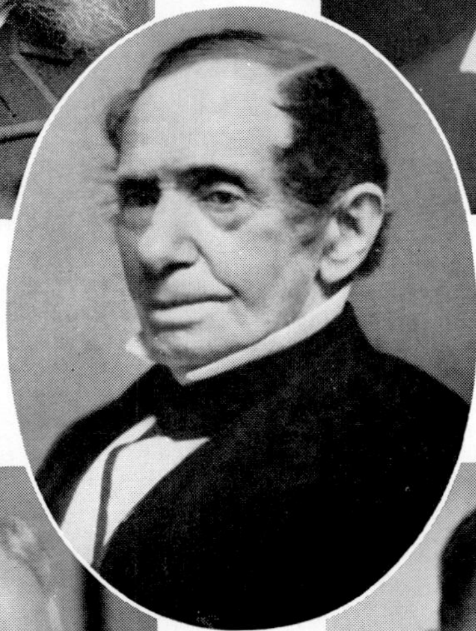
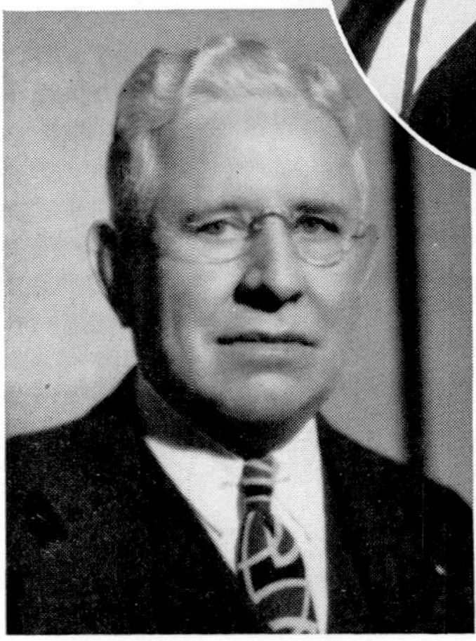
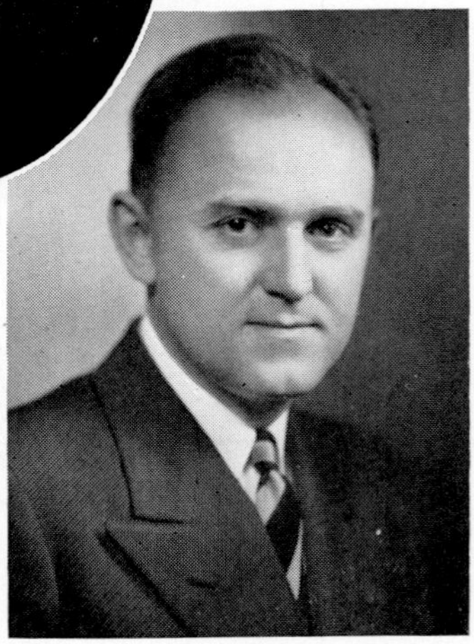

DANIEL C. GILMAN
Acting Director, 1889
ALUMNI FILES

HENRY M. HURD
Superintendent, 1889–1911
BACHRACH

JOHNS HOPKINS
The Founder, 1795–1875

WINFORD H. SMITH
Director, 1911–1946
CARLYLE STUDIOS

EDWIN L. CROSBY
Director, 1946–
BACHRACH

immediately sent for and dressed the fracture and swung the limb. He left him in an apparently easy condition."

Unfortunately the patient did not progress favorably. A suite of rooms was set up for his accommodation and on July 18 the construction records refer to the first "nurse" ever to care for a patient within the sacred precincts of the Johns Hopkins Hospital. *He was a man.* A second entry indicates the duration of his ministrations and his recompense:

> Mr. Sm'l H. Kerr entered upon his duties as Nurse to Bruff Friday July 18th 3 P.M. $8. Quit Monday Aug. 11th 3 P.M. Total paid $27.42.
>
> July 26th
Aug. 2nd
" 9th } 3 weeks 3 days

The final statement concerning this patient is: "Mr. Jno. K. Bruff left the Hospital about 9 o'clock this morning, Aug. 23rd. Saturday." This minor episode must surely have provoked one of Dr. Billings' rare but gentle smiles.

Within the next year or so his attitude toward the education of nurses seems to have become less positive and while there is no means of knowing why he changed his mind there is a distinct possibility that he may have been influenced by a report submitted in December 1878 by Mr. John Eaton to Mr. Carl Schurz, at that time Secretary of the Department of the Interior in the Federal Government. Mr. Eaton was a Commissioner in that Department, and his report was published by the Government Printing Office under the title of "Training Schools for Nurses. Circulars of Information of the Bureau of Education, No. 1, 1879." In a covering letter addressed to Mr. Schurz, as well as in the text of the report, Mr. Eaton submitted strong arguments in favor of the extension of nursing education:

"Several training schools for nurses established in our cities have vindicated the wisdom of their founders. They disseminate much useful information in regard to the care of the sick and by helping to shorten the period of suffering, save many lives. Moreover, by rendering women skilful, training schools for nurses secure for them employment they would otherwise be unable to find, and fitly supplement schools of medicine. The subject of the extension and management of these institutions has largely entered into the correspondence of this Office. The great superiority of well trained nurses, manifested in the late epidemic, has led to the hope that schools for nurses may be speedily established in many cities not yet supplied."

Mr. Eaton gave a list of schools which at that time were in operation in the eastern United States and adds this comment: "The Johns Hopkins University is considering similar plans in connection with its hospital in Baltimore." The very fact that Mr. Eaton and Dr. Billings both held appointments in the Federal Government in Washington may have brought them into touch with one another and Mr. Eaton's reference to the projected School at the Johns Hopkins Hospital suggests that he may have talked with Dr. Billings about it. In any event it seems probable that Dr. Billings did read the report, although it is doubtful whether at that time he would have been in full agreement with Mr. Eaton's assertion that "the training of nurses is substantially an educational work, and may be urged on purely educational grounds; that persons employed as nurses can best be fitted for this delicate and responsible duty by special training and instruction; and that nursing is not necessarily the work either of physicians or religious bodies, though done under the direction of the former and not subversive of the latter. To establish schools for training nurses is not antagonistic to either; it is rendered necessary by the times in which we live."

After all, the reasons for his change of heart do not greatly matter. The fact remains that Dr. Billings became the firm friend and strong supporter of the School of Nursing and at the opening of the Johns Hopkins Hospital spoke with deep sincerity and conviction:

"A word now on the fourth object kept in view of this Hospital—the training school for nurses. Some of you probably have had some personal experience of the difference between an educated, properly trained female nurse, and much of the old-fashioned sort; but if you have not, it would take much more time than I now have to describe it. I can only say that in many cases a competent trained nurse is as important to the success of treatment as a competent doctor, and that one of the greatest difficulties in treating well-to-do patients in their own homes in this city is the want of proper nurses. Affection and zeal may do much, but they cannot take the place of knowledge, and this kind of knowledge is not to be acquired in a day or in a month. It is a work best carried out by women, though not one woman in ten is fitted for it, or should undertake it. But the woman who is fit for it, who has physical health and strength, sound sense, loving kindness, patience and tact, and who has been thoroughly taught the art of nursing the sick, with all its thousand details, has the power of doing good and increasing happiness to a degree which few others possess. In a properly conducted hospital ward, she is a necessity, but her field of usefulness is by no means limited to that. She is needed outside the hospital—in the home of the rich, to nurse and care for the sick; in the home of the poor, to teach prevention as well as nursing. To gather here such women, to have them thoroughly instructed, to furnish them with the attractive and comfortable home which they deserve, and to send them where they are most needed, with provision for their return when the work is done, is the object of the training school of this Hospital."

Miss Nightingale Is Consulted

A BITTER controversy arose in 1882 among the Trustees of the Johns Hopkins University regarding the site upon which that institution was to be established. Eventually, it was decided that the grounds at Clifton would not be suitable and it so happened that the Hospital and the School of Nursing were the only buildings actually constructed where Johns Hopkins intended them to be, on the plot of ground bounded by Broadway, Wolfe Street, Jefferson Street and Monument Street. The happy inspiration of grouping the buildings around a garden with green lawns and fine trees came from the founder himself, and the roofs of the connecting corridors formed an open-air bridge that for many years was one of the most delightful amenities of the Hospital. Originally lighted by gas, the various units were wired for "incandescent electric lamps, when deemed best to adopt this system of lighting." There was telephone communication between all departments and a pneumatic system of clocks, "all driven by puffs of air sent through small iron pipes from a central apparatus in the administration building," thus assuring uniform timing even (it is noted) in the Nurses Home.

In some respects the buildings were not entirely satisfactory, even though they were far ahead of their time in others. In Dr. Hurd's opinion, Dr. Billings had been led by his European consultants to lay too much stress upon the theory that most forms of disease were due to emanations from the ground and that infection was air-borne. The fact that Baltimore had no system of sewage, and that excreta were discharged into privy pits and cesspools, may have prompted Dr. Billings to take fantastic precautions to prevent air from passing from one ward to another, and to forbid the installation of elevators since they would interfere with the meticulously planned ventilation system. From a nursing point of view, as Dr. Hurd pointed out, the ward units were decidedly inconvenient:

"The whole structure was too much upon the line of the army hospital. It was deficient in modern facilities for nursing and in the modern laboratories for studying disease. The sink rooms, ward bathrooms, linen rooms, etc., were too small and not arranged for the convenience of nurses. They seemed to contemplate the presence of the army orderly at every turn. There was also imperfect provision for housekeeping and store rooms and other conveniences which housekeepers love to plan and sometimes to use."

Nevertheless, the Nurses Home was far superior to any constructed prior to that time. Accommodation was provided for fifty nurses and the reception rooms had a grace and dignity that defied the passage of the years. The setting which Dr. Billings had taken so much pleasure in planning for the School of Nursing is best described in his own words:

"For this purpose the trustees have provided a large and handsome building, separated from the others, and exclusively appropriated to the female nurses, where each can have her own comfortable room, and where a common parlor, library, dining-room, bath-rooms, and, in short, the arrangements of a first-class hotel, are provided for their use. Here also is a training kitchen and a lecture room to aid in the work of instruction. The intention is that when the nurse has finished her six or eight hours of duty with the sick, she shall be quite away from the ward and all that pertains to it and take her rest and recreation in a totally different atmosphere, and special effort has been made to have this home attractive and pleasant."

The search for a competent staff for the School of Nursing may be said to have begun as early as 1875 when Mr. Francis T. King, president of the Board of Trustees, decided to pay a visit to Florence Nightingale. He was accompanied to London by his daughter Elizabeth who, twenty-five years later, in an address delivered before the Maryland State Association of Graduate Nurses, described this historic occasion:

"I will not apologize to this audience for asking you to recall the memory of my father, because it was he who first, when I was a child, spoke of trained nurses at a time when it seemed an almost unknown word. It is so many years that I hardly like to remember it myself, but I remember when a school girl hearing him say in the serious, collected, persuasive voice that bore conviction to many minds when he had new ideas to bring before them, 'I want very much to carry out this new idea of trained nurses at the Johns Hopkins Hospital and I hardly know where to go to hear more of it; I think I must go to England.' I, still as a school girl, was taken over with him to London where I experienced the wonderful glamor that the first trip abroad brings over everything, including your profession. He came home from visits to Miss Nightingale and Miss Lees, and they gave him the result of their experiences in England, and sat night after night talking over the developments which these women had carried out. I remember on one of his visits a huge mastiff appeared at Miss Nightingale's door, and he stood in imminent danger of his life until the English maid carried off the guardian, and he was welcomed. There might have been no trained nursing in Baltimore for some time, had he not been so discreet as to step forward until the obstacle was removed. They became so interested that long after midnight they sat with the plans of the Johns Hopkins Hospital before them while they talked of all the developments that were possible."

The "Miss Lees" who was present at these conferences was, of course, Florence Lees, a close friend and associate of Miss Nightingale. Mr. King was evidently so favorably impressed that later in 1875 Judge George Dobbin was authorized to ask her to take charge of the School of Nursing. Part of this correspondence has been preserved and is quoted in full:

The Lindens
St. Leonard's on Sea
England, March 24th, 1875.

Dear Mr. Dobbin:

I should have written to you before to acknowledge the receipt of my Handbook and your letter, but unfortunately I mislaid the latter, and am ashamed to say that I forgot whether *you* had written it, or Judge Brown.

Deciding that it was the *latter*, I asked Mr. Bonham Carter the Secretary of the Nightingale Fund, to forward to "Judge Brown, Trustee of the Johns Hopkins Hospital" a copy of Miss Nightingale's "Notes on Hospitals" for the use of the Trustees—thinking that the defects pointed out by her, in existing European hospitals might lead to your avoiding them in your new Hospital. For the Baltimore Hospital *ought* to be "a model" of its kind for imitation in American as well as European cities, and for this purpose the administrative, and college buildings might be as handsome and as permanent as you could afford, *but the wards for the sick* should be built on the barrack principle *to last only ten years.* Of course the furniture of each "baraque" need not be destroyed with the building.

When is your new Hospital to be begun and what rules have you made with regard to your Nurses' School or College? I am really sorry that it is not in existence *now* and then I would avail myself of your offer to take charge of the new School for Nurses, for two or three years, "to start it fairly."

They are very anxious in England that I should take charge of the new Training School that is to be started, in connection with the National Association for Providing Trained Nurses for the Sick Poor in their own homes (of which I am at present honorary secretary). But I am afraid that it will be many years before I can make the Committee see the necessity of a far higher *theoretical* course of Teaching for Nurses and I cannot take the superintendency of any Training School, when my firm convictions on this point are not carried out. And yet I am wearying for *work!* I have therefore serious thoughts of taking charge of the new Fever Hospital that is being built near London (having been promised the refusal of it) if there is any chance of its being completed by August or September.

Pray let me hear how your Hospital is progressing. Believe me, yours faithfully,

Florence S. Lees.

Judge Dobbin's reply to this letter gives proof that, in addition to the five medical consultants who were originally asked to submit their views to the Board of Trustees, a nurse—Florence Lees—was also invited to do so.

Superior Court of Baltimore City
Baltimore, April 13th, 1875.

Dear Miss Lees,

Your welcome letter of 24th ult. has been duly received, and Judge Brown has also received and delivered Miss Nightingale's book which you so kindly sent the Hospital Board. I avail myself now of the permission which is implied in your enquiry to tell you what we have been doing in the hope that we may interest you to the extent of giving us such views as may suggest themselves to you for the benefit of the benevolent enterprise we have in charge. We felt our first duty to be to visit such of the principal Hospitals of the Country as are within our reach and we accordingly inspected those of Boston, New York, Providence and Philadelphia, and learned what those who have them in charge had to say in their behalf. In no case did we find any one of them which seemed to satisfy the professional gentlemen at their head as being the best that could be done in the way of Hospital construction and management. In this contingency, we deemed it wise to take very deliberate advice upon the subject and to that end five of the most distinguished medical authorities were selected from different parts of the country to each of whom we addressed the circular letter a copy of which I send you with this. These gentlemen have severally undertaken to advise us fully upon the subject and from them we expect the most instructive information that can be derived from science and experience. As soon as this experience shall be received and digested we shall begin the actual construction of the buildings, and as the funds are in hand there is no reason why they should not be pushed to the earliest practicable completion.

If with the subjects of our needs before you as indicated in the papers sent with this, you will kindly add to the information we hope to receive by replying to this letter as if one of the five to whom it is addressed, which your wide experience most amply qualifies you to do, I hope I need not say that your contribution will be most gratefully received and availed of.

I sincerely deplore that we are not now at work and ready to take advantage of your present leisure by inviting you to take the headship of our Training School and such other direction of our work as you so usefully could. When the time arrives, we shall however assuredly press upon you the claims which our enlarged philanthropy may urge upon your benevolence in this new field of Christian labor.

In the again repeated hope that you may find it in your good heart to respond to the request that I have now made to you, I beg you to believe me, dear Miss Lees, faithfully yours,

George W. Dobbin

Miss Lees' reply to Judge Dobbin's request does not seem to have been preserved but there must have been further correspondence between them because, early in 1876, she wrote to him again. By this time she had become the superintendent-general of the Metropolitan and National Nursing Association for Providing Nurses for the Sick Poor.

Metropolitan and National Nursing Association
January 21st, 1876

Dear Judge Dobbin,

I have delayed replying to your note of November 27th in the daily expectation of the arrival of the book you so kindly said you were sending me. As it has not yet arrived at St. Leonards, I have thought it possible you might have deferred sending it to me until you heard from me.

I need hardly say with how much pleasure I am looking forward to it's perusal—and how gladly I will submit to you any suggestions that may occur to me. At present I am engaged in the organization of so large a nursing scheme for the benefit of our sick poor, that I have but little time at my disposal. But I often think of "the model Hospital of the world" that you propose erecting at Baltimore and of your "School for Nurses" in connection with it, and it will give me sincere pleasure if I can be of any service to you, with regard to the latter. Believe me, very sincerely yours,

Florence S. Lees

In the only remaining letter in this collection, Miss Lees puts forward the revolutionary suggestion that four or five Baltimore ladies might be persuaded to go to England in order to prepare themselves for the direction of the new School, but in 1876 the social tradition of the South would hardly have been in accord with so rash an adventure.

Metropolitan and National Nursing
Association for Providing Trained
Nurses for the Sick Poor
Central Home and Offices,
23 Bloomsbury Square, London, W.C.
May 1st, 1876

Dear Judge Dobbin,

At last I have received the book you so kindly sent me containing "the plans" submitted to the Johns Hopkins Hospital (I have also received "the review" of the same and drawings and I thank you warmly for both). I have not yet had time to read it, but I will promise to give it my best attention and so give you my "best thoughts"—such as they are, on the subject.

I am at present so over-worked, that I rarely have even half an hour in the day for anything not bearing on the work I have in hand. I enclose you a copy of extracts from my first report and I will mail you tomorrow a copy of The Standard containing a leading article on the nature of our work. I suppose you have seen Miss Nightingale's letter upon it, in The Times. If not, I should like to send you a copy.

Have you decided upon any plans with regard to the salaries etc. of your future Superintendent of Nurses? I wish you could persuade four or five Baltimore ladies to come over to England and train in the Nightingale School for Nurses!

With the Hospital you purpose to build, you ought to have the best procurable woman, to organise and start your Nursing School. And none but gentlewomen by birth and education are capable of such a work—at least, such has been my experience. I enclose you a letter from the Postmaster General, which I received concerning the book of plans you sent me, and which I have now received, I am happy to say.

Thanking you very much for the same, believe me, sincerely yours,
Florence S. Lees

Correspondence with Miss Lees (who later became Mrs. Dacre Craven) terminated at this point and no further attempt seems to have been made to select a superintendent of nurses until in April, 1888, Dr. Billings submitted a memorandum on the general organization of the Hospital and a committee was appointed to study the situation. On September 25, it was resolved that "the gentlemen of the Building Committee be requested to submit a plan of organization for the efficient working of the Hospital and also the name of a suitable person for the head of the Training School for Nurses."

In Search of Leadership

AFTER twelve years of planning and preparation, the Hospital was now almost ready for occupancy and it was feared that any further delay in opening its doors to patients might lead to criticism on the part of the public. It was at this critical juncture that Mr. Francis T. King who, as president of the Board of Trustees, had so long borne the heat and burden of the day, decided that he must seek relief and assistance. At his request, the Trustees persuaded Daniel Coit Gilman, president of the Johns Hopkins University, to act temporarily as the director of the Hospital and to undertake the organization of the medical and nursing staff. Early in January 1889 he tackled the problem so unexpectedly thrust upon him and his approach to it was thus described by Dr. Hurd:

"He entered upon his new duties immediately with all his usual ardor and energy. He familiarized himself with the literature of the subject and corresponded with experts at home and abroad. He visited hospitals and large hotels in other cities to see their method and details of management and studied their kitchens, laundries and linen-rooms. He even inspected such minor details as table linen and napkins. . . . He assisted in the selection of medical officers; he saw personally and recommended to appointment all subordinate officers and defined their duties and responsibilities; he familiarized himself with the proper sphere of the housekeeper, the purveyor and the superintendent of nurses, and set their bounds and thus secured harmony and co-operation. . . . He selected very wisely the first Principal of the Training School for Nurses and the first head nurses."

By the end of February, President Gilman was ready to present a memorandum to the Board of Trustees in which he outlined the principles upon which the administration of the Hospital should be based:

In all the chief departments of service there will be a recognized head, who will be responsible for those who come under his supervision. This officer will be responsible to the Trustees, through the medium of the Director, unless otherwise ordered. The heads of the different departments of service may be brought together for mutual counsel—under regulations to be hereafter determined; for example, the professional staff, the house committee, etc.

The principal officers of the Hospital, appointed or to be appointed by the Trustees on the nomination of the Executive Committee, are these:

Director
Consulting Director
Physician in chief
Surgeon in charge
Pathologist
Resident medical officer
Superintendent of buildings and grounds
Housekeeper
Steward
Two chief nurses

It will be noted that President Gilman recommended that there should be "two chief nurses" and, while there is no proof of what he had in mind, it seems reasonable to suppose that he may have intended one nurse to take charge of the hospital nursing service and the other to direct the school of nursing. In any event, Dr. Billings did not share his views and wrote vigorously opposing them: "I do not think that it will be wise to start with two independent head nurses in any case. One of them should be acting as temporary head." Dr. Billings may not have been willing to envisage the possibility that the School might be administered as an educational entity apart from the Hospital.

Certainly there was no dearth of candidates for the position of superintendent of nurses and several of them already held positions of considerable importance. Correspondence in the archives of the School of Nursing shows that Anna C. Maxwell, superintendent of nurses at the Massachusetts General Hospital, was willing to transfer her allegiance to the Johns Hopkins Hospital, and that Agnes Brennan, highly recommended as "having been in virtual control" at the Bellevue Training School for Nurses for many years, was ready to do likewise. Sophia Palmer, twenty years later to become the first editor of the *American Journal of Nursing*, wrote to the president of the Board of Trustees enclosing a glowing testimonial from a gentleman she described as an influential member of the medical staff of the Massachusetts General Hospital. Mary Agnes Snively was prepared to give up the position she had held for three years as superintendent of nurses at the Toronto General Hospital if her application was favorably considered. Yet another candidate presented herself—the woman destined to become the first superintendent of nurses and principal of the Training School for Nurses in the Johns Hopkins Hospital. The manner in which the choice was made was described many years later by Dr. William Osler in his own inimitable fashion:

"When we opened the Johns Hopkins Hospital, the question of a Lady Superintendent and the head of the Training School was a very difficult one. There were, I believe, some eighty applicants. A committee was appointed consisting of Mr. King, Dr. Billings, Dr. Welch, President Gilman and myself, to look over the candidates. It seemed a hopeless job and it was not one which I appreciated at all. We all looked to Dr. Billings and to Dr. Welch for guidance in these matters as they were older hands in this special work. The numbers were gradually reduced by a process of exclusion to three, it may have been five, and I remember perfectly that we made notes on the past history, the experience and the career of the candidates. The last one to appear was Miss Isabel Hampton. She entered the room looking like an animated Greek statue. Mr. Gilman looked at Mr. King and smiled; then he looked at Dr. Billings and he smiled again; then he threw a glance at Dr. Welch and he had no time to smile before he looked at me with a wider smile, and we knew that all was settled. It did not require anything further. Her certificates were looked at in a very perfunctory manner and the appointment was made in a very few minutes."

There is good reason to believe that the Committee's decision may have been less impetuous than Dr. Osler suggests. According to Dr. Hurd, the qualifications of all the candidates were closely studied by President Gilman "and he selected very wisely the first Principal of the Training School for Nurses." But even Dr. Hurd sufficiently departed from his customary reserve to admit that "when Miss Hampton entered the room, one member of the committee softly exclaimed: 'There is the woman for the position.' She was unanimously selected." Incidentally, Dr. Hurd states that in addition to the members mentioned by Dr. Osler, Dr. James Carey Thomas also served on the committee on selection.

On April 9, 1889, the appointment was ratified by the Board of Trustees as shown in this excerpt from the Minutes:

"The following report of resolutions from the Executive Committee was read and adopted with the concurrence of the director and the physician-in-chief: that Miss Isabel Hampton be appointed superintendent of nurses for a period of one year at a salary of $1000 per annum."

These Minutes also record the appointment of Caroline Hampton, Annie McDowell and Louisa Parsons as head nurses for a period of six months at a salary of $30 per month respectively. Rachel Bonner, who was not a nurse, was appointed matron of the Hospital at an annual salary of $800.

It so happened that Isabel Hampton could not immediately take over her new duties and the formal opening of the School had therefore to be delayed for several months. A conference was held between President Gilman, Dr. Osler, Dr. Halsted and Miss Hampton and it was decided that Louisa Parsons, as the senior of the newly appointed head nurses, should function as acting superintendent of nurses in addition to taking charge of the medical wards. Annie McDowell became head nurse in the private wards and Caroline Hampton took over the surgical wards and the operating room. The position of night assistant was assigned to Ida B. May, a member of the nursing staff of the Good Samaritan Hospital, in Baltimore. She had not at that time had formal training but later entered the Training School for Nurses as a member of the first class.

The opening ceremonies of the Hospital took place with due pomp and ceremony on May 7, 1889, although the first patient was not admitted until May 15. The wards filled rather slowly at first but before long the demands on the nursing service began to increase rapidly. Several years later, Dr. Osler gave high praise to the manner in which the staff responded:

"There are three women early associated in the work of the Hospital whom I would like to mention—indeed there is a fourth. Before Miss Hampton could come to take charge of the work, we had to make arrangements for the opening of the Hospital and for the general management of the house, and Miss Parsons, Miss Caroline Hampton (now Mrs. Halsted), and Miss McDowell took charge of the work during those first three months of the organization of the Hospital. I cannot say too much for the care and devotion and the energy with which these three women worked during those early and somewhat troublesome days. The fourth I would like to mention, as I was somewhat personally interested in securing her, is the woman I would like to call Sister Rachel—Miss Bonner—who came to us from the Pennsylvania Hospital. She was a friend of the Superintendent of the Training School at Blockley, and when I conferred with her as to the possibility of securing someone to take charge of the general housekeeping department here, she said: 'If you can secure Sister Rachel from the Pennsylvania Hospital, all will go well. She has all the necessary business capacity and she is, wherever she may be, a bond of peace.' "

The excellent morale which prevailed among the nursing staff in those early days was due in a large measure to Louisa Parsons herself. An administrator, rather than an educator, she had already had a successful career as an Army nurse during the British military campaign in the Sudan in 1883 and was said to have been the only nurse on duty in a hospital ship laden with wounded soldiers returning to England from the battlefields of Egypt. A woman of distinguished appearance, she never hesitated to exercise authority although she was seldom unduly severe. Her capacity for fearless leadership found full scope at the Johns Hopkins Hospital where she was expected to provide a reasonably good nursing service even though her staff was insufficient in numbers and for the most part poorly trained.

Ida B. May, who worked closely with Miss Parsons all through the first difficult months, told the present writer that she remembered her as an alert, intelligent and handsome woman who would herself have made an excellent superintendent. Dr. Osler also spoke of her in the highest terms: "She was a most devoted self-sacrificing woman and I can never forget the splendid work she did in putting the medical wards into shape. Trained in the Florence Nightingale School, at St. Thomas's Hospital, London, she brought an exact and thorough knowledge of nursing and of the methods of organization which were very helpful to us."

According to Dr. W. G. MacCallum,[1] Caroline Hampton was an aristocrat in the best sense, delightful to those whom she made her friends but a little intolerant with others. A niece of General Wade Hampton, she had enjoyed a typically Southern upbringing but when her family was impoverished by the Civil War, made up her mind to become a trained nurse. She first entered the school of nursing at Mount Sinai Hospital in New York but soon transferred to the New York Hospital School of Nursing from which she was graduated in 1888. Dr. John M. T. Finney once told an amusing story of which she is the heroine:

"Miss Caroline Hampton was operating room nurse. Dr. Halsted afterwards married her. . . . Miss Hampton had a delicate skin and developed an eczema of the hands from plunging them into carbolic acid and bichloride of mercury solutions. For some time she was obliged to remain out of the operating room tech-

[1] W. G. MacCallum, *William Stewart Halsted, Surgeon.* Baltimore, The Johns Hopkins Press, 1930.

nique altogether. Dr. Halsted tried to help her. At first he painted her hands with collodion but of course this failed because with the contraction of the fingers the collodion would split. . . . Halsted got his idea of using rubber gloves for Miss Hampton from Dr. Welch's autopsy gloves. He interested the Goodyear Rubber Company in making the gloves and they were successful. The gloves had long sleeves which came up to the elbow. Miss Hampton wore them with such success, that Dr. Bloodgood said, one day, 'What is sauce for the goose is sauce for the gander. Why should not the surgeon use the gloves as well as the nurse?' Really Joe Bloodgood deserves the credit of having thought of extending the use of the gloves to the surgeons but the Professor of course conceived the original idea for the protection of Miss Hampton's hands. So you see rubber gloves were introduced into surgery from the stimulus of the heart as well as the scintillation of the intellect, a case where Venus rendered great aid to Aesculapius."

By way of contrast, here is Dr. Halsted's laconic account of the same episode:

"In the winter of 1889 and 1890—I cannot recall the month —the nurse in charge of my operating room complained that the solutions of mercuric chloride produced a dermatitis of her arms and hands. As she was an unusually efficient woman, I gave the matter my consideration, and one day in New York requested the Goodyear Rubber Company to make as an experiment two pair of thin rubber gloves with gauntlets."

Annie McDowell, a native of Cork, Ireland, had been trained at the London Hospital and was a friend of Judge Dobbin and his wife who are said to have encouraged her to come to the United States. It is possible, therefore, that even after a lapse of fourteen years, Judge Dobbin still favored the appointment, as superintendent of nurses, of a woman who, like Florence Lees, possessed English training and background.

At first, the nursing staff and Miss Bonner lived in temporary quarters in the Hospital building and the administration of the nursing service was carried on in the Nurses Home which was not yet ready for full occupancy. They all got along very well with one another and especially with Miss Bonner who fulfilled the glowing expectations of Dr. Osler by rendering competent service as the housekeeper of the Hospital and also serving as "a bond of peace." As the work grew heavier during the summer months, three graduates of the Blockley Hospital School of Nursing in Philadelphia were added to the staff, namely, Marion Patison, May Richart, and J. Miller. Miss M. A. Selby, a graduate of the Nightingale School at St. Thomas's Hospital, was appointed night nurse in Ward C. She, like Miss Parsons, had served during the Sudan campaign and, according to one observer, was "all covered with medals."

The first pupil nurse to enter the Johns Hopkins Hospital Training School for Nurses was Marion Turner (Mrs. F. J. Brockway) who was accepted as a probationer on June 12, 1889. Many years later, she set down a lively account of her experience in which she said that her home was in Mount Savage, Maryland, and hearing of the impressive ceremony that marked the opening of the Hospital, she decided to make enquiries:

"Miss Parsons was in charge and sent for Dr. Osler. I can see him walking in, swinging a stethoscope. Miss Parsons introduced me as a young woman who was interested. He turned to me and said 'You don't want to be a nurse.' I said: 'Yes, I do, Dr. Osler.' He laughed and said, 'Alright, Miss Parsons, we will accept her.' Miss Parsons gave me a pattern for an apron and said to report on June 12, at noon."

Marion Turner bought the linen for her aprons and went home to break the news to her parents: "There was much conversation about disgracing every woman south of the Mason and Dixon line but I was firm and packed my trunk and left. The family hardly said good-bye." When she arrived at the Hospital, Miss Parsons led her to the men's medical ward, showed her how to use a clinical thermometer and left her in a small room off the ward to watch beside a delirious patient. One nurse who reported for night duty that evening seems to have been rather a picturesque character: "She was an attendant from Dr. Hunter McGuire's Sanatarium in Richmond, Virginia, and came on duty equipped with dozens of medical books and an accordion. When asked what she did with the accordion, she replied that she played tunes to awaken the patients in time to get their faces washed."

Miss Parsons resigned shortly after Isabel Hampton took charge, and became superintendent of nurses at the University of Maryland Hospital. Subsequently, she served as chief Red Cross representative in the islands off the Carolinas when in 1893 they were devastated by a hurricane and a tidal wave. During the Spanish-American war she took charge of the nursing staff in the hospital at Fort McPherson and later was recalled to England for military service during the Boer War. Her last days were spent in England on a farm near Reading and when her health finally broke down she had a great desire to consult Dr. Osler who, by that time, was Regius Professor of Medicine at Oxford University. "I feel that if anyone could help me he could" she wrote to a friend in America. Word was sent to Sir William (as he had now become) and he visited her and did all he could to comfort her. On November 16, 1916, she died and, as a member of the Reserve Nursing Staff of the British Army, was accorded a military funeral. Lady Osler wrote that "the coffin was carried to the Church on a gun carriage—a company of soldiers, buglers, and a firing party, rifles fired over the grave and the Last Post sounded by the buglers. Sir William went to the service; he sent a wreath with a card 'from the Medical and Nursing Staff of the Johns Hopkins Hospital.' "

It may truly be said of Louisa Parsons that she was a gallant representative of the military tradition in nursing. Although she did not actually participate in the organization of the Johns Hopkins Hospital Training School for Nurses, she nevertheless paved the way by initiating a nursing service characterized by the military virtues of courage, self-sacrifice, dignity and good manners.

Early in the summer of 1889, President Gilman announced that he had been successful in finding a physician qualified to become the Superintendent of the Hospital and, in August, Dr. Henry Mills Hurd was ready to take charge. He had previously served as superintendent of the Eastern Michigan Asylum, at Pontiac, Michigan, and had already acquired an excellent reputation as an administrator as well as a psychiatrist. Keenly interested in medical education, he had also had experience in dealing with the problems associated with nursing service. So far as President Gilman was concerned, release from the crushing burden of his dual responsibility to the University and to the Hospital did not come a moment too soon. His health was already seriously undermined and, in an interview with the present writer, his daughter, Elisabeth Gilman, recalled that her father had been on the verge of collapse—"and it was the Hospital that troubled him, not the University."

The University, the Medical School, the Hospital and the School of Nursing have every reason to cherish the memory of Daniel Coit Gilman.[2] When in 1875 he became its first president, he made known his determination that the Johns Hopkins University should offer advanced education of a quality previously unknown in the United States of America. He held firmly to this principle, especially in relation to medical education, and Abraham Flexner pays eloquent tribute to the good fortune which attended the authorities in finding leadership of so high an order:

"Thus precisely at the right moment, the University had set up a new pattern, meeting the country's need, and this pattern was copied by other academic institutions as rapidly as personnel was available and funds were obtainable. In the same way, the Trustees of the Hospital, at precisely the right moment and under precisely the same kind of leadership, set up a new pattern in medical education and in hospital-university relationships that has within fifty years become the ideal which medical schools and teaching hospitals throughout the country have striven to attain."

[2] Fabian Franklin, *The Life of Daniel Coit Gilman.* New York, Dodd Mead and Co., 1910

Isabel Hampton

According to Dr. Hurd, who was certainly in a position to know, President Gilman himself "selected very wisely the first Principal of the Training School for Nurses." It can, therefore, safely be assumed that her qualifications were subjected to a severely critical analysis. Character and temperament, family background, education and professional experience, were weighed in the balance and the woman thus chosen must have displayed unusual potentialities for leadership. Who was she, and what had been her preparation for so exacting a position?

Isabel Hampton's parents came of mixed Irish and Cornish ancestry, although both were born in Scotland. Samuel Hampton and his wife, Sarah Mary Lay, had come to Canada in a sailing ship and settled in Welland, a prosperous small town in the pleasant countryside of southern Ontario and here in 1860 Isabel was born. She grew up in a happy healthy family of four boys and four girls, well disciplined by their mother, a handsome red-haired woman, who looked well to the ways of her household and made a little money go a long way. Samuel Hampton was a successful merchant and a good provider, who seems to have been willing to let his wife dominate the home and whose customary response to any domestic problem is said to have been: "You had better ask your mother about that." He was, however, a highly intelligent man with a mind of his own and there was a close bond between him and his daughter Isabel who always went to her father when she needed help with her lessons.

Sarah Hampton had the local reputation of being "a natural nurse" who even vaccinated her children herself "from a very healthy cow" because she darkly suspected that the vaccine obtained from medical sources was not quite clean. Although she was always kind to her less fortunate neighbors, she never hesitated to scold them for such unsanitary practices as allowing the chickens to come into the kitchen. Her children were expected to help with the housework and Isabel is said to have disliked washing the breakfast dishes and cleaning out the porridge pot. Never a very good cook, she did learn to make a pie although her mother complained that "it would have tasted a lot better if she had kept her mind on it." She always seemed to be dreaming —and her mother was a little impatient with her.

One of Isabel's younger sisters, Mrs. Caroline Schofield, remembered her as a strikingly handsome girl, tall and well built, with fair hair and very blue eyes. Even as a child, she was rather independent and did not readily yield when opposed. Sometimes, she would lose her temper and fly into a sudden rage but bore no malice and was always ready to make friends again. She had a quiet sense of humor that seldom broke into laughter and although she could be sympathetic she rarely allowed her sympathies to affect her preferred course of action. The impact of her personality upon those with whom she came in contact made a profound impression upon her sister: "When Isabel came into a room, everyone in it was conscious of her presence. She had an influence over others which they did not resent. She could hold them until she made them understand. She once said that if she were a man, she wouldn't stop at anything—she would be Prime Minister of Canada. *She had a look of power.*"

Isabel went to school in Welland and later attended the Collegiate Institute in nearby St. Catherines in order to get a third-class teaching certificate that would permit her to teach for a limited period in a primary school. At the age of seventeen, she obtained a position in a one-room school in Merritton, a small manufacturing centre near St. Catherines. The school-house was a drab little building with no furniture except a few battered desks and a blackboard, and the children had the reputation of being rough and difficult to manage. In an interview with the present writer, one of her less turbulent pupils, Dr. Charles E. Smyth, recalled that his father, at that time a member of the school board, was amazed and gratified to find that this inexperienced girl could maintain law and order simply by the force and influence of a remarkable personality. Dr. Smyth still remembers the gentle and womanly sympathy with which she tended and comforted him when, as sometimes happened, he was not well. There was a maternal quality about her that he has never forgotten.

While she was teaching at Merritton, Isabel lived in St. Catherines and prepared for the examination leading to the second-class certificate that she hoped would qualify her for a better position. To her surprise and dismay she failed in one subject —mathematics—and as a result the current of her life took a new direction. She happened to hear two of her fellow teachers (none other than Mary Agnes Snively and Louise Darche) discussing the possible benefits of "a change of occupation." They had already obtained application forms from the Bellevue School of Nursing but had decided to postpone further action for the time being. It is said that acting on a sudden impulse, Isabel Hampton picked up one of the unused forms, filled it out and sent it in. She was quick to see that if she were accepted she could escape not only from the consequences of her failure but also from an environment that was becoming increasingly uncongenial to her.

The simple pattern of life in a small country town had never really satisfied her and while she sought the company of other young people she did not take part in their amusements. She loved the theatre and was thrilled by good music although she never had much opportunity of enjoying either. Reading was always a joy, especially a book she "could get something out of." Sometimes she used to drive all by herself, with the family horse and buggy, over the country roads that wound between the many-colored patchwork of the fields and orchards, and watch the clouds drifting against the blue Canadian sky. She had begun to long for a new horizon and her determination to seek it was strengthened when her family decided to leave Welland and to move westward to Manitoba. As soon as word came from Bellevue, she made up her mind not to accompany them. Her great adventure had begun.

In the archives of the Bellevue School of Nursing there is a precious volume entitled "The Training School, Bellevue Hospital, Record of Probationers." Entries are made in clear, flowing longhand and the first which concerns Isabel Hampton reads quite simply:

Addie Hampton
August 24, 1881
Single: Age 22
Canadian
Presbyterian

A subsequent entry shows that *Isabel* Hampton finished her course and received her diploma in October, 1883. All other documentary records concerning her training seem to have disappeared but these brief notes reveal that she had at last succeeded in getting rid of the pet name that she so cordially disliked. She had been named after her paternal grandmother, Isabel Adams Hampton, and proposed henceforth to answer to no other.

The Bellevue Training School for Nurses had been founded in 1873 by an indomitable group of public-spirited women who were determined to introduce a measure of cleanliness, decency and order into the nursing service of the Bellevue Hospital. The School was independent of the Hospital and subject to the direction of a Board of Lady Managers and, at the time that Isabel Hampton was in training, its superintendent was Eliza Perkins who, while not a nurse, has justly been described as "a New England gentlewoman whose high ideals, sterling character and wise leadership exerted a lasting influence on the nursing profession." In 1881, the total enrolment was 64 pupils, divided into two groups of 32 each in the first and second year respectively. During this particular year, no less than four hundred candidates had presented themselves so it is evident that Miss Perkins and the Board of Lady Managers had plenty of opportunity to pick and choose. At the end of the probationary term of one month, the aspirants were called upon to pass an examination in reading, penmanship, simple arithmetic and English dictation: "This amount of education is indispensable,"—a phrase which was destined to recur in most of the announcements of the earlier schools of nursing.

By a happy coincidence from an historical point of view, an article written by Franklin H. North which appeared in *The Century Magazine*, in November 1882 under the title of "A New Profession for Women," gives a vivid picture of the Bellevue School as Isabel Hampton must have known it. According to Mr. North, the nursing service in fourteen wards, of twenty beds each, was then carried on under the direction of the Training School for Nurses. This relatively large number of patients afforded opportunity for the nursing of men and women and gave some experience in medicine and surgery. This is Mr. North's description of the ward where Isabel Hampton, then in her second year of training, was in charge:

"Look in at the male surgical ward. These young women in white caps and aprons and blue and white seersucker dresses seem to have something of the training of the soldier added to that of the nurse. There is little talking and no laughing. When they do speak it is in subdued tones. Each seems to understand her duties. One of the house physicians enters, and, beckoning to a nurse, gives her directions regarding a particular patient recently visited. She listens attentively, makes no reply and turns at once to obey. A soldier pausing in his rounds, presenting arms to his superior officer and listening respectfully for orders, would not have more perfect discipline."

Instruction in theory consisted of courses of lectures, given by physicians, which included four lessons on hygiene, five on surgery, six on "diseases," four on obstetrics. During Isabel Hampton's first year of training the Board of Lady Managers announced with pardonable pride that "Dr. William Welch, a respected Microscopist, will give a practical course on the analysis of fluids." Isabel Hampton, dutifully taking notes, little dreamed that in a few short years the "respected Microscopist" would play a leading part in the development of the Johns Hopkins Medical School and that she herself was destined to direct the Johns Hopkins Hospital Training School for Nurses. All lectures were given in the evening and in later years Dr. Welch was to recall the painful impression left upon him by this group of girls so utterly weary after the long day on the wards that they could hardly keep their eyes open.

The hours of duty were from eight in the morning until eight at night with "an hour off for dinner and additional time for exercise or rest." One free afternoon a week was granted "when possible," as well as part of Sunday with the proviso that churchgoing was obligatory. Pupils were sent on twelve-hour night duty in the fourth month of training and were awakened to attend classes no matter at what time these were held. Those assigned to the care of private patients in their own homes were expected to take twenty-four-hour duty as a matter of course. If the patient were very ill and required continuous care for several nights in succession, the nurse "might be allowed six hours for sleep during the day." It is hardly surprising that Isabel Hampton should later speak of such assignments as "a pernicious practice" and should resolve to put an end to them.

Isabel Hampton tried hard to organize a study group among her fellow pupils who, like herself, missed the regular classes because they either could not be spared from the wards or were on duty in private homes. However, one of her contemporaries, Miss M. E. Cameron,[1] evidently did not think that these well-meant efforts were duly appreciated:

"Among her classmates there did not exist the same enthusiasm—small jealousy of her great personal charm accounts for this in part—but there seems to be an idea still in existence that there were nurses who folded clothes with more precision, and washed more dirty patients in a given time than Miss Hampton. She was regarded as a persistent nuisance by some of her classmates for the dogged patience with which she strove to extract from every class and lecture every atom of intelligence

[1] M. E. Cameron, "Isabel Hampton—Pupil Nurse in Bellevue Training School for Nurses," *American Journal of Nursing,* 11: October 1910

—comparing her own notes with those of others, following up the subject in any and every book she could lay hands upon, and questioning every doctor who lingered in the wards in the hope of some interesting conversation. That she worked to some purpose is shown in her passing her examination head in every subject. . . . One can easily imagine that such a nature would be regarded with impatience in a busy ward where instantaneous results are of paramount importance. . . . It is safe to say that the rather silent and unresponsive young woman, who needed constant pricking and goading to hurry with her work, was not wholly occupied, body and mind, with earning her head nurse's approval of a tidy row of bed patients."

Life in the nurses home seems to have been care-free and happy although a Lady Manager, making an unexpected tour of inspection, was dismayed to find "apple cores strewn about in the cupboards, and badly made beds." As a result of this shocking discovery, a book of rules was prepared which, among other stern admonitions, forbade cooking in the bedrooms. Since the residence offered little opportunity for recreation, Isabel Hampton took great pleasure in trying to see as much as she could of New York and, one fine day, set off down the Bay to Governors Island. On the ferry, and purely by accident, she made the acquaintance of Elizabeth Birdseye, a young girl of her own age. This chance encounter led to an ardent friendship and almost sixty years later, Elizabeth Birdseye (who had become Mrs. Percival Merritt) still spoke of Isabel Hampton with deep affection. She remembered her swift response to beauty, her love of flowers and especially of violets which she loved to wear and to give to her friends. In the romantic fashion of the day, the girls adopted special names for one another—Elizabeth became "Violet" and Isabel called herself "Rosamund." The years spent in training at Bellevue were greatly enriched by this friendship for there was now a delightful home to visit and, best of all, a beloved friend in whom to confide.

At about the time that Isabel Hampton finished her training, Miss Perkins was receiving "great demands from the large cities in different States for heads of hospitals and training schools. It is necessary for us to train more women of superior character and acquirements to meet these demands." More than once she may have thought of assigning Isabel Hampton to one of these exacting positions but fortunately refrained from doing so, and instead recommended her as a member of the staff of St. Paul's House, an institution conducted in Rome under the joint auspices of the Protestant Episcopal Church and the Church of England. Before sailing for Italy, Isabel Hampton served for a short time as substitute for the superintendent of nurses in the Woman's Hospital, New York, and Adelaide Nutting later recalled that even "in the few weeks of her stay there she found time to initiate a number of minor changes which she long after referred to, smiling rather tenderly at the recollection, as 'my first authority, you know.' "

Miss M. E. Cameron also gave a delightful glimpse of Isabel Hampton as she appeared when on the verge of her European journey:

"It was when she was starting for St. Paul's House in Rome where she spent the first two years after her graduation. Miss Perkins had summoned a probationer to her room for advice, counsel and, probably, penance, and the probationer went with considerable trepidation. In Miss Perkins' room there was a young woman of splendid proportions, straight and round, perfectly blooming with health. Her dress was a perfectly hideous pepper and salt grey wool—of which her hat, coat and dress were all composed—she wore neither feather nor flower, and no jewelry; despite the utter absence of aid in the way of dress she was a vision of loveliness."

The nursing staff of St. Paul's House was composed of American and English nurses whose services were made available to any wealthy travellers who might happen to fall ill during their sojourn in Rome. Evelyn Pope (Mrs. J. W. Lord) and Ruth Williams (both of whom graduated from the Johns Hopkins Hospital School of Nursing in 1891) were later on the staff at St. Paul's House and remember it as it must have been in Isabel Hampton's time. It was a large square villa with a beautiful yellow rose tree climbing over the front wall, but the domestic arrangements were far from comfortable, the heating system was perpetually out of order, and the sitting room so cold in winter that the nurses wore coats and gloves in a vain effort to keep warm. The beds were like sarcophagi and the sheets cold and damp and when the thin bedroom rugs were shaken ever so gently, clouds of fleas arose to torment the unwary. Ruth Williams had a lively recollection of the night she was attacked and tried in vain to pursue them by the light of her solitary candle.

The manifold discomforts of St. Paul's House troubled Isabel Hampton very little. After the bleak streets of the East Side, the soft Italian landscape seemed a dream of beauty. Fleas and damp sheets were forgotten when she walked in the Medici Gardens and gathered violets to send to the dear companion at home—their imprint can still be seen on the letter which carried them. The patients she cared for were very different to the poor derelicts at Bellevue. There was a young and beautiful Russian lady; there was the gay Lady Colin Campbell, who seems to have affronted Isabel's strict sense of propriety but of whom she grew very fond; there was even a mysterious bar sinister scion of English royalty. Last but not least, there was Mrs. William Astor, the wife of the American ambassador, to whom on several occasions Isabel gave nursing care.

Sometimes her duties took her to France or Germany and on one of these journeys she had an encounter that rather disconcerted her and which she related to "Violet" with considerable spirit:

"I came by the St. Gothard tunnel and from the time we reached Como and the Lakes, the Alps took any remnant of heart I may not have given to Rome. Only, to help me to remember that I was not altogether in the clouds but that the earth was still very near me, there was someone in the shape of a man. He was my adventure of the journey. He was alone. He made himself very agreeable—too agreeable. I got bored and told him so. The consequence was that he told me that I had made a fool of him but thanked me for the lesson all the same. I thought: 'Better the fool should be on his side.' Moral—never accept the attentions of a foreigner when travelling alone. No, I promise you, I never will again."

This minor passage at arms reveals one of Isabel Hampton's

most charming characteristics. She had no vanity whatever so far as her own good looks were concerned and was genuinely surprised and a little annoyed when people stared at her admiringly.

The whole European experience affected her profoundly and the vivid eager girl made every moment of the twenty-one months count. She studied Italian and German, visited art galleries, heard good music, learned how to dress, and conversed with men and women of the great world. It was at this time that she made up her mind to become a member of the Church of England into which she was later confirmed. She came nearer than ever before to the realization of her own powers and, on her return to the United States, she was ready for new and challenging tasks.

As so often happens, opportunity did not immediately present itself. For a short time, she practiced as a private duty nurse and during this uneasy interval cared for a member of the Conover family in South Amboy, New Jersey. Alice Conover, who was later to enter the Johns Hopkins Hospital Training School for Nurses, recalls that Mrs. Sidney Lanier of Baltimore was a guest in the Conover home while Isabel Hampton was on duty there and suggested that she should seek a position in the Johns Hopkins Hospital then in process of construction. It seems probable that Isabel Hampton kept this possibility in mind although she was first to undertake a different and difficult enterprise—the direction of the Illinois Training School.

This School had been organized and was conducted by a Board of Lady Managers composed of exceptionally able women who were striving to improve the nursing service in the crowded wards of the Cook County Hospital in Chicago. The general administrative pattern was similar to that prevailing at Bellevue where its first superintendent, Mary E. Brown, had taken her training under the supervision of Eliza Perkins. When Miss Brown resigned, Miss Perkins recommended Isabel Hampton as her successor although she may have had some qualms about the wisdom of doing so. According to Isabel McIsaac, who later became its distinguished principal, the early years of the Illinois Training School were clouded by poverty, prejudice and political corruption and Miss Perkins may well have wondered whether such a burden ought to be placed on the shoulders of a girl only twenty-six years old who had never had any administrative experience. Events were to prove that in this instance, as in others, Eliza Perkins was an excellent judge of character.

Isabel Hampton's faith in her own powers must have been shaken when upon her arrival in Chicago on a depressingly hot Fourth of July, the matron of the nurses' home at the Cook County Hospital, misled by her youth and freshness, mistook her for a new probationer. Her letters to Elizabeth Birdseye show how heavily her responsibilities weighed upon her during the first difficult days:

"Yesterday was such a long day and I was glad enough when night came and I could go to bed and forget. Of course I am running the gauntlet of many eyes but that troubled me little. This morning, I was up by six, had my bath and down to 6.45 a.m. breakfast. Miss Steere, the assistant, is very nice and I think we will work well together. . . . It strikes me that I'll get on here but, alas, I fear it will be forlorn enough. The outlook from my bedroom window is not pretty in any sense and everything has such an unfinished rough untidy look though the Hospital is very elegant and the grounds are fine."

Her next letter tells of her first administrative problem:

"You know the doctors here have never been particularly pleasant and they are beginning just the same with me. I've been in hot water with them once already—you see none of them have called at the office and I do not know one of them—so I've been having all my conversations with the head clerk—the Warden is away. The result of our talk was that the head clerk had something done to one of the wards that made the house-doctor there perfectly furious. He stormed to his head nurse about me, she came and told me how he felt and I at once sent for the said doctor. He came with wrath on his countenance but I was pleasant and after we had had a fair out-and-out talk he was alright, said he was sorry he had said anything and we are good friends. But the others still hold aloof and I suppose there will be more or less trouble."

Presently the absent Warden returned and she made a shrewd

appraisal of him: "The Warden came to my office to call on me and now has just gone. He is a very fascinating man—or at least has that reputation. I do not find him so only he has bonny blue eyes and in his fresh linen and suit of navy blue serge made a very pleasing appearance this afternoon."

Miss Hampton's mental reservations concerning this "very fascinating man" were justified by the fact that he later became involved in a political scandal and had to leave the country in order to avoid arrest.

Before long, she met with the petty and sullen rebuffs so often inflicted by those who resent authority:

"I all but lost my angelic temper this morning over a nurse. Shall I tell you? You see I sit at the head of a table-full of the oldest nurses, thirteen in all, and have to do the honors of helping the meat, vegetables, etc. This I am not fond of doing and besides, never having had to see after so many before, I felt I might neglect them sometime. So this I told them in the beginning and said to be sure to ask for themselves if they wanted anything more. On Friday I supposed I had supplied them all but they have a horrid way of passing things across the table and about half-way through dinner I looked up to see if anyone wanted anything more and to my horror found the nurse directly on my left making her dinner of cucumber, cabbage, and bread and butter without a plate. I at once asked her had she had no dinner? 'No.' I asked: 'Could you not ask for it?' Oh! I was furious!

"Scene no. 2 was this morning. I came down to second breakfast and had to wait on 22 plates. By the time that was accomplished nearly all the nurses at my table had finished and gone. But one remained and she sat looking straight in front of her and eating nothing. She is a night nurse and I asked her if she was very tired. For reply she said: 'I should like some coffee.' I then and there vowed I would end it and now I have breakfast and dinner alone. And so it goes."

As soon as the first strangeness wore off, there is even a hint that she was beginning to enjoy the exercise of authority for its own sake:

"You may guess it is no joke being the head of such a family. The housekeeper is responsible to me for the condition of things

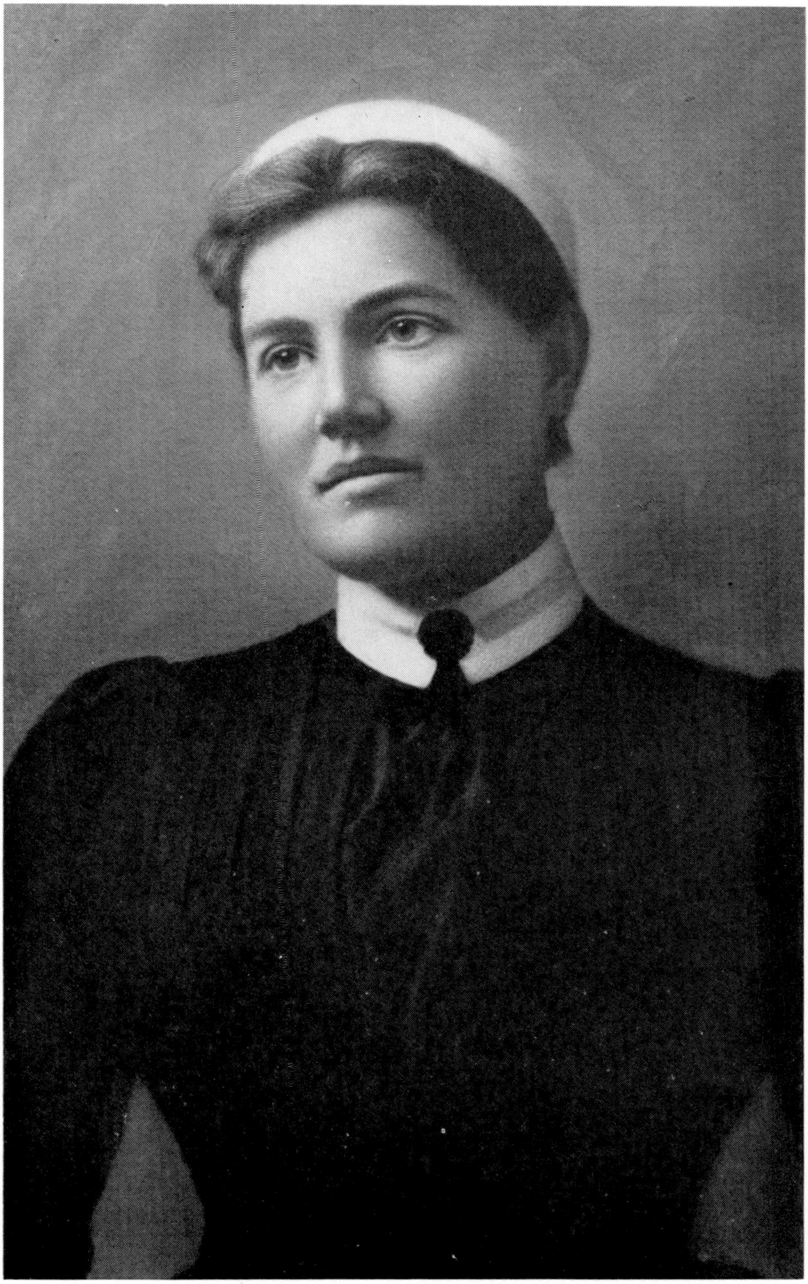

ISABEL ADAMS HAMPTON
Superintendent of Nurses and Principal of the Training School, 1889–1894

PORTRAIT BY SERGEANT KENDALL

in the home so I have done a lot of talking and putting to rights. The servants were doing much as they pleased and the way the dining room girls waited on the table was a sight—one might ring the table-bell for five minutes without getting an answer. I planned out more work for them and had them told how to behave. . . . Ever since, they have done splendidly but they think I'm an ogress."

In spite of these domestic preoccupations, Isabel Hampton did not neglect her educational responsibilities: "There are 55 pupils now and will be 60 soon. I commenced quizzes last week with a class of 21 pupils. . . . I am so sorry for the poor nurses. The wards are mostly about three times larger than Bellevue—for instance, 67 patients in a ward and the greater part typhoids. I went in one this morning and took their temperatures for them for they were so busy."

Then came a disciplinary problem more serious than any she had yet tackled:

"I took a head nurse to task severely yesterday and she'll go in two weeks time. I'll have her no longer. I know the older ones think I'm dreadful because I do not let them have their own sweet way. . . . I have the full say of keeping or dismissing nurses so there will not be any row."

She was mistaken. There was to be a row and a big one. She had yet to learn that "full say" usually has its limitations:

"I get many sullen looks and cold bows these days. The nurse went to the Committee about it. Just fancy! I never heard of such a thing being done all the time I was at Bellevue but eastern ways and manners are not like western ones. The nurse I sent away was most unreliable and I could place no confidence in her. It will pass over after a time I suppose."

It did pass over, but not without teaching her a lesson that she was not soon to forget although as time went on she became more and more absorbed in her plans for broadening the educational program:

"We are quite busy with lectures and the like. Three lectures for next week and a quiz by myself. There is to be a special meeting of the Board to discuss the advisability of taking two more wards. One is a surgical ward that we have wanted for a long time. . . . Do not feel uneasy about me. To be sure my eighth of a grain of common sense is very often worked hard (having such an owner) but usually I come out of it all some way."

Isabel McIsaac was one of Miss Hampton's probationers and freely admitted in later years that all these reforms were at first attributed to the rather irritating energy of the proverbial new broom that sweeps clean. Before her second year of training was over, Isabel McIsaac began to realize that she and her classmates should have been devoutly thankful for the new order of things and, after the lapse of years, she was filled with amazement at the intelligence, the discernment, and the undismayed courage which had brought it about:

"The methods of teaching and the division of time in a nurses' training which then prevailed in all schools for nurses, was still unsystematic and disorderly and Miss Hampton seems to have been the first superintendent to grasp the possibilities of reducing both the practice and the theory of nursing in the schools to a graded system. This task of reconstruction she accomplished within a year and in the second year, when Miss Hampton and the school had the assistance and teaching of Miss Kimber and Miss Draper, the school was as systematically taught as it is to-day."

In the early months of 1887, an especially spectacular political upheaval occurred at the Cook County Hospital. Seven members of the County Board were jailed on charges of misappropriation of funds and the Warden fled to Canada. While the School was in no way involved in the scandal, it suffered from the reaction and, for a time, the activities of the School were curtailed to some extent. However, the medical staff of the Hospital soon came to the rescue by petitioning the County Board for more nurses and insisting that the Illinois Training School was still the logical source of supply. This proof of confidence in the School meant a great deal to Isabel Hampton even though she was aware that she would soon sever her connection with it. The announcement of her appointment as superintendent of nurses at the Johns Hopkins Hospital did not come altogether as a surprise but it was received with sincere regret by all concerned and especially by the Board of Lady Managers who had given her such strong and steadfast support.

The Illinois Training School owed much to Isabel Hampton but she would have been the first to admit that she, in turn, owed much to the School and to the turbulent Cook County Hospital as well. Trials and tribulations had given her a direct and practical insight into many problems, disciplinary and otherwise, which was to stand her in good stead even in an environment that was entirely free from the menace of political corruption. Harassed by the unwarranted subordination of the educational needs of the School to the inordinate demands of the nursing service, she had come to realize that some means must be found of putting an end to it. Distressed by the meagreness of the teaching program, she had known the satisfaction of working out plans which would foster the exchange of new ideas and teaching facilities as well as enriching clinical experience.

Although she herself may not have been fully aware of it, less tangible but even stronger influences had been brought to bear on her. At the Illinois Training School, and for the first time in her life, Isabel Hampton found full scope for her native ability as a teacher and as an administrator. She encountered stiff opposition and learned not to be afraid of it. She realized now that she must deal with the consequences of her own mistakes as best she could. She knew that she must face the bitter loneliness which is the lot of those who are clothed with power and authority.

The Curtain Rises

THE CEREMONY that marked the inauguration of the Johns Hopkins Hospital Training School for Nurses took place on October 9, 1889, in the presence of a distinguished gathering. Mrs. Miles White, the only surviving sister of Johns Hopkins, was present and so was his business partner, Mr. Henry D. Harvey. Among the representatives of the Board of Trustees was Charles J. M. Gwinn who had drafted the Founder's mandate, now after a lapse of sixteen years at last to be fulfilled:

"I desire you to establish, in connection with the Hospital, a training school for female nurses. This provision will secure the services of women competent to care for the sick in the Hospital wards, and will enable you to benefit the whole community by supplying it with a class of trained and experienced nurses."

The Johns Hopkins University was represented by President Gilman himself and the members of the medical staff were out in full force. Among the guests of honor were Cardinal Gibbons and the Superior of the Mount Hope Retreat. Superintendents of nurses from various hospitals in Philadelphia came to share the rejoicings and "about one hundred ladies from Baltimore and the vicinity" lent an air of social distinction to the occasion.

After Isabel Hampton had been presented to the audience by the President of the Board of Trustees, Mr. Francis T. King, she delivered a notable address that proved to be a declaration of the proposed aims and policies of the School. This had been prepared at the request of the Trustees and revealed in almost every sentence that the young Principal had a firm grasp of the underlying philosophy of nursing education as well as clear insight into the problems of nursing service. A single paragraph indicated the general pattern of the course of training:

"The proposed plan of study is much like that in other large schools for nurses. The first year the pupils will be engaged in hospital work entirely, acting as assistants in the wards and, under the instruction of appointed head nurses, being changed from time to time from one department of work to another. In connection with this practical work, they will receive theoretical teaching, given systematically in classes, and by means of lecturers. In their second year, they are expected to be sufficiently taught to be able to assume more direct responsibility of patients in the hospital, and to undertake the care of patients in private families. In addition to this, a certain portion of each pupil's second year will be devoted to district nursing among the poor, in their homes, under a competent head nurse, where it is hoped that such nurses may not only leave their sick restored to health, but also leave behind them some good practical work and simple lessons in hygiene and right living that may result in better health and happier homes; and especially it is hoped that their presence for good may be felt in this city as it never has in any city in America, in the homes of those with moderate incomes who will be required to give in return for her services only in proportion to their means."

Miss Hampton also pointed out that training schools were already the victims of their own success and were being set up in connection with all sorts of hospitals, even in those devoted to the treatment of a single type of disease:

"When such graduates go forth, and undertake not only the kind of work they are qualified for, but also other branches that they are in almost entire ignorance of, they bring unjust criticism on all who call themselves by the same name. It is a cheap method of securing hospital nursing, but fair neither to the woman they receive nor to those who spend many more months and much greater labor in the large hospitals, fitting themselves for the work of caring for any and all kinds of maladies. . . . The question arises would it not be better if an arrangement could be made whereby one large school could do the nursing in several small hospitals?"

The importance of providing nursing service for all classes in the community was brought sharply into focus:

"Up to the present time, the usefulness of schools of nursing is recognized chiefly from three standpoints. They have answered the question of how to properly care for the sick poor in our large charity hospitals and infirmaries, and have made it possible for private and church hospitals to give their patients skilled care. The rich can also secure the same service in their homes. For women, they have created a profession which is unquestionably womanly; thus far they have ministered to the rich and the very poor.

"The trained nurse is almost an unknown quantity to the poor in their homes, and to the great majority of people with only moderate incomes, who are obliged to struggle thro' with their sick as of yore, as best they may, for the simple reason that a nurse is too great a luxury, as she in some instances costs more than the modest income amounts to, and cannot very often afford to render her services for less. How to bring the services of the trained nurse into just such homes is a problem that has caused and is causing food for thought in many minds."

As her address drew to a close, Isabel Hampton spoke with deep feeling and sincerity of what she conceived to be the duty of each and every Johns Hopkins nurse, and of her own vision of the future destiny of the School:

"It is not so much the great amount of work that she can accomplish practically that is desired, but the kind of work, and to render unto each patient under her care nursing in its best and truest sense; and as the University and the Hospital are looked to from all quarters for what is best in science, so may it follow, that as time goes on, and women go forth as graduates of the Johns Hopkins Hospital School for Nurses, this School may be looked to for what is best in nursing, and her graduates uphold their part of a grand work with all faithfulness."

The exercises ended with an address by the superintendent of the Hospital, Dr. Henry Mills Hurd, in which he dwelt at length on "what the Hospital has a right to expect from the pupils of this School." However, it is only fair to admit that he did redress the balance by acknowledging that the Hospital also had some obligations toward the School:

"It is an organic part of the Hospital foundation, as much a part of it as any of the wards or numerous departments of the establishment. It is not under the charge of any outside governing body, but is under the fostering care of the Trustees. It is not here by sufferance. It has a right to be here; and a recognized position in all work of the Hospital. . . . In the eyes of the Trustees, nursing is not to be considered a trade but a learned profession. . . . Its course of study should be more thorough and systematic than that of any other school in the land, and it must inevitably feel the influence of the great University to which the Hospital is so nearly allied."

Dr. Hurd's address unquestionably reflected the attitude of the Board of Trustees toward the School and in one respect had a special significance. The lines of authority were sharply drawn and it was made clear that whatever other rights and privileges were granted, that of independence would be withheld. "It is not under the charge of any outside governing body, but is under the fostering care of the Trustees."

There is no means of knowing what Isabel Hampton thought about the wisdom or otherwise of conducting the School of Nursing under "the fostering care of the Trustees." At the Illinois Training School, the Board of Lady Managers had been her loyal supporters without whose help the sinister influence of a corrupt hospital administration could not have been overcome. In Baltimore, the administration of the Hospital was in the hands of men who without exception were gentlemen and scholars. Several were members of the Society of Friends and all were prominent in the business and professional life of the city. Out of a total of twelve, nine were also Trustees of the University and there was something stable and dependable about the group as a whole. The president, Mr. King, had even been in direct communication with Florence Nightingale herself and was known to be in sympathy with her views.

The School of Medicine was not yet in operation but Dr. William Osler had already been appointed professor of the theory and practice of medicine at the University as well as physician-in-chief of the Hospital. Then there was Dr. William Welch, professor of pathology at the University, whom Isabel Hampton remembered as the "respected Microscopist" of her Bellevue days. Dr. William Halsted was associate professor of surgery and acting surgeon-in-chief, and Dr. Howard Kelly was gynecologist and obstetrician in the Hospital. These men were destined to go down in medical history as "the Big Four" and, while she was not yet fully aware of their real stature, she did realize from the beginning that she was in the presence of men who were not only skilled physicians but great teachers as well.

She knew, of course, that shortly after his appointment as superintendent of the Hospital Dr. Hurd had made a brief tour of observation during which he visited the schools associated with Bellevue Hospital, the New York Hospital, the New Haven Hospital, the Massachusetts General Hospital, the Boston City Hospital and the Pennsylvania Hospital. The text of the report which he submitted to the Trustees has fortunately been preserved and affords a valuable insight into the conditions then prevailing in contemporary schools of nursing. It dealt with such general topics as the age at which pupil nurses were admitted; the duration of training; the nature of theoretical instruction; the hours of duty; money allowances; contractual arrangements; the assignment of pupil nurses to private duty outside the hospital, and the use of their services as district nurses.

The age of admission he found to be practically the same in all six schools, namely from 25 to 35 years with occasional exceptions in special instances. At Bellevue Hospital, he was told that pupils might be accepted who were only twenty-three years of age: "It is, however, the opinion of the Acting Principal that it is unwise to receive any person less than twenty-five years of age, as there is always danger that younger persons may not endure the labor of nursing. It also seems important that the would-be nurse should be old enough to have gotten through with the fickleness and frivolity of youth."

The duration of the course ranged between eighteen months and two years and schools offering the shorter course usually required the pupil to remain in the service of the hospital for at least six months after its completion. All pupils were required to sign contracts binding them to remain for the period of time agreed upon but in three schools this commitment was not rigorously enforced if it involved genuine hardship. Money allowances of from $10 to $16 monthly were granted and board, lodging and laundry were provided. A probationary period of from one to two months was required.

There appears to have been no lack of candidates and in the Bellevue School of Nursing no less than a thousand candidates had presented themselves for sixty-four vacancies. Many of them must have been quite ineligible since of the few who did qualify for entrance, about a third were rejected either during the probationary period or later in the course. Severe working conditions may have had something to do with this wastage for Dr. Hurd had found that in all six schools day duty extended over a twelve-hour period. Only one hour off duty was granted daily, one free afternoon weekly and part of Sunday, but all free time depended upon the demands of the service and upon the hours set aside for class and lecture. The New Haven Hospital stated that a vacation of one month was allowed during the training period: "but notwithstanding this, nurses frequently break down in health."

There was a strong similarity in the general arrangement and content of the program of theoretical instruction in all six schools and weekly recitations were given during the first year, followed by didactic lectures during the second year. Dr. Hurd noted that some attempt was made at Bellevue to teach invalid cookery "but the amount accomplished is not great for lack of conveniences. It seemed to me that the Acting Principal was somewhat inclined to undervalue didactic instruction and to lay too much stress upon the practical side of nursing. Instruction is given in bandaging but nothing is done in bacteriology. It is not thought necessary to have head nurses in charge of wards." At the New York Hospital School of Nursing, didactic instruction included recitations, lectures and demonstrations and the pupil nurses spent three weeks in the diet kitchen. Graduating exercises were held upon the completion of the course and a diploma was granted. Head nurses were selected from the graduating class and the practice was said to be a good one. At the Massachusetts General Hospital the program was much the same except that there was little or no practical work in cookery. The head nurses in this school were also selected from the graduating classes. All six hospitals found it difficult to obtain the services of orderlies and the New York Hospital authorities stated that attempts to train male nurses only led to their becoming medical students.

Dr. Hurd seems to have taken special pains to investigate the desirability or otherwise of permitting pupil nurses to care for private patients able to pay the hospital for their services and also made inquiries about assigning them to district nursing in the homes of the poor. At Bellevue Hospital he was told that: "In view of the fact that all the nurses which the school will accommodate are required for the services in Bellevue Hospital, it has been found impossible to do private or district nursing. It is also thought that the superintendent of nurses in any event could not get sufficient time to supervise this work."

At the New York Hospital, the assignment of pupil nurses to private duty, as a means of increasing the income of the School, was not permitted. There was no clear statement of the policy of either the Massachusetts General Hospital or the Boston City Hospital but in both institutions the demands of the nursing service seemed to preclude any other assignments. The New Haven Hospital frankly admitted that pupils were assigned to private duty as a means of earning money for the Hospital. Four schools had tried to make arrangements for pupil nurses to obtain experience in district nursing but in no case had it been possible to spare them from their work in the wards.

Dr. Hurd's recommendations were as follows:

"As a result of the above examination I would present the following conclusions:

1st.—That neither private nursing nor district nursing should be attempted for at least one year. It may in fact be better to wait until after the graduation of the first class. The conclusion is irresistible that district nursing is fraught with difficulties. In my judgment it could be best combined with a system of district medical visitation, as in Boston. As to private nursing the creation of income for the school should be a minor consideration. It is a question whether either should be attempted by non-graduate nurses. If private nursing or district nursing among the poor are attempted they should be assumed by pupils only because they promise to develop the school and increase the efficiency of its pupils.

2nd.—That the most acceptable ages for pupils are between 25 and 35 years.

3rd.—That careful attention should be given to the more purely intellectual part of the nurse's training to the end that nursing may be elevated into a profession and raised as far as possible above the standard of a mere practical trade. It is desirable that recitations and lectures be graded, systematized and extended beyond what is at present attempted in any existing school.

4th.—That nurses should take their meals at a Nurses' Home and enjoy as far as possible a family and home life there. Their duties being often extremely taxing and arduous they should have an opportunity to go entirely away from the atmosphere of the Hospital when their hours of service are completed.

5th.—That the School should form an organic part of the Hospital and become fully identified with its work. Wherever a school is not a part of the hospital and responsible to its governing body, experience has shown that a spirit of disloyalty develops which robs the Hospital of the most enlightened services of the School, and the School of the active co-operation of those physicians who are connected with the Hospital."

These recommendations were important because they were to set the pattern for the organization of the Johns Hopkins Hospital Training School for Nurses. To begin with, they demonstrate that Dr. Hurd's conception of the aims and scope of nursing education was far in advance of that commonly held by the physicians and hospital administrators of his time. In this respect, as in many others, he was doubtless influenced by President Gilman whose spacious and far-sighted educational policies made a profound impression upon him. The recommendations are also revealing because they clearly reflect the attitude of the administrative head of the Johns Hopkins Hospital toward the School of Nursing. The fifth and last recommendation betrays his strong and deeply rooted conviction that the School should be an integral part of the Hospital rather than an entity in itself.

One aspect of the situation gave Isabel Hampton cause for some anxiety. Upon her arrival in Baltimore during the latter part of September and prior to the formal opening of the School, she discovered that although the Trustees had announced their intention of limiting admissions this good resolution had not been carried out and the reception of patients had been left to take its natural course. The total nursing staff consisted of two head nurses, four graduate nurses, and nine probationers. The nursing load was heavy, so heavy indeed that already it threatened to interfere with the teaching program. Was she to find that in the Johns Hopkins Hospital, as in the Cook County Hospital, the educational interests of the School were to be sacrificed to the exigencies of the nursing service?

Things began to look a little brighter as soon as the Nurses Home was sufficiently furnished to permit the transfer of the nursing staff from temporary quarters in the Hospital. Jessica Glenn, a graduate of the Boston City School of Nursing, arrived to take charge of the newly-opened dispensary and Florence Macrae, a graduate of the same school, became head nurse in the surgical wards. The latter appointment made it possible to limit Caroline Hampton's activities to the operating room and from this time on she was no longer subject to the general authority of the superintendent of nurses, a situation which was soon to become difficult from a disciplinary point of view. She never got along well with Isabel Hampton, possibly because she herself had hoped to be appointed superintendent of nurses. Perhaps it was inevitable that she would clash with any woman set in authority over her, especially when that woman happened to be what Dr. MacCallum described as "a Northerner with a very different background."

During the latter part of October, six more probationers were accepted for their trial month and Isabel Hampton made an historic entry in her monthly journal: "On the 15th, the first weekly class was held and again on the 26th and 28th." The regular course of lectures began on the first day of November and during the month four classes were held and five lectures given. At long last, the School was underway.

The First Year

AT THIS point it seems appropriate to take a look at the pupils themselves. Who were they? What were they seeking? What had been done to determine their fitness? To begin with, each candidate had been given a circular of information together with "a paper of questions" bearing on age, health, previous education and freedom from family responsibility. The text of the circular appeared in the first number of *The Johns Hopkins Hospital Bulletin*, published in December 1889 but no copy of the "paper of questions" seems to have been preserved although its general trend is indicated by the replies that it elicited. The candidate was evidently not required to fill out a printed form but was instructed to write a letter which would not only answer specific questions but would also shed some light on her social background and her reasons for wishing to become a nurse.

The circular gave the candidate a fairly clear idea of what would be required of her. She must be of "acceptable age," that is to say between twenty-three and thirty-five years old, sound in health and of good moral character. During the month of trial, and previous to being accepted as a pupil in the School, "the applicant must be prepared for an examination in reading, penmanship, simple arithmetic, and English dictation. The examination is to test the applicant's ability to read aloud well, to write legibly and accurately, to keep simple accounts, and to take notes on lectures. This amount of education is *indispensable* for a member of the School, but applicants are reminded that women of superior education and cultivation will be preferred."

Pupils were warned that "the Superintendent will decide as to their fitness for the work and the propriety of retaining or dismissing them. She can, also, with the approval of the Board of Trustees, discharge a pupil at any time in case of misconduct or inefficiency." In the event of their acceptance, pupils would be required to sign a formal agreement: "I, the undersigned, do hereby agree to remain two years from date a pupil of the above-named institution; and promise during that time to faithfully obey the rules of the school and the hospital, and to be subordinate to the authorities governing the same."

It was stated that: "The course of instruction will be given by visiting and resident physicians and surgeons at the bedside of the patients, and by the Superintendent and Head-nurses. A regular course of lectures, recitations and demonstrations will be given, with examinations at stated periods." In addition to these educational advantages, the pupils were to be provided with board and lodging, and with free care in illness subject to the understanding that "time so lost must be made up." Upon acceptance, the pupil received an allowance of eight dollars per month, increasing to twelve dollars during the second year. It was explained that this allowance "is not given as pay for services rendered, as the teaching and the profession acquired are considered to be an ample equivalent, but is allowed for uniform, textbooks, and other expenses incidental to their training."

The pupils were told that they would be required "to serve for the first year as assistants in the wards of the Hospital, the second year they will be expected to perform any duty assigned to them by the Superintendent, either by service in the Hospital, or to be sent to private patients on application or to district nursing among the poor." The normal working day was to extend over a twelve-hour span: "The day nurses are on duty from 7.30 a.m. to 7.30 p.m. with an hour off duty for dinner, and additional time for study, exercise, or rest. Unless in an emergency they are also given an afternoon during the week, and half of Sunday, and a vacation of two weeks is allowed each year. Pupils are not placed on night duty until they have been in the School three months."

It was conceded that when the full term of two years was ended: "the nurses thus trained will be at liberty to choose their own field of labor, whether in hospitals, in private families, or in district nursing in the homes of the poor. On leaving the School, they will, upon passing an examination, each receive a diploma, and will be expected for the next few years to make an annual report to the Superintendent."

Undaunted by these stern conditions, the members of the first class set down their answers to "the paper of questions" and even after the lapse of more than sixty years these letters still have an extraordinary freshness and vitality.

First of all, there was Marion Turner who had been educated in a private school. Mary Gross had enjoyed "a good common school education, including languages, music and painting" at Miss Woodward's Seminary in Harrisburg, Pennsylvania. She had previously entered the training school of the Philadelphia General Hospital and explained that: "My parents were extremely opposed to my going to Blockley and when they heard that I was expected to serve for six months in the Insane Department they brought me home two weeks after I left." Then there was Kate Emory who had been "a teacher in schools and kindergarten," and Nora Anthony who had taken a musical course at Lebanon Valley College. Tillie Spencer and Anna Hudson both laid claim to a good plain English education and Anna Rutherford had had "three years at a seminary." A letter from Emma Cleaver, written in beautiful copper plate handwriting, stated that she held the degree of Master of Arts from Ripon College, Ripon, Wisconsin. She had taken the classical course, "three years in Greek" and her average standing had been 97 per cent. For five and a half years, she had been teaching in the public schools.

Ida May had left school at fourteen but had already done good work at the Good Samaritan Hospital. Susan Read's brief letter written in the third person and in a strong hand, gave the assurance that she had been well educated in private schools in Baltimore and Philadelphia. Mrs. Mary Emory was a widow, thirty-five years old and the mother of five children, who had been a member of the staff at All Saints Home. Gertrude Hammerel stated that she had received an excellent German education and could speak some English and a little French. Her handwriting is a joy to behold. Ruth Williams had rashly applied elsewhere "but when I saw the account of the opening of the Johns Hopkins Hospital I withdrew." Evelyn Pope proudly said that she was a graduate of the Roland Academy and her letter was endorsed by Mr. Francis T. King, the President of the Board of Trustees. Georgia Nevins had received her education in a school at Mount Holyoke, Massachusetts, and at Clare Place Seminary in Warsaw, Kentucky. She had previously applied at Bellevue but was refused "because of the number of applicants before me."

The letter from Elvina Hartley had a quality all its own for it was written in the "plain speech" of the Quakers: "The list of questions which thee kindly sent me has been received, for which please receive my thanks." She had been a member of a Quaker household in Baltimore where "the family were all Friends and regular attendants at their meeting, taking their children with them." Elvina Hartley was to carry her Quaker serenity into her training. No matter what turmoil there might be in the ward, she pursued the even tenor of her way and disregarded all interruptions. On one occasion, she was told to hurry with a basin and towel for the use of the impatient Dr. Halsted. She gravely watched him wash his hands and then looked up at him with her gentle smile and said: "Shall I dry them for thee?" The reply to this innocent request has not been recorded.

There was one letter which was subtly different from all the rest. It came from a Canadian, Mary Adelaide Nutting.

Waterloo East, P. Q.
Canada.
September 6th, 1889.

My dear Madam,

I have received the circular you kindly sent me concerning your Training School for Nurses, and wish to apply for entrance. I submit the information you ask for in regard to myself and hope you may find it satisfactory.

I was thirty years old on the first day of November last, am five feet, five inches in height, weighing one hundred and twenty-nine pounds. Though not remarkably strong, I have a good deal of endurance and have not had an illness of any importance since childhood. I have no diseases or physical defects of any sort that I am aware of. I have been educated almost entirely at home, and spent some years studying music, with the hope of going on with it elsewhere, which I was obliged to abandon for lack of means.

I am single and as I live with my brother who is married my family ties are not binding. My mother is dead and my father though elderly is not an invalid. I have never been a nurse elsewhere, but I applied to Bellevue, New York, some days ago, from whence I have as yet received no reply. Hearing since then, that their replies are often delayed many weeks and sometimes months, I decided to apply to you, being anxious to avoid suspense, and also to begin work at the earliest possible date. I enclose copies of letters from my clergyman and physician and should you wish for further information regarding me, beg to refer you to the Hon. G. G. Stevens of this place and to the Hon. Sir Hector L. Langevin, K.C.M.G., Minister of Public Works, Ottawa, Ont.

Tho' aware that I am applying very late for this year I earnestly hope that my application may be accepted and that I may be further fortunate in securing an early entrance.

Believe me, dear Madam
Very truly yours
Mary Adelaide Nutting.

Unlike Bellevue, the Johns Hopkins Hospital Training School for Nurses did not keep Mary Adelaide Nutting in suspense:

Waterloo East
September 15th, 1889

Dear Madam,

I have just received your letter of the 9th telling me that my application has been accepted.

I shall make the preparations you require without delay, and you may rely upon my being in readiness to go, whenever you send for me.

Believe me
Most sincerely yours
Adelaide Nutting

Incidentally, it is worth noting that within the compass of a single year Georgia Nevins and Adelaide Nutting were lost to

Bellevue and claimed by the Johns Hopkins Hospital Training School for Nurses.

The members of the first class were admitted at irregular intervals and were immediately placed on duty in one of the wards. Georgia Nevins thus describes her own abrupt initiation:

"Never having seen a trained nurse or the inside of a hospital, I was cordially greeted by Miss Hampton and happily impressed. Next morning, I was sent to the men's medical ward. The head nurse bade me put the linen room in order. She returned later, found the blankets were not folded properly and that was her opportunity to say what she thought of a stupid probationer. It reminded me of the initiation of students in fraternity houses.

"This incident was soon forgotten for my work increased by leaps and bounds. Susan Read was in that ward for a number of months where I could witness daily to her exquisite care of her patients. . . . Typhoid fever was rampant. One of the treatments was baths at the bedside for high temperatures. . . . On day duty, it was a mad rush to have everything in readiness for Dr. Osler's rounds for he was sure to appear leading a number of assistants, promptly at ten o'clock.

"Hours were long, the number of patients increased rapidly, there weren't enough nurses, and we were often too weary to prepare properly our theoretical work which, by the way, would bring a smile to the present day student, so much less was required. Miss Hampton was an interesting teacher, and she saw to it personally that our patients were given the best possible care. . . . Perhaps we didn't realize how fortunate we were in working with Dr. Osler, Dr. Halsted and Dr. Kelly, and never shall we forget Dr. Finney's kindly teaching in the Dispensary."

The adoption of a school uniform gave rise to animated discussion and according to Marion Turner, was finally decided upon at a conference in which even the pupil nurses took part:

"After Miss Hampton arrived, she called those nurses who were there to help decide what sort of a uniform we should wear. The blue dress and the cuffs were copied from the Blockley Training School uniform. The apron was presented by Miss Tillie Spencer and was from the one used in the English hospitals. The cap was presented by Miss Susan Read and was a modified copy of the

Philadelphia Episcopal Hospital cap. Later, Miss Hampton decided what sort of collar we should wear."

Another and somewhat different version of the origin of the cap is attributed to Mary Gross (Mrs. J. M. T. Finney) who, like Marion Turner, was a member of the first class:

"It is believed the model finally determined upon was a combination of a Bellevue and a New York Hospital cap, with many alterations and improvements. To Mrs. Finney and Mrs. Thayer, then Susan Read, was entrusted the actual making of the first cap. Mrs. Thayer particularly was a most meticulous needlewoman and after long and patient effort the cap evolved exactly like the one we wear today, except that every cap at that time was made large enough to cover all the hair of the nurse, which was its original purpose."

During the greater part of the year, Isabel Hampton herself wore a simple black china silk uniform, cut on flowing lines. The cap, collar and cuffs were made of fine lawn and the cap is said to have been inspired by one that she had seen worn by an ecclesiastical dignitary in Rome. When the weather was very hot, she wore white, but she liked the black dress better. Its extreme simplicity, almost severity, suited her perfectly.

The development of the teaching program went steadily forward although in her first formal report of the activities of the School, Isabel Hampton made a somewhat disquieting statement: "Owing to the School being still in a state of organization, changes from month to month have of necessity taken place according to the needs of the Hospital." In other words, the exigencies of the nursing service had already taken precedence over everything else. Under the circumstances it could hardly have been otherwise since eight divisions of the Hospital were already open for the reception of patients. These included D and E, the male and female surgical wards; F and G, the male and female medical wards; B and H, the private and public gynecological wards; and C, the medical and surgical private wards. The daily census had risen as high as 116 patients, the dispensary was very active and so were the operating rooms, not to mention a special ward for "patients who required isolation or seclusion."

In January 1890 the total nursing staff consisted of six head nurses, four staff nurses, and seventeen pupil nurses all of whom were in their first year. The four staff nurses took charge of the wards at night and the pupils acted as "assistants" to the head nurses during the daytime, carrying on in their absence as best they could. It is hardly surprising that the teaching program was somewhat desultory even though Miss Hampton did her best to give her "regular weekly recitations." A considerable amount of informal teaching was done in the wards by the head nurses and this informal instruction was remembered by one of the pupils as more valuable than the meagre classwork: "At least it did prepare us to deal with difficult situations without much help or direction."

The transfer of pupils from one ward to another was recorded in a series of bound books encased in heavy linen covers. Brief entries indicated the nature of the service and served as a record of the time spent by each pupil on day or night duty or as nurse in charge of a ward. The first assignment to night duty seems to have occurred about the beginning of the sixth month of training, and its duration did not usually exceed six weeks. The total time spent on night duty during the entire two-year course was seldom more than four months. The division of time between the various services appears to have been haphazard and there were complaints that pupils were assigned to the private wards for too long a period. Several pupils in the first class were placed in charge of wards as early as the eleventh month of training. Others, with less executive ability, served for shorter periods. Time lost by sickness was also recorded and opposite these entries there frequently appeared two melancholy words—"sore feet."

One assignment was regarded as terrifying by every pupil who had to face up to it. To quote Ada Carr:

"The isolating ward was a good deal of a trial in those days; many and terrible tales could be told by our early nurses who—after the ward had been entirely closed for weeks—would be called in the dead of night to convey a delirious patient to those haunted halls, re-echoing to their lonesome tread, of which the official description of Ward I says with pride, 'All these rooms open on a corridor through which the wind is always blowing'—with no companion except the telephone and that quite often out of commission. We have delirious patients nowadays but none such as those, and certainly our present day nurses would consider themselves somewhat abused if they were called upon to confront the conditions the early nurses accepted stoically."

In the fifth month of her training, Adelaide Nutting was sent to "the isolating ward" to care for an insane patient and was alone on duty there for three long weeks. It was an experience that she was long to remember:

"This building, known as Ward I, was the isolating ward, and its use for the purpose of caring for those patients who developed infectious diseases while within the Hospital had been slight and irregular. It had also proved useful for instances of sudden acute mania, arising under the same conditions, and probably some nurses of the earlier days have tolerably vivid remembrances of times when they found themselves alone on duty with patients of this description and no friendly voice or helping hand within reach. Such experiences are undoubtedly developing, but they do not furnish cheerful memories. No one who has ever been on duty in the Ward I of those days can ever forget it. It was a gloomy looking structure, cold bare and forbidding, without and within."

The schedule of formal lectures given by physicians from November 1889 to June 1890 appears to have been consistently carried out even though the demands of the nursing service continued to be heavy. It appeared in printed form and its full text was included in a report submitted by Dr. Hurd to the Board of Trustees.

Few schools of nursing can ever have been blessed with so distinguished a faculty—three of "the Big Four"—Dr. Welch, Dr. Osler and Dr. Kelly—not to mention other famous men. Dr. Osler's solitary lecture dealt with typhoid fever and had a direct clinical application since the wards were full of it. The six lectures on ventilation were intended to explain the management of the elaborate system of fans and air ducts by which the Hospital was supposed to be protected against air-borne infection. Dr. Hurd's lectures on psychiatric nursing included references to "occupation for invalids and the convalescent"—a topic that did not figure on most programs until much later. It seems a little

Schedule of Lectures: November 1, 1889 to June 26, 1890

Subject	*Lecturer*	*Number of Lectures*
Ventilation:	Dr. Alexander Abbott	6
Anatomy and Physiology:	Dr. W. T. Councilman	6
Elementary principles of aseptic and antiseptic surgery and the care of surgical patients:	Dr. F. J. Brockway	13
Elementary Principles of medical nursing:	Dr. H. A. Lafleur	8
Materia medica, common remedies, poisons and antidotes:	Dr. H. A. Lafleur	10
Fever nursing:	Dr. William Osler	1
Disinfection:	Dr. William Welch	1
Nursing in diseases of the eye and ear:	Dr. Samuel Theobald	3
Nursing in diseases of the throat and nose:	Dr. J. N. Mackenzie	3
Nursing care of gynecological patients including operating room technics:	Dr. Howard A. Kelly	5
Nursing care of infants and children in health and in disease:	Dr. W. D. Booker	4
Nursing care in diseases of the skin:	Dr. R. B. Morison	3
Application of electricity:	Dr. Thomas	2
Care of the nervous and insane and occupation for the invalid and convalescent:	Dr. Henry M. Hurd	3

incongruous that two lectures should have been given on "the application of electricity" and only six on anatomy and physiology and that Dr. Kelly should give five lectures on gynecological nursing but not one on obstetrics. At that time, however, the Hospital did not have an obstetrical service and although the pupils did receive a few lectures in their second year, Marion Turner recalled that "Dr. Kelly very kindly marked my paper 100 though I had never seen a case."

The teaching program was considerably strengthened in April 1890 when the cooking school was organized under the direction of Mary A. Boland, a graduate of the Boston Cooking School. Isabel Hampton had always believed dietetics and invalid cookery to be of paramount importance and had persuaded the authorities that suitable space in the main building should be converted into a diet kitchen. She thus described the general arrangement of the course:

"The organization of the cooking school resembles that of a ward with its head nurse and pupils, the teacher corresponding to the head nurse. Two pupils are sent to her for a month at a time. . . . The first hour and a half of the day is spent in the two private wards, where each pupil takes charge of the preparations for breakfast, makes the toast, arranges the trays daintily and gets everything in readiness for the breakfast which arrives from the general kitchen at eight o'clock. They then serve the trays and leave the wards at 9 a.m., going directly to the cooking school kitchen which is in a small room conveniently situated and easily accessible to all the wards. There they meet the teacher and the day's instruction begins. . . . The method of preparing about 150 different articles of sick diet is taught during the month and each article is made at least three times by the pupils themselves. . . . The afternoon hours are devoted to theoretical teaching."

Practical, oral and written tests were given and, in addition, Miss Boland gave three formal lectures on dietetics to the whole School. Ada Carr claims that this was the first instance in which a resident teacher of dietetics was ever employed in a school of nursing. Some of the pupil nurses remembered this particular course as better organized and more effectively taught than any other formal instruction that had come their way.

On June 15, 1890, Isabel Hampton had the satisfaction of recording in her monthly journal that the School "had taken over the nursing at the Thomas Wilson Sanitarium." This institution served as a summer home in the country for infants and children. Some mothers left their children just for the day and took them home at night but there were cottages where they might remain for as long as two weeks. There was also a large frame house with a bedroom for the use of the nurses and two smaller bedrooms for the accommodation of children who might be ill. Miss Hampton appointed Miss W. Miller as head nurse, "and a staff of three pupils to remain for three weeks and not all to be changed at once." Ada Carr has vividly described the weird experience of the nurses who had to wander among the scattered cottages at night, carrying baskets of milk bottles, and lighted by the dim rays of a lantern in the intervals of the frequent thunderstorms of the Green Spring Valley.

As yet, the Hospital had no pediatric service and Isabel Hampton evidently thought that even a meagre experience in the nursing of children was better than none at all. At any rate, she had a chance to experiment with an affiliation in the hope that its usefulness might be demonstrated from both an educational and an administrative point of view. All summer long, she made biweekly visits of inspection and managed to spare enough pupils to keep the scheme going until the Sanitarium closed for the winter.

The setting up of a diet school and the establishment of an affiliation within a few months of the opening of the School were distinct achievements and may have compensated Isabel Hampton for frustration in other directions. She had never been satisfied with the general pattern of education which prevailed in contemporary schools and yet she had been constrained to follow it much more closely than she wished. Much against her will, she still had to assign pupil nurses to duty in private homes and the working day remained far too long. Although the teaching program had to be suspended during the summer months, the members of the first class were given their first preliminary examination in September: "The surgical examination was conducted by Dr. F. J. Brockway, House Surgeon, the medical by Dr. H. Lafleur, House Physician. The examination was oral." Mary Gross headed the class with an average of 96.5 and Adelaide Nutting came out fifth with an average of 94. Everyone, in fact, did very well.

Meanwhile, the fame of the Johns Hopkins Hospital and its Training School for Nurses had been spread abroad in the land and had attracted a stream of observers that has never slackened from that day to this. The first to make her appearance at the Training School for Nurses was Mary Agnes Snively, superintendent of nurses at the Toronto General Hospital, and before long she was followed by Louise Darche, superintendent of the New York City School of Nursing. It was only eight years since Isabel Adams Hampton, Mary Agnes Snively and Louise Darche had taught school together in the pleasant Ontario countryside. Feeling an urge toward "a change of occupation" they had pondered over the application forms of the Bellevue School of Nursing. All three had come a long way since then.

Lavinia Dock

In November 1890 just as the School was entering upon its second year, Isabel Hampton recorded in her journal that: "On the first, Miss Lavinia L. Dock was appointed Assistant Superintendent, and the instruction of the first year pupils was put under her care. It was arranged to divide the pupils into three classes, one senior, one middle, one junior, and classes to be held Mondays for seniors, Tuesdays for middle and Fridays for juniors from 3 to 4 p.m."

Born in Pennsylvania, in 1858, Lavinia Dock belongs to a family of distinguished scholars who are well known in the field of education. She was educated in private schools and graduated in 1886 from the Bellevue School of Nursing. She quite early manifested the intellectual brilliance and indomitable spirit that have since found expression in a variety of social and political crusades and has been aptly described as "mildly socialistic in theory, in practice an ardent philanthropist; by choice an apostle of the democratic idea, really a spiritual and mental aristocrat; and perfectly independent in every action." Although she was directly associated with the School for only three years, Lavinia Dock was destined to exercise a profound influence over its development.

A small notebook has been preserved which affords a glimpse of the organization and content of her first classes. The principal topics were anatomy and physiology, materia medica and practical nursing. The subject matter, while quite elementary, was systematically arranged and well tied in with the more advanced lectures given by the physicians. There were references to collateral reading and to oral reviews and written examinations. One class in each subject took place every week and the schedule shows a marked advance over the first year when Miss Hampton's "recitations" were held only once weekly. The notebook also contains a few headings that were evidently intended for a talk on ethics:

"The nurse is a soldier. Absolute and unquestioning obedience to a superior officer is the fundamental idea of the military system in order that responsibility may be rightly placed. . . . There is a necessity for drill in producing quickness, skill and quiet. Criticisms are not accusations. Strictness and exactness produce better nurses."

Every pupil nurse in the School felt the impact of the magnetic personality of Lavinia Dock and one of them, Adelaide Nutting, had this to say of her: "They will remember her as an unfailingly generous friend and helper, if occasionally as a frank and merciless critic; as one who gave them new conceptions of duty, loyalty, justice, and new ideas of the value of human life and the worth of human labor." One of her other pupils told the present writer that she "learned more from Lavinia Dock than from all the others put together."

From the very beginning, Isabel Hampton and Lavinia Dock were in complete accord so far as the broader issues of nursing service and education were concerned. On Sunday mornings they used to have breakfast together, a little later than usual, and talk about what might be done to broaden the education of nurses, not only at the Johns Hopkins Hospital Training School for Nurses, but all over the world. The exploits of "the Big Four" interested them enormously. Dr. Osler would drift into Miss Hampton's office, talking discursively about this and that and occasionally giving an impromptu rehearsal of one or other of his famous addresses. Miss Dock still remembers an occasion when he was trying to awaken the citizens of Baltimore to a belated sense of responsibility for municipal sanitation: "He wandered in as usual and told Miss Hampton what he meant to say, she making no reply to any of it. In my small office I could hear every word. As he went out of the door, he turned and with unusual intensity of feeling said: 'I am going to let myself go.' And he did, indeed. This address turned out to be a picture of his remarkable personality, based as it was on the most complete humanitarianism."

In an interview with the present writer, Miss Dock recalled other memories of those early days and confirmed impressions which she had set down many years previously:

"It was while I was on duty as night superintendent at Bellevue that I first met Miss Hampton. I remember that, it being rather late in the morning, she reproved me for being out of bed, with that serious, dignified, sympathetic yet restrained manner so characteristic of her, which instantly struck me as the perfection of bearing for a nurse. I did not see nor hear of her again until she wrote offering me the position of her assistant at the Johns Hopkins.

"The three years that followed were the most delightful possible. The hospital was new, and though the fortune bequeathed to it had been gathered by the most unlovely business methods, the trustees, who were all men of the highest aims, framed a noble ideal of its mission. It was designed to be a centre of liberal teaching and instruction and to radiate the pure light of science for truth's sake. A fresh and inspiring atmosphere did indeed permeate the whole place, and there was not then the rush of work that has now fallen upon it. In contrast to the vast and crowded Bellevue, it struck me at first as being nearly all hospital, and very little patient.

"Life in the training school was cheerful and simple. It was Miss Hampton's custom to read prayers just after breakfast, in the parlor, and with military discipline every nurse attended. It was always a new sensation to see her, serene and beautiful, enter the room with her prayer-book in hand after the whole staff had taken its place and this impression was not lessened when I learned later that she had sometimes dressed in three and a half minutes. We had a hymn, which I played on the piano, then it was our custom to go with the nurses to the door and watch them go down the corridor. When I think of the Hospital now, it is always this picture that I see—the nurses streaming down the corridor, the green lawn, and young trees outside in the sunshine (the sun always shines in Baltimore), and Miss Hampton's caryatid-like figure, clad either in black or white, her large eyes radiant with pride and joy in her flock. Never was any mother prouder. Almost always, as we turned away, she would say to me with perhaps a little squeeze of the hands, 'Docky, aren't they nice?'

"Baltimore had never before known the trained nurse, and Miss Hampton took from the outset the gracious yet commanding position which fixed the nurses' status in the community as a dignified and respected one, both professionally and socially. The hospital attracted a superior set of women, and the city accepted them readily but she herself had not a few amusing tilts with the lords of creation who were unaccustomed to see a nurse hold any command. She had a scrupulous insistence on her own sphere of authority. There she permitted no encroachment, but respecting others' boundaries, demanded equal respect for her own.

"She was capable of a righteous indignation and of a most salutary anger which, one felt, was held in perfect control. Unlike most people, she was superbly beautiful when angry; her brow remained clear and her features tranquil, but her color rose, her eyes blazed and grew larger, and her pose became indescribably expressive.

"No one else, I think, so well as I, knows the truly original and creative character of Miss Hampton's mind, for during the three years we were together there I saw her conceive and develop all the various ideas which are now embodied in living groups of persons and in broad lines of organization. We were quite secluded in our work—there was not the excitement and stimulus of a metropolis, where ideas are generated one knows not how and spread mysteriously, so that in a moment everyone is thinking the same thing. Miss Hampton's mental visions of future nursing growth and development came as a sort of picture, hazy at first, with outlines more or less indefinite, gradually taking form until the whole was clear and vivid, filling her with joy and enthusiasm, eager interest and an untiring energy. Thus long before a national association had been thought of, she saw all its groupings, powers and activities, and rejoiced over its great possibilities; so, too, the course at Teachers College showed itself to her in long vistas of certainties. She saw the women at work, knew what they would do, and what would come of it. It was this reality to her of visions of the future that made her so delightful to live with and gave her her great fascination, for even if one did not always get clearly the drift of her talk, which was often impressionistic and suggestive, ignoring details, one could not but be stimulated and thrilled by her rich vitality.

"She had a wonderful feeling of the solidarity of women; her devotion to her profession was based on great loyalty to the cause of women's progress. She believed women to be the superior moral force and was impassioned for every advance which brought them upward. Along with her large grasp and insight she had a certain childlikeness and simplicity. Banalities and superficial witticisms often left her bewildered, not understanding their drift. But her sense of humor in real human things was keen. Many times has she come into the office after rounds, convulsed with laughter over some ludicrous happening in the wards."

A set of the textbooks which were in use in the School at this time was later presented to the School of Nursing by Marion Turner. This set included *A Textbook of Nursing for the use of training schools, families and private students*, compiled by Clara S. Weeks, a graduate of the New York Hospital Training School, and at one time superintendent of the Training School for Nurses, Paterson, New Jersey. In the preface, she indicated that she made no claim to originality but that the book was "a compendium with a few practical points added." The appendix contained questions for use as a quiz, as well as a vocabulary and index. Another text was *A Treatise on Physiology and Hygiene for Educational Institutions and General Readers*, by Joseph C. Hutchinson, M.D., described as "the late President of the Medical Society of the State of New York." This text was illustrated and emphasized the practical application of physiological and hygienic principles. Marion Turner also mentioned the use of "a book on materia medica, by Potter," but this particular volume does not seem to have been preserved.

Both Isabel Hampton and Lavinia Dock were aware of the need for more and better nursing texts and Miss Dock had already completed the manuscript of her famous *Materia Medica for Nurses*, most of it written while she was still night superintendent at Bellevue. Isabel Hampton made up her mind to provide something more far-reaching than the compendium of Clara Weeks and forthwith undertook to write *Nursing—its Principles and Practice*, a volume which was to remain a classic for several years to come. They also tried to compensate for the lack of textbooks by fostering interest on the part of the staff and pupils in current periodicals. Early in 1891, the Nurses Journal Club was organized "to promote an *esprit de corps* among the members of the School, to keep in touch with what is being done in other schools and hospitals by means of reports and discussions drawn chiefly from English and American weekly and monthly nursing magazines, and to ensure the reading of such papers by all." At the first meeting, Isabel Hampton gave an address on "The Scope and Aims of the Johns Hopkins Medical School," a choice of topic which at an earlier date might have astonished Dr. Billings considerably.

He does not seem to have been disturbed, however, when a few months later Miss Hampton was elected a charter member of the Women's Fund Committee, a militant band "whose avowed purpose it was to raise a sum of money sufficient to establish the School of Medicine and to offer it to the Trustees of the University on condition that women be admitted on the same basis as men." This ambitious undertaking seems to call for a word of explanation.

A large proportion of the Johns Hopkins estate consisted of stock in the Baltimore and Ohio Railroad and, in 1887, the railroad got into difficulties. As a result, the income of the University was sharply reduced and the opening of the Medical School had to be postponed. This blow came at a critical juncture since the Hospital buildings were nearing completion and appointments to the staff of the Medical School had already been made. At this point, five women quietly deployed their forces and moved into action. They were Mary Garrett, Carey Thomas, Elizabeth King, Mary Gwinn and Julia Rogers, all of whom, through their respective families, were well aware of what was going on both in

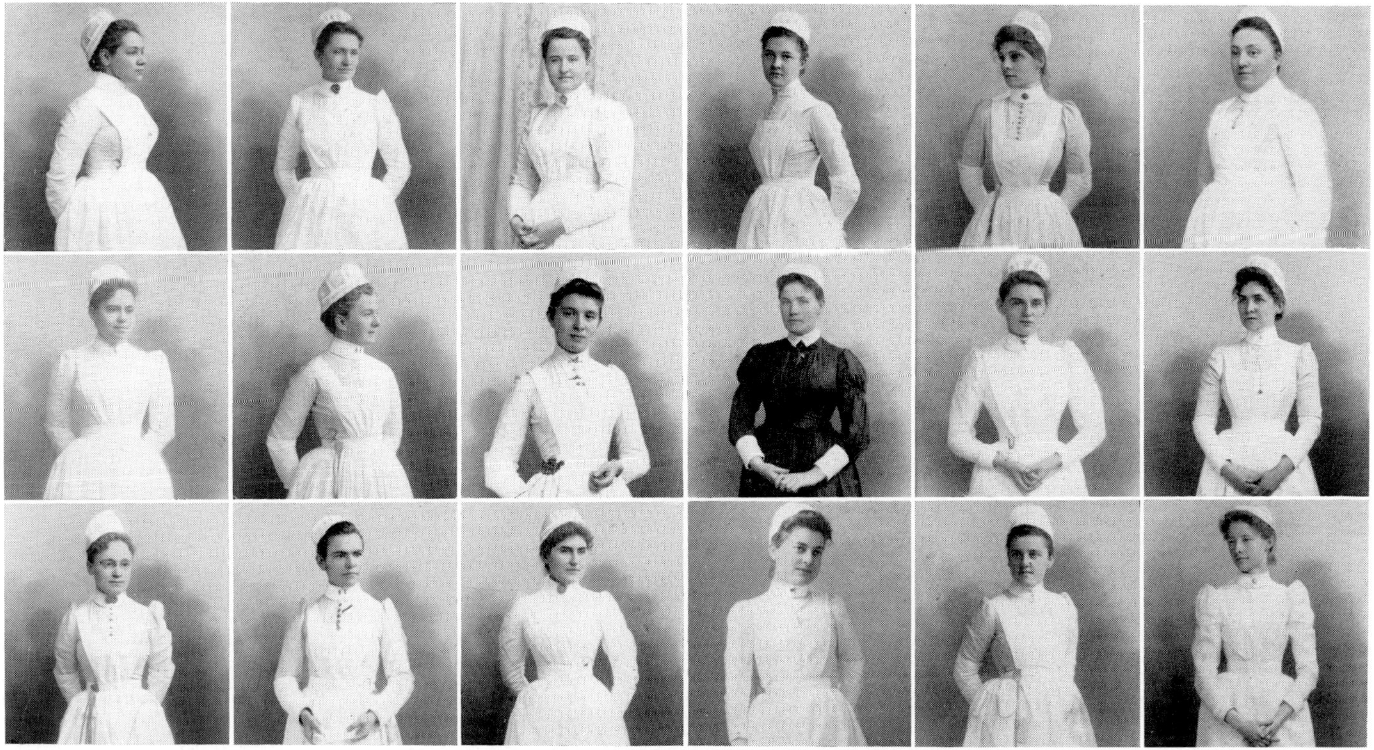

The First Graduating Class, 1891

IDA MAY	KATE EMORY	MARION TURNER	MARY GROSS	SUSAN READ	ELVINA HARTLEY
ANNA HUDSON	NORA ANTHONY	GERTRUDE HAMMEREL	ISABEL HAMPTON	MARY A. NUTTING	MRS. MARY EMORY
TILLIE SPENCER	EMMA CLEAVER	EVELINE POPE	RUTH WILLIAMS	ANNA RUTHERFORD	GEORGIA NEVINS

the Hospital and the University. Elizabeth King, as the daughter of Francis T. King, the president of the Board of Trustees, occupied a particularly strategic position and it was at her home that on May 2, 1890, the Women's Fund Committee was organized. The records show that Isabel Hampton was present.

Mary Garrett and Carey Thomas were the moving spirits in the campaign and Miss Garrett started the ball rolling by donating a substantial sum and promising more if the Trustees could raise a corresponding amount. Carey Thomas was then Dean of Bryn Mawr College and was soon to become its president. She had earlier been a graduate student at the Johns Hopkins University and had keenly resented the unfriendly attitude of the authorities towards women. Her biographer, Edith Finch,[1] thus describes the general strategy:

"Learning of the dilemma from their fathers, who were connected with the university and the hospital, the five friends saw their chance to open another door to women. It seemed to them that, if they could collect a sufficient sum of money toward the endowment of the school, the university trustees might be forced to accept with the gift the condition that women be admitted to the school on the same footing as men; in view of its ends, a highly respectable form of bribery. They formed committees for propaganda and the collection of money in large cities, wherever they could find in the United States one or two women whom they could interest in the scheme."

This feminine incursion into the affairs of the University was not relished by the authorities but the financial position had now become so acute that they were forced to seek help from some source. Dr. Welch regarded the presence of women in medical classrooms and laboratories as decidedly embarrassing and even Dr. Osler seems to have had misgivings. Nevertheless, within eight months, the indefatigable Committee had raised a hundred thousand dollars and Miss Garrett was ready to do even more if the Trustees could be spurred into greater activity. To quote Miss Finch:

"Carey Thomas's carefully planned maneuvers had reached their intended climax and the women were at last in a position to

[1] Edith Finch, *Carey Thomas of Bryn Mawr*, New York, Harper and Brothers, 1947

dictate terms. They must, nevertheless, while dictating, provide the money and, as usual, Mary Garrett came forward, this time with the whole remaining sum needed to make up five hundred thousand dollars accompanied by a letter in which the conditions of the gift were outlined unequivocally and the high standards of the school as well as the position of women in it thoroughly safeguarded."

As a matter of fact, the Women's Committee had not actually formulated these unusually high standards although it heartily approved of them. Several years previously, Dr. Welch had already set forth the terms of admission to the Medical School and Miss Garrett had obtained this document through her lawyer, Mr. Gwinn. Dr. Welch ruefully remarked: "She naturally supposed that this was exactly what we wanted. It is one thing to build an educational castle in the air at your library table, and another to face its actual appearance under the existing circumstances." The high entrance requirements were ultimately agreed upon although, to quote Dr. Simon Flexner: "Osler expressed the general feeling when he said: 'Welch, we are lucky to get in as professors, for I am sure neither you nor I could ever get in as students.' "

Neither Isabel Hampton nor Lavinia Dock took any active part in the campaign for funds but they both did a great deal toward creating a receptive attitude within the Hospital itself. When the Board of Trustees invited the embattled ladies to visit the Hospital, luncheon was served in the Nurses Home and "members of the Training School" acted as guides during a tour of inspection of the remarkable clinical facilities which the Hospital was ready to offer to medical students. After a prolonged struggle, the right to enter the School of Medicine was granted to women and the conspirators rejoiced that one more door had been opened to women—even though it yielded only to a golden key.

The final examinations for the first graduating class of the Training School for Nurses began during the first week of May 1891 and continued throughout the month, averaging two a week and lasting from one and a half to two hours. "Five questions were set in each of the following subjects; nursing in surgery, medical, hygiene, gynecology, materia medica, children, dietetics, urinalysis and massage. The examiners were Dr. A. C. Abbott in hygiene; Dr. Osler, medical; Dr. Finney, surgical; Dr. Robb, gynecology; Dr. Kelly, obstetrics; Dr. Booker, children; Dr. Meredith Reese, materia medica; Dr. Lafleur, urinalysis; Mary Boland, dietetics; Isabel Hampton, massage."

The entire class survived the ordeal although several were dangerously close to failure. The total required pass mark was 70 per cent and some of the examiners were not easily satisfied, notably Dr. Lafleur, who advised answering two of his questions by the use of a diagram. Mary V. Emory stood at the head of the class with an average of 96.7 per cent; Mary Gross came a close second with 96 per cent; Ruth Williams obtained 94.9 per cent and Adelaide Nutting came fourth with 94 per cent.

The first graduation exercises were held in the rotunda of the administration building of the Hospital on the afternoon of June 5, 1891. It was a dignified and gracious ceremony and the authorities of the Hospital and the medical staff were present in full force. The pupil nurses, seated on the winding stairs leading up to the famous Dome, made an enchanting picture of youth and freshness as one looked upward. The diplomas were presented by the Superintendent of the Hospital, Dr. Henry M. Hurd, and in the engraving which appears on each parchment, two tiny figures may be distinguished—they are Marion Turner and Mary Gross, standing on the porch of Ward C. As each graduate received her diploma, she was given a bunch of roses by Mrs. Daniel Coit Gilman. These flowers had been provided by Dr. Osler who was to make a more notable contribution to the occasion by delivering his famous address "Doctor and Nurse," now become a classic.

Mary B. Dixon (Mrs. Thomas Cullen) was an eager and interested witness of that historic ceremony: "At an impressionable age, I was deeply thrilled to think of the steadfast courage of these young women, so thrilled in fact that I was irritated and irked by the persistent prophecies that romance, not nursing, would soon claim the class of 1891. Adelaide Nutting was a member of that class seated on the steps. Let us be thankful that nursing was her romance and remained her romance throughout her life."

In 1948, the present writer talked with William Edward

Thomas, the Negro doorman, who had served the Hospital continuously since it opened in 1889 and, by way of proof, proudly wore a blue and silver enamel medal inscribed with his name and the legend "JHH—1889 to Heaven." He said that he would remember that summer afternoon as long as he lived for it was he who "had the honor of opening the door for Miss Hampton and her nurses—she was a most beautiful lady."

Major Objectives

THREE major objectives seem to have been in Isabel Hampton's mind from the beginning. These were the extension of the duration of the course of training from two years to three; the reduction of the working day to eight hours; and the abolition of the cash allowances made to pupil nurses in order that the money thus saved could be devoted to the improvement of educational facilities. Changes so drastic and far-reaching obviously could not be made in a hurry, but she lost no opportunity of trying to persuade the authorities that they would be benefical to the Hospital as well as to the School. The establishment of a three-year course was her primary aim, and in his report for the year 1891 Dr. Hurd had so far yielded to her persuasions that he made the following recommendation to the Board of Trustees:

"It is becoming more apparent that the term of instruction ought to be lengthened for those nurses at least who intend to devote themselves to teaching, so that they may have an opportunity to familiarize themselves with methods of instruction, the routine of administrative work, and the higher branches of the work. It is also pretty evident that the course as at present planned taxes the time, capacity, and strength of the pupil nurses severely and leaves little opportunity for collateral reading in the studies of allied branches. If, therefore, a period of six months or one year could be added to the term of instruction, it is quite sure that nurses would gain materially by this change. Such a course would also render the nursing in our private wards more uniform and satisfactory."

The last sentence betrays the lure with which Isabel Hampton so cunningly baited the hook—the financial advantage to the Hospital of assigning pupil nurses to special duty with private patients under treatment within the Hospital. Such assignments were already a routine practice and pupils were still being sent occasionally to private homes. Ada Carr recalled "being on duty all day and all night and on into the next day," and when at last she did return to the Hospital, she was promptly sent back to ward duty "until someone discovered that I was rather sleepy and I was relieved." This pernicious practice, as Miss Hampton herself described it, was gradually discontinued but pupils were to be assigned to special duty with hospital private patients for several years to come. It should be remembered, however, that such experience was regarded as valuable from an educational point of view, especially when the necessary supervision could be provided and the hours of duty kept within reasonable limits.

In their usual deliberate fashion, the Trustees delayed action for the time being with respect to Dr. Hurd's recommendation that the course be extended to three years although it early became evident that the seed had fallen on fertile soil and was soon to germinate. Miss Hampton was less successful so far as the reduction of the length of the working day was concerned. The hours of duty remained far too long and in her journal there were fairly frequent references to absence from duty due to "rheumatism of the feet," an euphemism that deceived nobody. In one instance, this condition was so severe that a pupil was granted her diploma on compassionate grounds before she had completed her full two years of training. With regard to vacations, Miss Hampton held her ground and though the day book shows that it must have been difficult to staff the overcrowded typhoid wards, a holiday of two weeks was granted each summer to every pupil nurse. She seems to have realized that the time was not ripe to proceed with the withdrawal of the cash allowances and did not press the matter further.

One of Isabel Hampton's most baffling problems was the strife which inevitably arose among head nurses, drawn from a variety of schools, each with her own fixed idea of how nursing procedures ought to be carried out. As they were transferred from ward to ward, conflicting orders so bewildered the unhappy pupils that they hardly knew what to do next and the resulting confusion led Miss Hampton to seek at least a measure of uniformity by avoiding, as far as possible, the employment of "outside" nurses. As early as October 1890 she noted in her journal (probably with a sigh of relief) that with the exception of the head nurse, Alice Chase, "the entire night nursing is now done by pupils." Seniors who were soon to complete their course of training were placed in charge of wards as vacancies occurred and afterwards remained as members of the graduate staff. Adah Patterson, a member of the second class, was appointed as head nurse in "Dr. Kelly's operating room" while she was still in training, and pupil nurses sometimes substituted for the head night nurse. Immediately upon graduation, Georgia Nevins became head nurse in Ward B, and Evelyn Pope "succeeded Miss Moore as head nurse in the Dispensary."

These relatively inexperienced young women were necessarily called upon to assume what would now be regarded as alarming responsibilities, and Dr. Halsted's laconic statement: "Here, we try things" must have had terrifying implications for some of them. Mistakes were made and sometimes things went wrong, but even when they did, Isabel Hampton never failed to stand by her nurses. Furthermore, she refused to allow any interference on the part of the medical staff so far as the placing of the nurses in various services was concerned and listened quite unmoved to bitter complaints when they were transferred from one ward to another. She took the position that, since she had trained these young women, she was the best judge of their needs and abilities, although in one instance she was forced to yield. Dr. Halsted had never acknowledged her authority over the head nurse in his operating room and after some minor but disconcerting incidents had occurred, decided to dispense altogether with a head nurse and to appoint a member of his medical entourage in her place. He may have seen nothing out of the way in such an action since it followed the accepted German practice to which he had become accustomed during his prolonged studies abroad. His retinue consisted of four internes, one extern, three assistant residents and a resident surgeon. From among this group he selected James T. Mitchell, who took charge until two years later the breach was healed and a graduate nurse was found who was acceptable to both Dr. Halsted and Miss Hampton. This odd arrangement worked out better than might have been expected and Emily Baechtel, a member of the class of 1894, told the present writer that Dr. Mitchell was always kindly and helpful toward her and other pupil nurses who were assigned to the operating room service.

In the autumn of 1891, the nursing load had been somewhat lightened by the termination of the agreement with the Thomas Wilson Sanitarium. Miss Hampton had previously recorded in her journal that "the pupils had suffered from severe colds due to exposure to the inclement weather" and that it had, in any case, become almost impossible to spare a sufficient number of pupils to maintain the service. Moreover, steps were already being taken to provide separate accommodation for children in the Hospital and wider clinical experience in pediatric nursing would shortly be available.

Meanwhile, steady progress was maintained so far as instruction in theory was concerned. New lecturers and new subjects were added to the teaching program and the original courses were strengthened and enriched. The course on the mechanics of ventilation was expanded into a series of lectures dealing with water supply and elementary hygiene in general and Dr. Osler gave four lectures on symptomatology instead of his single discourse on typhoid fever. Each year, Isabel Hampton herself gave a series of lectures to the senior class on such diversified topics as ethics, ward management, private nursing and district nursing. She made daily rounds in the wards to make sure that the patients were receiving proper care and, as Grace Baxter recalled, occasionally demonstrated nursing procedure:

"Her class teaching was often of the clear and commonsense

kind that remains indelibly impressed upon a scholar, and leaves a complete picture in one's mind of the subject treated. She never needed to explain a thing twice over. And her practical advice to individual nurses in the wards—for superintendents did not live on Olympus in those days—was of the same invaluable quality. I remember her to this day taking me, a raw probationer, into an isolation backroom to nurse a baby with virulent gonorrheal conjunctivitis. She did not need to touch it; in clear words she explained the technique minutely, the danger to be incurred, and my responsibility to myself as well as to the child, and after assuring herself that I understood the significance of each act, she watched me do the first dressing. I listened to her talking to the baby's mother, and I realized that for the first time I had seen the ideal of a trained nurse."

As a matter of fact, Isabel Hampton stood in need of all the courage and good humor she could muster. As time went on the demands of the nursing service became more and more exigent and the pupil nurses were sometimes too tired to benefit by the broader instruction she tried so hard to provide for them. Duty on the typhoid wards was almost a nightmare and one round of tub baths was hardly over before another began. The incidence of this disease among the pupils was rather high, although as one of them put it, "it was considered to be a disgrace and your own fault if you contracted it." However, the morale of the School remained excellent and the prevailing conception of nursing as a sacrificial profession led to the tacit acceptance of hard work and long hours without much protest or grumbling.

The general set-up of the nursing service gradually became more or less standardized, and in most of the wards the staff consisted of a graduate head nurse, a senior pupil and two or three junior pupils, one of whom was usually a probationer. The senior pupil served as "chart and medicine nurse" and cared for one or two of the very ill patients. She also accompanied the head nurse on medical rounds and was responsible for assisting the patient, adjusting bed clothing and so forth. All this had to be done quickly and deftly: "Sometimes we were nervous and clumsy about it. Then we heard from the head nurse later on." Nevertheless, attendance at rounds was a highly-prized privilege, because it afforded opportunity for contact with the chiefs of the various divisions: "Their influence pervaded everything and their attitude toward the pupil nurse was always kind and considerate. We learned far more during medical rounds than we ever did from lectures."

No matter how hard the work on the wards might be, there was one abiding consolation—life in the Nurses Home was happy and congenial. Probationers were assigned to comfortable airy rooms on the ground floor, each of which contained four beds. Later on, they were promoted to double rooms on the upper floors. The luxury of a single room was accorded only to those who had attained the dignity of being placed in charge of a ward. The dining room was a large pleasant room where Miss Hampton at first presided over a single large table until, as the number of pupils increased, she and Miss Dock shared a small table in an alcove formed by a large bay window. In keeping with their lowly estate, the probationers were relegated to tables near the door. The food was plain but reasonably well cooked and the only serious complaints came from the night nurses whose midnight meal does not appear to have been particularly attractive or satisfying: "We each picked up a little wicker basket which was placed on the radiator in the hall of the Nurses Home, summer and winter. This contained a sandwich, raw fruit such as an apple, or sometimes cooked fruit. As we often had not time to eat it, the sandwich usually got pretty dry." It was not until October 1899 that a Minute passed at a meeting of the Trustees authorized the provision of hot meals for night nurses.

Informal parties were held in the reception room of the Home and Miss Hampton herself attended the occasional dances and thoroughly enjoyed them. Dr. Osler entertained in his customary hospitable manner and Miss Hampton encouraged attendance at concerts and the theatre. The president of the Board of Trustees, Mr. Francis T. King, did all in his power to secure recognition for the School in the exclusive society of Baltimore and immensely enhanced its prestige by so doing.

There was yet another activity in which Isabel Hampton took a leading part. Alumnae associations were already being formed in connection with schools of nursing in various parts of the country as a means of keeping their graduates in touch with one another and with their respective schools. There had been a proposal, with which she was very much in sympathy, that a national association should be formed and that the alumnae associations should be its constituent elements. It was obviously desirable to make sure that when the time was ripe the Johns Hopkins Nurses Alumnae Association should be in a position to participate and even to assume leadership. On June 3, 1892, a meeting of the graduates of the first two classes was held in the Nurses Home, with Georgia Nevins as temporary chairman. Helena Barnard was elected president; Adelaide Nutting, vice-president; Georgia Nevins, secretary and treasurer; and Susan Read, corresponding secretary. Subsequent meetings dealt with the setting up of bylaws and before long the Association was engaged in the first of the manifold activities which through the years were to be a source of strength to the School as well as an inspiration to its members.

Flowers from Miss Nightingale

In spite of all other preoccupations, Isabel Hampton maintained a lively interest in the developments which were taking place in the national and international fields of nursing. In the early summer of 1893, the International Congress of Charities, Correction and Philanthropy was held in Chicago under the auspices of the World's Columbian Exposition. Dr. John Billings was chairman of the section dealing with Hospitals, Dispensaries and Nursing, and appointed Miss Hampton as chairman of a sub-section on nursing. The redoubtable Mrs. Bedford Fenwick, president of the British Nurses Association, had paid a flying visit to Baltimore in connection with arrangements for the Congress and it is unfortunate that there is no way of knowing exactly what happened during this brief encounter. Conversations between Ethel Gordon Fenwick, Isabel Hampton, Lavinia Dock and Adelaide Nutting, all four then in the first flush of youth and enthusiasm, would have been well worth recording.

The program for the sessions of the sub-section on nursing included an address, entitled "Sick Nursing and Health Nursing," by Florence Nightingale, although she herself did not attend the Congress. Lavinia Dock spoke on the relation of training schools to hospitals, Isabel McIsaac described the potential values of Alumnae Associations, Louise Darche outlined the proper organization of training schools in America and stoutly maintained that "it was soon proved that nursing under a distinct management and head could and *did* work harmoniously with the hospital management and to the mutual benefit and advantage of both," a bold statement which must have affronted both Dr. Billings and Dr. Hurd if they happened to be listening.

In her capacity as chairman of the sub-section, Isabel Hampton had the privilege of addressing the general session of the Section on Hospitals, Dispensaries and Nursing, and chose "Standards for Nurses" as her subject. It is illuminating to compare the content of this address with that delivered at the opening ceremonies of the Johns Hopkins Hospital Training School for Nurses. It displays deeper insight and more mature judgment but the underlying educational principles and the main objectives remain the same. During the discussion of a paper on "The Necessity of an American Nurses Association," given by Edith Draper, Miss Hampton pointed out that the organization of alumnae associations and the formation of a superintendents' society must necessarily precede organization on a national basis and urged that action be taken "before the Congress adjourns and while the English group are here to give advice." Mrs. Bedford Fenwick naturally lost no time in acceding to this request and the first steps were taken, then and there, to organize the American Society of Superintendents of Training Schools for Nurses of which Isabel Hampton was later to become president.

Taking it all round, the Congress was a triumph for both the Johns Hopkins Hospital and its Training School for Nurses. Dr. Hurd described the glories of the Hospital itself, Dr. Billings explained the principles which guided its construction, Mary Boland gave an able address on the handling of food in large institutions. The contributions made by Isabel Hampton and Lavinia Dock were acknowledged to be outstanding although it had to be admitted that it was Dr. John Billings who had given them this golden opportunity to demonstrate before a distinguished international gathering that nurses could think and plan and build for themselves.

Toward the end of 1893, and after all this excitement was over, a vague sense of uneasiness began to make itself felt in the School of Nursing. Miss Dock took over the direction of the Illinois Training School and Adelaide Nutting succeeded her as assistant superintendent of nurses. This transfer had just been made when another and more disconcerting change began to loom on the horizon. It was rumored that Isabel Hampton would soon give up her professional career and become the wife of Dr. Hunter Robb. The pupil nurses, with the uncanny prescience of youth in such matters, "had seen it coming." On June 12, 1894, her resignation was accepted at a meeting of the Board of Trustees and the following tribute was incorporated in the Minutes:

"She has had broad views as to the education of nurses and has labored to realize them zealously and efficiently by voice and pen. Her influence and example have contributed much toward awakening an interest in nursing in the community. Her departure is a severe loss to the Hospital and the School."

The wedding took place in London, at St. Margaret's Church, Westminster, and an account of it appeared in *The Hospital Nursing Supplement*, an English nursing periodical:

"A stormy night and cloudy morning were succeeded by a gloriously bright noon on July 11th, the wedding day of Miss Isabel A. Hampton.

"Miss Hampton's brilliant career is well known to nurses, and the organization of the training school for nurses at Johns Hopkins Hospital, Baltimore, remains a permanent memorial of her administrative abilities. . . . Miss Hampton, herself the busy head of a model school, has yet spared time to write a book for the aid and guidance of superintendents and nurses, which is quite a unique work, dealing exhaustively with every branch of skilled nursing. Setting before her sisters a high ideal, she shows a lofty standard, which must be attained and not lowered by those following in the footsteps of so able a teacher and guide.

"Hearing of her long years of noble work it was almost a surprise on Wednesday to see the fresh fairness and youth of the gracious and stately bride who entered the quiet old church at Westminster on the arm of Mr. Merritt who, with his wife, had come purposely from Scotland to be present at their friend's marriage.

"Dr. Hunter Robb, of Cleveland, Ohio, was accompanied by his two brothers, and English as well as American friends awaited the bride and bridegroom, with Miss Rogers and Miss McLean of Baltimore, who came to England with Miss Hampton three weeks ago, Mrs. Bonham Carter (a fellow-countrywoman), Miss Amy Hughes, Mr. Mrs. and Miss Burdett, Lady Colin Campbell, and others.

"The ceremony was performed by Archdeacon Farrar, D.D., rector of the parish. Mrs. Merritt gave away the bride, whose dress, of bluish grey tint was very becoming. It was trimmed with russet velvet, and the bonnet corresponded with it, but the delicate white bouquet, with long white ribbon bows, gained more attention than any other detail, for everyone in the church knew that Miss Florence Nightingale had just sent it. A long interview took place on Sunday between the latter and Miss Hampton, and the meeting cannot have failed to interest both.

"After the wedding ceremony was over most of those present repaired to the vestry to convey their congratulations to the bride and bridegroom, who were starting to Oxford. Cliveden has been lent by Mr. Astor to Dr. and Mrs. Robb for their honeymoon, and they will inhabit the bridal suite of apartments which the Duke of Westminster placed at the disposal of the Princess Christian on the occasion of her Royal Highness' marriage. Cliveden is too famous a palace to need any eulogies, and is, indeed, too beautiful in itself and its surroundings to be easily described.

"Miss Hampton's time in England has been too short and too fully engaged to allow of her seeing more than a small proportion of those who would gladly have made the acquaintance with such a leader of nursing. However, it has caused much pleasure to many of those who admire and love her for her work that she should have chosen to be married in the heart of London, and if our American sisters regret the arrangement we trust they will not grudge us this small part of Miss Hampton's time, as she and her husband are returning in the autumn to make their home where Dr. Robb has been appointed professor of gynecology, at the Western Reserve University, Cleveland, Ohio."

It all reads like the conventional happy ending of a mid-Victorian fairy tale. Elizabeth Birdseye Merritt, who gave the bride in marriage, was none other than "Violet," the friend and confidante at Bellevue and the Illinois Training School. The chatelaine of the palace at Cliveden was Mrs. William Astor who, like the gay Lady Colin Campbell, had shared those halcyon days in Rome. And then, for good measure, there was the wedding bouquet, presented with such superb assurance by Florence Nightingale. According to Mrs. Merritt, the bridegroom's flowers had been received before Miss Nightingale's gift arrived—they were gently but firmly put to one side and as always the Lady of the Lamp had pride of place.

It would be idle to pretend that the marriage met with the approval of Isabel Hampton's professional associates. Among the unyielding ranks of the feminists it was regarded as a defection. By one or two, it was considered to be a tragic anti-climax—why should any woman so obviously destined for leadership be content to relinquish so promising a career? A Canadian physician who had known Isabel Hampton for many years had a short and simple answer to that question: "Perhaps she just wanted a home, and a husband—and children."

Adelaide Nutting Takes Command

NINE YEARS after her marriage, Isabel Hampton Robb was invited to address the graduating class of 1903 and in the course of her remarks, recalled her profound sense of satisfaction in the appointment of Adelaide Nutting as her successor:

"For the graduate of today, that first class must needs have a special interest, for early in its formation there came into its ranks one who was destined to become a few years later the chief executive of your school. From probationer to junior, from grade to grade, she worked her way up until there was no form of nursing within her reach she had not done, no nursing position the hospital had to offer she had not held. Thus year by year she went on with perseverance, unconsciously training mind and hands, so that when the time came there was no need for the hospital authorities to look beyond their own graduates for a principal for their school for nurses, since they had readily to hand one who was in every way capable of assuming a position of responsibility and trust equalled by few and excelled by none open to members of your profession. And it should be a matter of no small pride and pleasure to all Johns Hopkins nurses that with the exception of the first few years they have held within their own hands the welfare of the nursing department of their own hospital, and at the same time have contributed superintendents for similar positions to other hospitals in a greater proportion for the length of years it has been in existence than perhaps any other school in the country."

No other candidates were considered and the appointment of Adelaide Nutting was a foregone conclusion although the Board of Trustees proceeded to make it with their customary deliberation. For the first few months, she served as acting superintendent until on November 13, 1894, she was formally appointed superintendent of nurses and principal of the Training School "as from September 1st, 1895." The months that intervened between her appointment and the assumption of her duties on September 24, 1895, were granted as leave of absence in order that she might visit schools of nursing in the United States and abroad. Helena Barnard, a member of the class of 1892, was appointed to take charge during her absence.

Helena Barnard was "a New Englander, positive and delightful, who possessed a tranquil indifference to praise or blame, an entire candor and directness, together with an unfailing sense of humor." She was a woman of thirty when she entered the School of Nursing and had already acquired the poise and maturity that the situation required. Even as a pupil nurse, she displayed considerable executive ability and served acceptably as head nurse on Ward C. Immediately after graduation, she took a course in obstetrical nursing in the Columbia Hospital, Washington, which, while far from satisfactory at the time, proved useful later on at Johns Hopkins. Early in 1894, she was offered a position in the Royal Victoria Hospital at Montreal and was thus engaged when she was recalled by Adelaide Nutting whose capacity for enlisting the talents of other people had already come into play. As an administrator she had only one fault—the exercise of authority did not greatly appeal to her—an indifference that did not please Miss Nutting who, on one occasion, indulged in a little judicious prodding. Helena Barnard's reaction to this stimulus must have come as a surprise if not a shock:

"You and I are as opposite as the poles—what is to you a stimulation as of wine, is to me an effort if not a pain. I am not a public woman in thought or deed or feeling. I shrink from public meetings, and reporters and all that kind of thing with a mental and physical dread. What it is apparent Mrs. Robb and Miss King and yourself enjoy, I only seek to avoid—it is my nature, my ego. I am not discussing whether it is admirable, it simply *is* and with hundreds and thousands of modern progressive women crowding into print and speech and action why poor little me has to be thrust into the arena I fail to comprehend. I never want to fail to support desirable measures much less to discourage—but that is different from leadership. You know we think differently on almost every subject, which does not prevent my feeling respect and admiration and affection for you. If you would only realize that I am different and then you would not be disappointed for something—responses or whatsoever—and fail to find it. My youthful training and environment have made me what I am—not what I wish I might have been. Try to remember that one cannot fit square pegs into round holes, and believe that it is not contrariety on my part, and do not try to measure me by very modern twentieth century standards."

Adelaide Nutting usually destroyed personal letters but she kept this one all her life.

The administration of the nursing service and the School of Nursing was carried on so smoothly and efficiently by Miss Barnard that Dr. Hurd formally expressed his complete satisfaction in a report to the Trustees. Then, in September 1895 the monthly journal of the principal of the Training School contained the following entry: "The superintendent of nurses, Miss Adelaide Nutting, returned from her prolonged vacation and took up her work on September 24 and Miss Helena Barnard, acting superintendent in her absence, left the Hospital at the end of the month."

No record is available of what happened during this "prolonged vacation" beyond the fact that Adelaide Nutting did visit schools of nursing in the United States and abroad. During this interval she must have given much thought to the task that awaited her and may even have pondered her own fitness for it. Unlike Isabel Hampton, she had no previous experience as a superintendent of nurses and had never faced obstacles such as those which Miss

Hampton had surmounted in the Illinois Training School. Neither had she had any formal training as a teacher, a fact of which she was painfully aware. Nevertheless, she believed, and with good reason, that her family background and general education were in themselves a firm foundation upon which to build. With characteristic clarity and reticence, she once set down a brief account of those earlier days:

"I was born on November 1st, 1858, in Waterloo, a small village in the beautiful Eastern Townships of the Province of Quebec, Canada.

"My parents were both born and brought up in the same part of the Province, in Bolton, about twenty miles from Waterloo. On both sides they came from Loyalist stock, from families who had come to Canada shortly after the Revolutionary War, had been given grants of land, and had settled there. My mother's name was Peaselee.

"In this small village of Waterloo, newly settled, and made up largely of English families, or of those who like ours had come from the New England States bringing their strong loyalist convictions, I grew up under English ideals, customs and traditions. Our house was a small one, surrounded by a few acres of land reaching down to the river. My father held a small municipal office, and our narrow resources called for some industry on the part of every member of the family, and for constant self-denials. There were five children, Charles, the eldest, followed by Arthur Knowlton, then James Peaselee, the two youngest being girls, myself, and my younger sister, Harriet Armine.

"Life in those early Canadian homes, amid simple surroundings and few luxuries, and with the long and severe winters, and a remoteness from the amenities and cultural opportunities of cities, had yet its own social structure and activities, interesting, wholesome, happy and developing to character. But there was an epic quality running through all life.

"My formal education was slight. It began at the age of six or seven years in a village academy, under the instruction of a group of teachers of quite remarkable ability, character and personality. At the age of fourteen as I remember it, I spent a year at a Convent in the nearby town of St. John's, studying French and music and the following year I attended a private school in Montreal, known as Bute House, situated on Sherbrooke Street just opposite McGill College. It was typical I suppose of the private schools of that day, in devoting much attention to accomplishments, though there were some very good teachers on the staff. I particularly remember our teacher of music, Monsieur Ducharme. The next year, I spent a winter with some relations who lived in Lowell, Mass., devoting the entire time to the study of music under a private teacher and to a course on design at an Art School. For the next few years I stayed at home with mother who needed me in the care of our household, devoting my spare time to continued study of music and drawing.

"Later we gave up our house in the country and moved to Ottawa, and there I was fortunate enough to come under the instruction of a very gifted young English musician, who opened up a new world in music to me. I also attended the Art School there both day and evening classes for some time. After my sister became the Principal of the Cathedral School for Girls in Saint Johns, Newfoundland, I spent a year with her introducing music into the School (or rather trying to).

"My mother died in 1884, and a few years later in 1889 I entered the Johns Hopkins Hospital School of Nursing, which opened that year in Baltimore, and became a member of its first class. I chose the School because it seemed to offer unusual opportunities for training in nursing, but also because the Principal of the School was a Canadian, and because two other Canadians, Dr. William Osler and Dr. Henri Lafleur were on the hospital staff.

"After graduating from this School in 1891 I remained two years as head nurse, first of Dr. Osler's Men's Medical Ward, then of the Men's Surgical Ward, and later of one of the private wards. In 1894 I was invited to become Assistant Superintendent of Nurses and, after holding this office one year, was asked to undertake the office of Superintendent of Nurses and Principal of the School, because of the resignation of Miss Hampton."

As a young girl, Adelaide Nutting thoroughly enjoyed the social amenities of the Canadian capital and was duly presented in all the glory of a white satin gown at a Drawing Room held by the Governor General, the Marquess of Lorne, and his wife, Princess Louise. Among Miss Nutting's papers at the time of her death there was a letter from the secretary of the Ottawa Rowing Club thanking her for contributing to "the vocal and instrumental portions of the Club's recent moonlight excursion on the steamer, 'Peerless' " and, in the same container, a certificate signed by William H. May, the gifted young English musician whom she mentions in the brief sketch of her life. He commended his pupil as "a young pianist of unusual talent, fine technique, intelligence in rendering good music, and in every way competent to teach the Piano Forte in all its branches."

As the years slipped by, she began to realize that the teaching of art and music would never be a genuinely satisfying career. There was more than one offer of marriage and possibly a brief engagement, but she seems never to have been able to accept the sacrifice of personal independence that marriage would have involved. Once she made up her mind to enter a school of nursing she never looked back—she had found her true vocation.

The years spent as a nurse-in-training proved to be happy and satisfying though by no means free from strain. It was fortunate that Isabel Hampton perceived from the outset that although Adelaide Nutting possessed an excellent mind and potential capacity for leadership she was not physically robust and might not be able to perform heavy tasks or to endure long hours of duty. Miss Nutting left some pencilled notes that show that she was aware of this solicitude and was grateful for it:

"I received a warm greeting from Miss Hampton when I arrived at a late hour from New York after a long journey from Montreal, and she asked the Matron to get me something warm to drink. A few weeks later, she invited me to go with her to see a new play. Incidentally, this was probably to help her in sizing up a new probationer—a good idea. It was several weeks before she placed me on night duty. She came down the ward on her morning rounds and bent over me at the table where I was making my patient's chart and said quietly: 'You are to go on night duty tonight. I have kept you from it as long as I can.' She knew how hard I would find that kind of solitary responsibility—long wards full of very sick people and no night superintendent in the early days of the Johns Hopkins Hospital."

A brief note to her father, written shortly after her arrival at Johns Hopkins, reveals her steadfastness of purpose: "A few weeks ago I said goodbye to you and started out on my career. I vowed I would succeed and (D.V.) shall do so in whatever I undertake."

Another letter, written during her second year of training, reflects her misgivings about her chances of success:

"My final exams come off early in June—and I find myself so ill-prepared that my heart goes down to my boots whenever I think of it. I want to come out very well and have studied pretty hard but my competitors are very formidable, three of the class having been teachers—one having taken a degree at College and nearly all of them being physically stronger than I. The very utmost that I can expect is that I shall come out sixth.

"I am in new work today—general surgery—after five straight months of medical. I never expect to like surgery as well as medical, which just exactly suits me, but of course a general training in everything is necessary before one makes a choice. After a month or two of this ward I shall probably go to the operating room and dispensary and then there will be little left for me beyond the necessary months of private nursing which I hate the very thought of.

"The grounds around the Hospital are looking very beautiful this year and I often envy the patients sitting out under the trees hour after hour with such a nearly perfect climate as we have here at certain seasons of the year. There are days here during April and May and September and October when there is something in the atmosphere I never can find words to describe. It makes me feel that it is good to be alive, no matter how weary the physical part of me may be. The flesh is a nuisance anyway, and a perpetual drag and hindrance to the spirit. If I had as much strength as spirit, there is nothing I would be afraid to undertake. . . . I realize, however, fully that this work is carrying me farther and farther from my old life and those dear to me."

A little later she wrote again:

"I like Baltimore very well and it has grown to mean something like a home to me. My work takes all my time and strength and spirit but yet in some mysterious way I have come to know several Baltimore people. . . . They are most hospitable and had I any leisure I might go about a good bit. . . . I generally manage to get to every good concert. . . . I have not absolutely settled about going to Rome in November although I am sure I shall go sooner or later. Miss Hampton seems to think I ought by and by to take a hospital of my own and for many reasons I would like to do so as soon as I feel myself to be quite fitted."

Evidently Miss Hampton had suggested that she should join the staff at St. Paul's House and thus have an opportunity of sharing her own happy experience in Italy, but the project fell through and on March 6, 1892, she tells of her experience as a head nurse:

"The wards are full and there are a good many serious cases requiring each a special nurse so that many of the wards (like mine) are running with a short staff of nurses and only those at the helm know what that means. So great is the demand for nurses in the Hospital as well as outside that they are talking of building an annex to the Nurses' Home which has already fifty-seven bedrooms. It shows conclusively that this profession, at all events, is not over-crowded. This is the dearest old Hospital in the world and I offer up perpetual psalms of thanksgiving that I came here instead of elsewhere. The work never loses its interest nor the place its charm and tho' it is undeniably hard it is not uncongenial and hard work as you know seldom does any permanent injury. Whenever you think of me, let it be as contented and happy in my lot."

A letter written early in October 1893 reflects her attitude towards the new responsibilities that she knew she must face when she succeeded Lavinia Dock as assistant superintendent of nurses:

"This work is so important and I am so determined to stick to it and make a success of it that I have to let everything else slide. It is the only way to get along. My life and work to an outsider present a low level of monotony which while interesting to me, because steadily leading to something higher, leaves me little to say to anybody. . . . The winter's class work has just begun.

I had my first class in anatomy on Tuesday afternoon and shall start on my second class today. It is no joke to take thirty very wide-awake young women and try to teach them something of which I am only indifferently sure, but I shall be very severe and rigid and they shall have good discipline if nothing else."

Then, in a little outburst of homesickness: "If I lived here fifty years, I should still be the warmest kind of a Canadian."

A subsequent letter shows how stimulating the new opportunities for teaching were to her:

"My work is much easier and more satisfactory than ever before. It is easier in this one way that I do not have to walk or stand about so many hours—otherwise it is harder—and it is more satisfactory because I am, in preparing for my classes, steadily acquiring a great deal of useful knowledge. I have now a class of twenty-six bright young women who are here for the purpose of getting everything possible out of the training—and it taxes my mental capacity to its utmost to be able to furnish them at all times with the information they wish. . . . I shall always believe that teachers are born and not made."

While she was serving as acting superintendent after Miss Hampton's resignation, a letter betrays both strain and fatigue:

"There is not such a thing as a free moment for me from early morning until anywhere along about midnight and I have reluctantly come to the conclusion that this is in a large measure due to my lack of executive ability or else to slowness in working out ward management. The correspondence in itself is so large that I should need to sit at my desk for from four to six hours daily in order to attend to it satisfactorily. Then the classes, lectures, interviews, over-seeing of ward work and the thousand and one details take up the other minutes and so it is always. My very own, just because *they* can wait, are daily pushed aside for the demands of this work. Of course, I am happy and my surroundings are very pleasant and much more than merely comfortable. My rooms are beautiful and everybody is considerate but the work is too great for any but a very strong woman—I mean to ask for a second assistant."

Eight months of comparative leisure were to give Adelaide Nutting the necessary opportunity for analysis and reflection.

She already had a firm grasp of the main issues and was quietly confident that she could deal with them effectively but, as her letter to her father shows, she was also aware of her inability to cope with the problems of ward management. The discipline and morale of the School were excellent although it had to be admitted that this happy state of affairs was due in some measure to Isabel Hampton's "passion for uniformity," a sentiment that she did not altogether share. The reputation that the School had acquired for giving skilled nursing care was a deep satisfaction to her and it was gratifying that Dr. Hurd should report to the Trustees that the efficient administration of the School of Nursing was an important factor in the development of clinical teaching in the Medical School.

She had always been in complete agreement with Isabel Hampton as to the three major objectives that the School should first strive to attain. The extension of the course from two to three years had already been approved in principle and now the time might be ripe to withdraw the allowances paid to pupil nurses and to devote the money thus saved to improving the educational facilities. Owing to the rapid extension of the hospital services, it was evident that reduction of the hours of duty would have to be deferred although the three-year course would make it possible to devote more time to theoretical instruction. When it came to ultimate goals in nursing education, however, she was less sure of where Isabel Hampton really stood, especially when (to use her own words) she was "dreaming true," and yet no one realized more keenly than Miss Nutting that this mysterious process had sometimes produced remarkable results:

"One of the strongest and most obvious of Isabel Hampton's characteristics was what we might call the organizing faculty, . . . planning, initiating, directing and controlling,—such activities provided for her an atmosphere in which she moved with the greatest of ease and freedom. She was in every sense of the word, a leader, by nature, by capacity, by personal attributes and qualities, by choice and probably to some extent, by inheritance and training: a follower she never was. . . . It seems easy, almost inevitable, in fact to trace in the rich full-glowing nature of Isabel Hampton, the unison of qualities at once progressive and conservative, practical and prophetic, which gave her so remarkable a power, and so inexhaustible a charm. For while, on the one hand, her plans might be of great magnitude, extending far into the future, and vastly comprehensive in grasp, seeing and covering the whole field of possible action and not occupying herself with any section or division of it, on the other hand, she would throw herself with ardor and also with steady patient industry, into small practical details, so as to seem for the moment entirely oblivious to and unmindful of larger issues."

This tendency to lose sight of the ultimate goal troubled Adelaide Nutting and, indeed, nothing could have been in sharper contrast to her own far-sighted, deliberate intellectual approach. Yet she was quick to see how fruitful Isabel Hampton's intuitive response had been to an environment such as that afforded at Johns Hopkins where "her practical genius had full sway and could create standard, precedent and tradition at will under conditions which were at that time little less than ideal." Here Adelaide Nutting touched upon the *genius loci*—the spirit of the place—that in those early days cast a spell over all that were exposed to its subtle influence. She herself was profoundly affected by it and it was intensely invigorating to watch the rising tide of enthusiasm and enterprise in the Medical School and to ponder how its impact might be used to favor the fortunes of the School of Nursing. To work with and for such men as Osler, Welch and Flexner was both a challenge and an inspiration, and among the Trustees there were men to whom she knew that she could look for understanding and support when the time came for enlarging the scope of the educational program. A sense of exhilaration swept over her as she took command.

Declaration of Rights

ADELAIDE Nutting's first important official action was to submit an outline to the Board of Trustees for the three-year course which had been one of Isabel Hampton's major objectives. She recommended that "the School should be divided into three classes: junior, intermediate and senior" and that one class only should be admitted each year. Further recommendations dealt with the withdrawal of money allowances, the reduction of the working day to eight hours, and the establishment of scholarships. The Trustees set up a special committee and on April 14, 1896, the following entry appeared in the Minutes: "The report of the Committee upon the three-year course for nurses was adopted and the Superintendent authorized to carry out the recommendations therein contained at such time as may seem to him most feasible after consultation with the superintendent of nurses and all parties interested."

The text of the committee's report closely corresponded to the outline presented by Miss Nutting and was put into force immediately, although seven probationers who had not yet been accepted as full-fledged pupil nurses objected strenuously. Feeling ran high and an appeal was made to the Trustees. Five of the seven were assured that they would be permitted to graduate at the end of a two-year period and the other two decided to complete the full three years. In spite of this flurry of opposition, the course was safely launched and the money allowances were done away with. No mention was made of the reduction of the length of the working day and this recommendation continued to be more honored in the breach than in the observance. A new circular of information for candidates, drafted as soon as the three-year course was authorized, indicated that the probationary term had been increased from one month to two. No definite academic requirements were set up other than the following general statement:

"If approved, applicants are received into the school for a period of two months on probation. Classes are formed and pupils are received in the spring but application should be made at least three months in advance. During the months of trial and previous to being accepted as a pupil in the School, the applicant must be prepared for an examination in reading, penmanship, simple arithmetic and English dictation. The examination is to test the applicant's ability to read aloud well, to write legibly and accurately, to understand mathematics as far as fractions and percentage and to take notes of lectures. This amount of education is *indispensable* for a member of the School, but applicants are reminded that women of superior education and cultivation will be preferred."

It is interesting to note that these educational requirements are almost identical with those which were in force in the Bellevue School of Nursing in 1881 at the time that Isabel Hampton was a pupil nurse. The remaining regulations were just as explicit, not to say authoritarian, as those set forth in the original Johns Hopkins circular and the form of contract was retained word for word except that the duration of the course was defined as three years instead of two. This document evidently had teeth in it, for during Miss Hampton's regime a pupil who left the School without permission was mentioned in the records as having "absconded." Several years later, Miss Nutting herself was to report that "a member of the senior class asked to be released from her contract and allowed to go home owing to her engagement and probable marriage before the three years of her training were completed.

This was not considered a sufficient reason for breaking her contract and she left the School without permission and therefore dishonorably."

The new circular also made it clear that the pupil nurses must still be prepared to perform any duty assigned to them by the superintendent of nurses and that they would be required to be on duty not less than eight hours daily in addition to two hours devoted to lectures, classes or study. There was a stern warning that "except under exceptional circumstances, failure to pass the examination at the end of the first year is considered a sufficient cause for the termination of the pupil's connection with the school."

The general program for the three-year course was arranged as follows:

Medical:	6 months	Infectious:	2 months
Surgical:	6 months	Diet School:	1 month
Gynecological:	6 months	Gynecological operating room:	1 month
Obstetrics:	2 months	General operating room:	6 weeks
Children:	2 months	Dispensary:	1 week
Private wards:	6 months	Vacations:	9 weeks
	Total:	36 months	

First year:

Practical teaching and training in medical, surgical and gynecological free wards. Demonstrations and classes in practical work weekly.

Class work:

Elementary materia medica:

Anatomy, physiology and hygiene:

Cookery and dietetics, practice and theory.

Intermediate year:

Continued practical teaching and training in medical, surgical and gynecological work in free and also private wards, children's ward, infectious ward, and dispensary.

Class work:

Care of medical, surgical and gynecological patients:

Care of infectious diseases:

Analysis of urine:
Massage.

Senior year:

Practical work in operating room and dispensary; private wards; maternity and children's wards; further training in whatever direction it is evidently more needed. Seniors may be placed in positions of responsibility when their progress and ability render it advisable. Lectures and classes will follow the work of the year.

Several points in this general program need clarification. Six months in the private wards may seem like an unduly prolonged assignment until it is remembered that pupils were frequently placed on special duty for relatively long periods. This experience was regarded as having both educational and practical value since at this time private duty offered more opportunities than any other field. It was also considered justifiable, even from an educational point of view, to place senior students in charge of wards and thus to save the salary of a head nurse. The withdrawal of money allowances was looked upon as sound in principle and economical as well, since it cost the Hospital far less to provide the pupils with free uniforms and text books.

The establishment of scholarships is dealt with as follows:

"Though the object of the School is to educate and to train those best fitted to receive such education, irrespective of their necessities, it is thought that it would be well to establish scholarships to meet the needs of those poor but desirable women who might not otherwise be able to receive the training. I would suggest, therefore, the establishing of a certain number of scholarships to assist those who could not otherwise obtain this teaching. The need or hope of obtaining such a scholarship would be an incentive to the pupil to put forth her best efforts. These scholarships should be awarded for general excellence in work, and should be held for the year following the appointment. Four of these might be awarded the first year, each $100; four the second, each $150; or there might be three given each year for the full three years:

1st. Those whose work in the wards about their patients has been uniformly of an excellent character.

2nd. Those who stand first in their classes.

3rd. Those whose conduct and influence in the School have been above criticism.

"These scholarships might be so bestowed as to be forfeited by subsequent bad work, unworthy conduct, or anything which would necessitate the nurses' leaving the School. Those who wish for the benefit of other pupils to return the sum of the scholarship should be permitted to do so."

The three-year course was an immediate success and Dr. Hurd told the Board of Trustees: "This change has worked well, and the School has never been more prosperous and efficient than at present." Miss Nutting was more guarded in her appraisal of the results but she, too, appears to have been reasonably well satisfied:

"These changes were instituted after much careful consideration of the best methods of providing a better and more thorough training for our nurses, but were nevertheless purely experimental. At the end of the first year, it is too early to estimate the full value of these changes or to make any definite statements concerning them, but I am glad to be able to report that so far our results have been satisfactory. The work of teaching has been carried on slowly, but very thoroughly, and with much attention to detail, and the shorter hours have given the pupils time to study and have enabled them to receive the full benefit of their teaching, while the record of good health for the year exceeds any record we have been able to present in previous years.

"The withdrawal of the allowance of money has not been followed by any marked decrease in the number of applications, or lowering of the high standing of those who have heretofore applied."

Miss Nutting had, of course, realized that the retention of the pupils for a third year would lighten the nursing load for a time, but she was also aware that it would not be long before the steadily rising demand for service would again encroach on the teaching program. A reduction of the hours of duty must be brought about before she could hope to introduce the broader educational scheme that she already had in mind. Little reference to this basic problem appears in her journal or her reports at this particular juncture but she evidently decided to make an indirect approach to it. In February 1896 a favorable opportunity presented itself

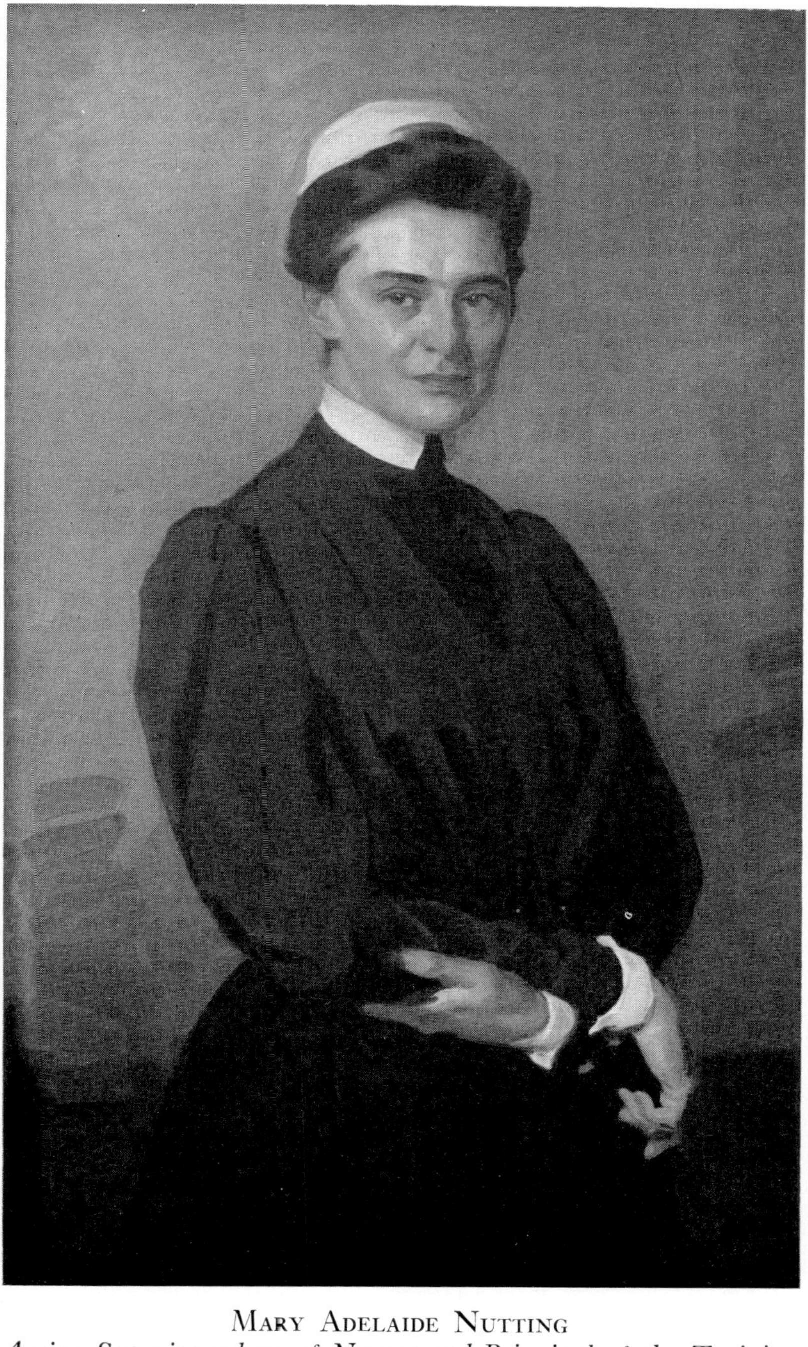

MARY ADELAIDE NUTTING

Acting Superintendent of Nurses and Principal of the Training School, 1894–1895

Superintendent of Nurses and Principal of the Training School, 1895–1907

PAINTING BY CECILIA BEAUX

and she delivered a pungent and succinct address entitled "Hours of Duty for Nurses," before the American Association of Superintendents of Training Schools for Nurses. By way of preparation, she had laboriously assembled first-hand information "from all the larger hospitals of the country of which I have any knowledge and from many smaller ones. They range from Maine to California and from Illinois to Louisiana." The replies to this enquiry formed the substance of an indictment which was all the more penetrating because it was presented without exaggeration and with characteristic clarity, force and brevity. A few excerpts indicate its general trend:

"There is no other work sufficiently like nursing to serve adequately for purposes of comparison, but to take the first that comes to mind it may be said that from fifty-six to sixty hours a week are generally considered fair working hours for the laboring man. I believe I am right in stating that few industries require their employes to work more than ten hours daily, and their Sundays are usually free. We cannot actually compare industries with training schools, nor wage-earners with pupils receiving their training in an educational institution, but we can state that a pupil in a training school may work harder to receive her training than a laboring man to support his wife and family; for here we find in one of the most difficult and responsible careers a woman can undertake, that her only method of receiving a certain kind of education is not to work sixty hours per week, but a number of hours varying from that number to 105 hours.

"In those schools in which the very shortest hours are adopted, nurses are working at least nine hours a day at work which taxes the physical strength even of the strong in no small degree; of the moderately strong, to the utmost. After nine hours of hard physical labor, the nurse comes off duty—to what?—to rest? To get out of her uniform and away from the trying atmosphere of the sick-room, and into the fresh air? Not at all, but to go to her room which may perhaps be shared by a stranger, and try to bring the energies of a tired mind resident in a tired body to bear upon whatever problems her theoretical work may present. Having thus taken up her hour or hours supposed to be for rest and recreation, are her evenings free? We find that they are not. For here a class, or a lecture, or possibly two of each, or perhaps relief work in a ward while a member of another class is at lecture, occupies her, and thus two or three, or it may be four, evenings in a week are taken up. If this be the picture of a day in a school in which the work is thought to be easy, what must be that in those schools where the working day is not nine, but eleven, twelve or thirteen hours long, and where study and attendance at lectures or classes are still compulsory.

"Now what are training schools? Are they charitable institutions? Is it a condition of employer and employee? When we read in some circulars of nurses' wages, one might think it. They are really, however, educational institutions, and it is time that this fact be better appreciated. It should not be forgotten that the long hours of duty in the wards may reduce pupils to a condition of servitude. In many instances it is not for the purpose of giving them more and better training that they are kept on duty so long, but rather that the amount of service rendered to the Hospital may be increased, and that the working force of the institution may for economy's sake be kept small. These long hours render it nearly impossible for a nurse to profit by the teaching for which her services are supposed to be given, and with such long hours the teaching offered as an advantage to attract applicants is not really deserving of mention. If we look for an explanation of the origin of these long hours of service, it may be found in the fact that, as a rule, provision has not been made for a sufficient number of pupil nurses. Such attempts at economy are far-reaching in their effects, and detrimental to the best interests of patients, as well as of nurses.

"What we should do, and what if we fail to do others who come after us will do, is to open our eyes and our minds to the actual state of things about us. Let us look into the matter and satisfy ourselves as to the fair amount of physical labor required for the necessary training, which can be done without over-fatigue, and without infringing upon other duties. Let us plan out a suitable amount of mental work and give our pupils time to do it thoroughly, and see to it that they are in a condition physically to do so. Let us give time for a proper amount of healthful exercise and diversion, that spirit and enthusiasm, and the 'merry heart which doeth good like a medicine,' may not be utterly lacking. Finally, let us provide the needful time for sleep.

"To sum it up, including, first, the number of hours on duty in the wards; second, the number of hours taken up with class or lecture, and third, the amount of time expected or necessary to be devoted daily to study, and calculating how much time each day, or even in a week (under the most favorable circumstances and conditions), can be secured for necessary rest and healthful diversion, the following conclusions are inevitable:

"1st. The working hours in the wards being but a portion of the day's work, are now in almost all hospitals too long. They should be so arranged as under no circumstances to exceed nine hours, and should, when possible, be limited to eight hours.

"2nd. The hours set apart for rest and recreation are now necessarily and frequently infringed upon by class, lecture or study, in order that the pupil may perform the work required of her. This should in no case be done, but these hours should be reserved for the purposes for which they were intended.

"3rd. When an increase in the theoretical course of instruction becomes necessary or advisable, it should on adoption be followed up by a certain corresponding decrease in the amount of practical work required, if necessary, increasing the total length of the period of training."

The delivery of this address marked an important milestone in the professional career of Adelaide Nutting as well as in the history of the Johns Hopkins Hospital School of Nursing. From this time on, with quiet assurance and perhaps a touch of arrogance, she took her rightful place as a leader and educator not only in her own School but in the nursing profession at large. She had long meditated upon and then clearly stated the fundamental problem with which every school of nursing in the country was confronted. She knew, and had the courage to tell those in authority, that the education of nurses could not be carried on as it ought to be unless the exploitation of pupil nurses could be stopped, or at least kept within bounds.

Although the meeting at which Miss Nutting spoke was held in Philadelphia, reverberations were distinctly heard in Baltimore. The Trustees must have realized that they too were vulnerable even though they could take comfort in the assurance that their own School stood foremost in the front rank. To their everlasting credit be it said, they allowed Miss Nutting to submit the whole text of her address as an integral part of her annual report, thus giving it tacit endorsation as well as wide distribution among the medical staff and other persons of influence in the community.

The impact of this declaration soon made itself felt throughout the hospital and nursing world, and, although its conclusions were not immediately accepted or clearly understood, they became, and for many years remained the Magna Charta of the nursing profession—a goal toward which the leaders pressed forward. The very fact that she was the head of so distinguished a school gave Adelaide Nutting prestige and authority that she might not otherwise have possessed. If her recommendations seemed somewhat startling, that was to be expected. Had not Dr. Halsted already said of the Johns Hopkins Hospital: "Here, we try things"? She had been afforded an incomparable laboratory in which to work out experiments in the education of nurses, and her immediate task was to strengthen and consolidate the three-year course. When that was done, it would be time for the next forward step.

The Preparatory Course

THE DEMAND for increased service from the School of Nursing was not long delayed since the expansion of the Medical School created a need for additional clinical facilities which in turn placed an added burden on the School of Nursing. An "outside obstetric service" was organized in 1896 under the direction of Dr. J. Whitridge Williams, and an intern, accompanied by a medical student and a nurse (usually a pupil) attended each patient in her own home, the nurse remaining with her for at least eighteen hours after delivery. The rapid growth of this service soon made it necessary to provide an obstetrical ward to which patients who required special attention could be admitted and the south end of the isolation ward was transformed for this purpose:

"Upon the first floor a comfortable ward for waiting women was provided and furnished with eighteen beds; also a dining room, kitchen, lavatories, bathroom and examining room. The place was made not only habitable but quite attractive by the lavish use of paint and bright linoleum. Upstairs, by a judicious removal of partitions, two operating or delivery rooms, a disinfecting room, and a nursery were provided, as well as several small, bright, airy rooms for the recovery of the mothers. A room with bathroom attached was set apart for the head nurse of this ward, and the first one to occupy it and to give most valuable help in starting the work upon a satisfactory basis was Miss Helena Barnard." The postgraduate course at the Columbia Hospital had proved useful after all. At about the same time, the building formerly used as a bath house was transformed into a children's ward "containing fifteen cots and equipped with a large airy playroom" and a senior pupil nurse was placed in charge.

In the light of these and other developments it was obvious that enrolment would have to be increased but although there were plenty of candidates the Nurses Home was so crowded that there was no room for them. Miss Nutting bitterly complained that "the nurses have been subjected to inconveniences which are incompatible with the best work and the hurtful influences of these upon comfort, order and proper discipline have been distinctly felt." The Trustees finally took action even though finances were at a rather low ebb:

"The two floors of bedrooms over the Officers' Dining Room and Pharmacy were set aside for the use of the School. There are eight rooms on the first floor and ten on the second floor of this building, excellent bedrooms, and these properly furnished and equipped form what is known as the Nurses Home Annex. Later, the third floor of this building was finished and arranged for the use of night nurses, and ten small bedrooms were thus placed at our disposal for that much needed purpose. While it may seem that by these additions every need is supplied, we must add that every room now in both Home and Annex, except those reserved for officers and head nurses, is occupied by two pupils or by two of our very large staff of special nurses."

Ada Carr had served as assistant superintendent of nurses since 1894 but the administrative duties now became so heavy that in October 1896 Georgina Ross, a member of the class of 1894, was appointed second assistant "and placed in charge of the Junior Year," a task that was soon to have new implications.

Even while the three-year course was still in the early stages of development, Adelaide Nutting took over yet another task that made heavy demands upon her time and strength. At the outbreak of the Spanish-American War, the Associated Alumnae of Trained Nurses of the United States and Canada immediately offered its services to the Government, and its president, Isabel Hampton Robb, promptly sought an interview with the Surgeon General. She was told that Army nursing had been given into the charge of the Daughters of the American Revolution and that a woman physician, Dr. Anita Newcomb McGee, had been appointed as its director.

In December 1898 a conference was held at the New York Hospital Training School for Nurses between a number of influential lay women and the executive committee of the Associated Alumnae of Trained Nurses. Plans were made to submit a Bill to Congress that would provide for a permanent Army Nurse Corps, directly responsible to the military authorities, free from the control of any voluntary organization, and under the direction of a nurse rather than a physician. Miss Nutting was appointed secretary of a sub-committee which (to use her own words) had a three-fold purpose: "to get committees of nurses organized in various States throughout the country, to keep them informed about the progress of the Bill, and to urge them to acquaint their Members and Senators with the need for a properly organized Army Nurse Corps." She soon found that: "this work grew to such dimensions that it took up almost my entire time for the better part of the winter. There was a good deal of opposition, some of it from medical men and some from medical women, for of course Dr. Anita Newcomb McGee's friends rallied to her support and made the usual objections to giving nurses any authority over their own work."

A formidable lobby was organized in Washington in support of the Bill and Miss Nutting persuaded the Board of Trustees of the Johns Hopkins Hospital to pass a resolution in favor of it, based on evidence obtained from graduates of the School: "Twenty-three of our graduates offered their services and were sent to the various camps and hospitals. Four were in charge of hospitals. In the majority of instances, our nurses were in charge of the work to which they were assigned and notwithstanding peculiar difficulties and many untoward conditions, they have been able to do good work." The Bill came before Congress in 1900 and Miss Nutting afterwards recalled that: "The last act I remember was that of summoning the committee to a hearing before the Committee on Military Affairs in Washington and asking other persons to join us in urging our claim to proper legislation. Dr. Welch came and made an excellent speech for us."

The Bill was finally passed in 1901 and Miss Nutting was careful to record her sense of obligation not only to the nursing leaders who had worked with her but also to the distinguished lay women who were its sponsors: "The New York Committee was an able, energetic and influential body of women and I always thought we owed the Bill to them and that the efforts of the nurses alone, at that time, could not have assured its passage although we all did our best."

Meanwhile, the teaching program underwent expansion and modification in order to provide suitable instruction for the third-year pupils. New courses were introduced and there was a general rearrangement of subject matter. Then, in 1899, there was a distinct innovation described by Miss Nutting under the caption of "studies of social conditions."

"Recognizing the wisdom of bringing into the education of nurses some study which would prepare them for more intelligent and active usefulness in the community, a brief course of lectures was given during the year on various public and social questions. These were interesting and valuable and we hope to be able to include such lectures as a definite portion of the third year's study. The program is appended:

Organization of charities:	Miss M. E. Richmond.
The rescue of children from unfavorable environment:	Miss Mary Wilcox Brown.
How to relieve the needy:	Mr. John Cary.
The place of the home in modern society:	Mrs. Ellen Richards.
The Church as a factor in modern progress:	Mr. Jeffrey Brackett.
The functions of the municipality and the State:	Mr. Jeffrey Brackett.
The meaning of education:	Miss E. T. King.

A letter to Miss Nutting from Elizabeth King shows that she not only took part in the series but also acted as a consultant:

"I like your titles on the whole but if I were you I would get Mr. Cary to talk on Preventive Charity instead of his present title. I cannot think of a better title for myself—so put me down for plain education unless you can think of something better than 'The relation of education (or training) to life.' . . . Next Fall I wish you would give an address at the Club on the *profession* of trained nursing and its relation to institutions. We will have it fully reported and the public can get a glimpse of what are the possibilities beyond caring for sick patients.

"To change the subject, won't you go with me to hear Lohengrin and help my ignorant musical soul to appreciate its beauty?"

This letter, brief as it is, sheds light on a many-sided friendship that meant much to both women and, incidentally, to the School of Nursing as well.

Miss Nutting herself gave classes in ethics but other opportunities for direct contact with the pupil nurses were confined for the most part to her morning and evening rounds in the wards. "It was a distinctly educational process," said one of them with a smile, "and I think I might have learned a great deal if I had not been too terrified to profit from it." There is a story (possibly legendary) that on one occasion Miss Nutting was talking to Dr. Osler in the corridor when a pupil nurse hurried by. Miss Nutting stopped her and asked: "What did you learn on the ward today?" The poor girl gazed at her hopelessly, vainly tried to think of an answer, and then rushed on without replying. "Sister Adelaide, Sister Adelaide," murmured Dr. Osler reproachfully, "over-wrought and over-taught—over-wrought and over-taught!"

Although she must have known that her pupils admired and respected her, she also knew that many of them (though not all) were afraid of her. It was not that she was unduly severe for in some ways she was lenient. From the beginning, the pupils had been subjected to strict discipline and those who rebelled were dismissed from the School. Isabel Hampton would fly into one of her sudden rages and scold an unhappy victim unmercifully and yet no one seems to have been afraid of her. Why should they fear Adelaide Nutting? No one has ever given any clear explanation. She never raised her voice to convey a rebuke—its subtle scorn was sufficient. Her calm level gaze was a reproach in itself. She was (or seemed to be) cold, remote and unapproachable.

In September 1897 a particularly difficult disciplinary situation arose. A case of leprosy had been admitted to the isolation ward and the second-year pupil nurse who happened to be on duty there had refused to give nursing care. The record shows that "she was given until the beginning of the year to reconsider the matter and informed of what the consequences of refusing to nurse this patient must be. When detailed for duty in Ward I this month (January) she refused again to go if there was any chance of being required to do any service for the patient in question. She was therefore allowed to leave the School." In the annual report of the School of Nursing, she is mentioned as having been dismissed for "disobedience of orders." Her case had been referred to the Board of Trustees and the decision of the head of the School had been upheld. Such was the Spartan discipline of the time.

There is good reason to believe that this and similar incidents may have troubled Adelaide Nutting profoundly. A letter written to her sister betrays her sense of isolation: "Nothing is really unbearable if there are loved ones to share it. Loneliness is the only truly awful thing. I know—and I have had about a thousand years of it." As yet, she did not realize that her own greatness inevitably set her apart, but, as one of her classmates put it: "We knew from the very beginning that she was different from all the rest and that she was destined to go far beyond any of us." Fortunately, there was little time for brooding and before long she wrote in quite another vein: "I suppose I have had a share of life to be grateful for—the chance to work and to grow and as much freedom and power as I have had the sense to use."

Now that a strong plea for shorter hours had been made and the three-year course was well under way, the next forward step could be taken. In 1899, in a report to the Board of Trustees, Adelaide Nutting made these recommendations:

"In my judgment, the course of instruction for the first year should be so altered as to permit of a certain preliminary training of the pupil before she enters the wards of the Hospital. This training might cover a period of six months with distinct advantage to the pupil, and should embrace a practical study of household duties and administration and of cookery for invalids.

"All necessary study of anatomy and physiology, of hygiene, and of materia medica, should form the earliest training and instruction given to a pupil. Such a change would be a further development of the educational ideals in the training of nurses which this School has at all times advanced. It would in some measure correspond to the generally accepted methods of teaching in other professions, notably that of medicine, where it is considered neither wise nor safe for student or patient that theory and practice should begin together."

Reform was distinctly overdue, for conditions had hardly changed since the early days when pupils were placed on duty in the wards as soon as they arrived, and left to sink or swim as best they could. Elsie M. Lawler had a lively recollection of her experiences during the first months of her training:

"On my first day, my room-mate took me over to report for duty. We went to Ward E by a devious route and I was presented to the head nurse who said: 'This is how to strip a bed and this is how you make it.' I was then told to make up the other beds in the ward, struggling with the mitred corners as best I could. . . . Each ward was supposed to have twenty-eight beds but sometimes a row of extra cots had to be placed down the middle. These were very low and required a great deal of stooping thus making it difficult to care for surgical patients especially. There was no office for the head nurse and a table out in the middle of the ward served as headquarters. The linen room was frequently used for taking the night report—close quarters for the entire ward staff.

"The eight-hour day was supposed to be the rule but it simply could not be adhered to because there were not enough nurses available. We worked on broken time and were 'staggered' so as to take care of the rush hours. The night nurses were on duty for eleven hours, usually for two months at a time. They were recalled to the ward even after they had gone to bed if the head nurse found any evidence of neglect or untidiness. Candles were used when treatments or catheterizations were done at night. I do not understand why no one was ever burned to death. Sometimes an extra pupil was assigned to heavy wards to help out but we took a pride in getting along without her. There was one night supervisor for the whole hospital who was on duty from 9 p.m. to 7 a.m. every night. She never got a whole night off—just an evening occasionally."

Preparatory instruction obviously could not be carried on satisfactorily unless pupil nurses could be kept off the wards entirely during the early part of their training and Miss Nutting was obliged to admit that under these circumstances their services would be lost to the Hospital for several months. The financial situation was far from prosperous and it could hardly be expected that the Trustees would approve of any scheme that would involve expense. The three-year course had helped by augmenting the nursing service but the preparatory course would do just the opposite, and some means must be found of persuading the Trustees that it was safe to embark upon this new venture. Was there any way in which the course could be made to pay for itself in terms of service rendered?

It so happened that the domestic management of the Nurses Home, at that time under the direction of the Matron of the Hospital, was not giving entire satisfaction. At a meeting of the Trustees held on October 19, 1900, a recommendation was made by the Superintendent of the Hospital that there should be "a reorganization of the domestic work in the Nurses Home whereby all branches of it should be placed under the direction of the superintendent of nurses." A month later the Superintendent of the Hospital was authorized to make such structural changes in the basement of the Nurses Home "as would facilitate the preliminary training of nurses in housekeeping." As usual, Adelaide Nutting gained her point although she had to promise that maintenance costs would be reduced by utilizing the services of the pupil nurses. She made certain, however, that the control of the preparatory course remained in her hands and in February, 1901, made this entry in her monthly journal:

"In accordance with plans which had long been under consideration and which had finally been approved, the Nurses Home was on February 1st, removed from the charge of the Matron of the Hospital and placed under the control of the Superintendent of Nurses. This step was taken in order that conditions in the Home might be improved, particularly with reference to the food, and that a preparatory course of instruction might be given to the probationers.

"It had originally been intended to begin the instruction of the probationers during this month but owing to the necessity of organizing the whole household, training in the new maids and getting matters into perfect order and discipline it has seemed wiser to defer this instruction until the autumn with the second division of the Class, entering on October 15th. It is expected by that date the arrangements will be perfected and the work divided and arranged with reference to class teaching."

By December, 1901, Miss Nutting was satisfied that a good beginning had been made:

"Those of our graduates who are interested in the development of the Training School will probably learn with pleasure of the preliminary course of six months' training to probationers which has recently been established in the School. The idea is by no means a new one, a somewhat similar course of instruction having been in existence in some English Schools for several years, and also to a certain degree in the Waltham Hospital, Waltham, Mass. In all other professions but nursing it is the invariable rule that instruction precedes practice. It seems curious that anything so vitally important as nursing should be the one exception to this rule. By the present plan of work probationers enter twice yearly, in classes of sixteen to eighteen, at the beginning of each six months. They are placed on duty in various departments of the Training School, where they learn by practical experience the most careful methods of housekeeping, of selecting, cooking and serving foods—everything, in fact, which properly comes under the head of household science. They are also on duty in the surgical supply rooms, where they learn the preparation of all kinds of dressings, afternoons are largely devoted to classes and study. The full course of anatomy and physiology, covering about nine hours a week, is completed within the six months. Hygiene, materia medica, the elements of practical nursing, are all taught and the subjects completed within this period. Older graduates will remember that the food in the Nurses Home was cooked in the general kitchen and merely served in the Home. With a view to this teaching, however, the Home has been fitted up with a model kitchen, and all food served to the nurses is cooked in the School, largely by probationers, under the instruction of teachers. The work is going on admirably, and the need of such instruction for the average probationer is demonstrated daily. The nurse will enter the wards at the end of the six months carefully trained, even if for a short period, in habits of neatness, order and method. Familiar with her anatomy and physiology, she will begin her work over her patients with some understanding of the situation, while they will profit by her greater knowledge. Her knowledge of drugs and their uses will enable her to give out her medicines and observe their effects free from the harassing anxiety which every young nurse set at such a task without previous study must feel. Her thorough study of foods and cooking will make the serving of meals, the selection and preparation of special dishes, an easy and a pleasant duty.

"Miss Ross is in charge of the Home and of the practical instruction of these probationers, and instruction in foods and dietetics is given by Miss Emma Smedley, a graduate of the Drexel Institute, and Miss Mary Peacock, of the same institution."

One of the reasons why the Trustees yielded to Miss Nutting's persuasion and finally consented to the establishment of the course was later disclosed by Mary Bartlett Dixon (Mrs. Thomas Cullen), a member of the class of 1903:

"What a shock she gave my ego when I talked with her about my desire to enter the School of Nursing: This is about what she said with such frankness I could not help admiring it: 'I may accept you for one reason. I cannot develop our School unless I have the understanding and active support of the Board of Trustees. Your father is President of the Board and through you, as a student of this School, I believe I can demonstrate the reasonableness of one of my most important plans. I speak of the basic training of students over some months before they are called upon to assume ward duties and responsibilities. If you are accepted as a probationer, the morning after you arrive you will have to go to a ward completely unprepared for the work that will confront you. I am sure you will encounter great difficulties and I am equally sure your head nurse will encounter, through you, even greater difficulties for she is a very busy woman and has not the time to teach you.' Miss Nutting was correct. I must have been a first-rate Exhibit A. for as soon as possible Miss Nutting received the Trustees' consent to establish a preparatory period of six months training for students before they assumed their duties and responsibilities on the wards."

There can seldom have been so innocent or fruitful a conspiracy.

Trials and Tribulations

TIRED OUT by all these exertions, Adelaide Nutting was forced to seek rest and change of scene and in 1902 sailed for Europe with the intention of visiting Grace Baxter, a member of the class of 1894, who was then beginning a remarkable piece of pioneer work in connection with the development of trained nursing in Italy. On her way to Naples by sea, Miss Nutting had an amusing encounter that provoked one of her mildly satirical comments: "I have a *compagnon de voyage*, a charming creature who wears not only pink corsets and pink undervests and pink-beribboned underpinnings but gets hold of my towel by accident occasionally and, owing to imperfect ablutions, leaves a gentle smear of pink on the corner. I hate my sex when I look at her."

In the autumn, after she had visited Venice and had the delight of discovering the glories of Venetian painting and sculpture, she returned to Baltimore, refreshed and invigorated. Some major problems awaited her. It had already become evident that the preparatory course was not going to pay for itself even though it had been possible to dispense with paid workers in certain departments and to replace them with pupil nurses. The cost of food services had been materially reduced and the nurses were better fed than ever before but the sum total of these economies did not offset the expenditures associated with teaching and supervision. The finances of the Hospital continued to give cause for anxiety and it was evident that something must be done if the preparatory course was to continue. In October, 1903, Miss Nutting made this entry in her monthly journal:

"The following change in the regulations governing the work of the School is advised: the establishment of an entrance fee of $50; this should be paid by each student to help cover the cost of preparatory instruction. It should be returned at the end of the year to those students who have not been accepted."

This recommendation was accepted by the Trustees with alacrity although Miss Nutting herself seems to have had some mental reservations concerning certain aspects of it:

"All things considered, there seems to be little reason to doubt that the establishment of preparatory courses of instruction within the hospital, but outside of the wards, does mean a definite increase in expense varying with the work of different institutions and the manner in which the instruction is carried on. The idea that it shall cost anybody anything to give nurses a proper education has been for so many years unthinkable that we cannot wonder if it stands for some time in the way of better development for training-school work. It is not so many years since in most hospitals the entire teaching of all classes as well as the really great executive work of such institutions was placed upon the shoulders of one woman. The idea that a regular, definite system of instruction had any place in a training-school for nurses has taken form and substance quite within the memory of the youngest member present. As for paying for lectures when they can be had for nothing—perish the thought! So I think we need not shiver on the brink unduly, but make the plunge and say, 'Yes, the education of nurses if properly done *does* cost, and it should.' All good education anywhere costs, and it is a bad day for our schools, for our nurses, for physicians, and for sick people everywhere, when the first question is always, 'How little can we do it for?' rather than, 'How well can we do it?' In a medical school which comes under my observation, where the students number less than three hundred, their instruction is carried on by a staff of over eighty professors, associate professors, clinical professors, assistants, and instructors, and the services which have been rendered in instruction by about fifteen other men are duly acknowledged (to say nothing of the teaching constantly given to the medical students by the nurses in the wards), yet in a training-school of about one hundred and thirty students the actual instruction may be in the hands of a bare one-half dozen people, all of whom are occupied many hours daily in executive duties. Comparisons are odious, I admit it. They are made in this instance not with the view of claiming great similarity of needs, but to point my moral, which is, that a good education always costs. The question is, who shall pay, the hospital or the student? There seems to be a tendency to settle this in a measure, so far as preparatory instruction goes, by calling upon the student for a tuition fee, which, while at present in no instance large, probably well covers the actual cost of additional instruction."

In the meantime, the preparatory course not only flourished but also made possible a gradual rearrangement and expansion of the teaching program throughout the entire three years. Miss Nutting was particularly pleased with the introduction of a course in anatomy given by Dr. Percy Dawson who incidentally was paid the sum of three hundred dollars, thus vindicating Miss Nutting's contention that lecturers in schools of nursing should not be expected to give instruction on a voluntary basis. The course was held "in a small room specially fitted up for the purpose and partially equipped as a laboratory" and was acknowledged to be a model of its kind. Subsequently, the course was given for several years by Dr. Florence Sabin who always manifested a lively interest in the School of Nursing. The teaching of materia medica was later enriched by assigning the pupils to the Hospital pharmacy for three hours daily over a period of four weeks "during which they were taught in the handling of crude drugs and in becoming familiar with their appearance, peculiarities, methods of preparation, etc." It was also recorded that "a very pleasant and interesting feature of the winter's work in the Training School had been a fortnightly class in the History of Nursing which had been carried on by the officers and teachers of the School."

Georgina Ross gave excellent instruction in "the elements of nursing" and by way of practice, the pupils were assigned "to the clinics of the outside dispensaries to give assistance to the doctors in charge, helping to prepare patients for examination and for minor treatments and receiving their introduction to the problems of the patients whom they would later have to care for." Later on, the pupils went on duty in the wards for two hours daily and all along the line, a strong effort was made to link up theory and practice. The preparation of surgical supplies was organized, gathered together from the various wards and brought into a central surgical supply room, where the raw materials were kept and daily prepared for use in wards and operating rooms. Methods of making such supplies, of sterilizing them, and of preparing the various antiseptic materials required, was carried on by the students for about four weeks, concurrently with instruction in bacteriology, disinfection and sterilization.

Written notes on the lectures still had to be handed in for correction though Miss Nutting was less enthusiastic about this method of teaching than was Isabel Hampton. Even Miss Hampton's faith must have been shaken when, during one of her recitations, she asked the pupils to set down what they remembered about a lecture given the previous day. One unhappy girl could recall only a single isolated statement and spent the whole hour in writing it out over and over again. Strange to say, she was never rebuked for this audacity.

For the most part, the pupil nurses enjoyed the preparatory course, although some were not particularly happy during their assignment to the kitchen and serving room of the Nurses Home: "We were not required to do heavy work, such as peeling potatoes, but we washed mountains of spinach and cut up huge joints of meat, and struggled with boiling cauldrons filled with large slippery vegetables such as cabbages and beets." A future leader of nursing, precariously perched on a ladder, dusting a fanlight, is said to have murmured plaintively: "My mother never expected me to do work like this—it just *isn't* nursing." It was not until November, 1905, that Miss Nutting was able to announce that there would be better opportunities in future:

"A change in the preparatory department was rendered necessary by the crowded condition of the Nurses Home, the kitchen of which had been used for teaching cookery and household economics. In the beginning this was a fairly satisfactory arrangement for that was in reality but an experiment, and during the four years of work in this kitchen good teaching was given and valuable experience obtained. It was felt that if food could be prepared for the sick, still more valuable work could be done and better teaching given, and with this object in view the former bath-house which had later been fitted up for a small orthopedic ward, was transformed into a Diet School, where food can be prepared for the private wards and for private patients in the maternity or other wards, and where special orders for food can be filled. Probationers were placed on duty in the Diet School in November last and the entire service of food for the private wards is now carried on there in a highly satisfactory way."

The development of the preparatory course was watched with eager interest in the hospital and nursing world, and as early as November 1901, Miss Nutting reported that "already a committee of American and English superintendents of schools for nurses has been formed for the purpose of considering the best way of introducing this method of teaching into the larger schools." She must have been proud that this bold experiment in the education of nurses was being carried on in the School of which she was the head, but she did not fail to point out that too much should not be expected from it:

"It is affirmed that the work over the patients is done from the beginning with some skill and intelligence, and that every act in the work of the ward is done with a due appreciation of its importance or possible consequences, that the pupils are observant and attentive, that they are careful and cautious. It is considered that the whole character of the pupils' work is different and better —so much better than that of the average pupil at the same period of instruction under the old system, that in one school it was suggested that the next effort should be to bring the character of the work and teaching of the wards up to the thorough and careful standards of that done in the preparatory department. My own observation is that there is some tendency to expect too much of the preparatory department. A pupil who has just passed out from there into the hospital ward is an instructed, informed, intelligent probationer, but she is not a senior nurse and is, as an actual fact, just taking the rank of a junior. It should be noted that the very best standards of work are a little difficult sometimes for a beginner to apply to the needs of a busy hospital ward. She has been taught good methods, but to use them well under pressure of time and a diversity of seemingly urgent duties is one of the lessons which only experience teaches."

Just when things seemed to be going particularly well, a grave misfortune befell the Hospital. On the morning of February 7, 1904, "a generalized conflagration swept over the city of Baltimore and proved most disastrous to the real and leasehold property of the Hospital. During the fire, the sixty-four stores, warehouses and office buildings, widely separated and having an assessed value of more than a million and a quarter dollars were destroyed." This heavy loss was only partly covered by insurance and came as a crushing blow at a time when the financial situation was already precarious. Fortunately, no damage was done to the Hospital buildings although clouds of smoke and showers of sparks swept over them all night long from the flaming city below.

Elsie Lawler was assistant superintendent of nurses at the time and well remembers the glowing spirit of loyalty and devotion that prevailed when, on that wintry morning, prayers were held as usual in the Nurses Home. Every pupil nurse was eager to do all that she could to help and the graduate members of the staff offered their services to the Hospital free of charge for as long as might be necessary. This prompt and generous response meant a great deal to the authorities: "The Trustees of the Hospital, in the misfortune of the recent fire, received no word of hope and faith which so pleased and touched them as the voluntary offer of several of the physicians and nurses of the Hospital to surrender their salaries for a greater or less time, or to assume the expense of laboratories, in order to maintain unimpaired the usefulness of the Hospital." Substantial aid was to come swiftly from another source and therefore there was no need to accept this willing sacrifice. Within a few weeks, a grant of half a million dollars was made by Mr. John D. Rockefeller and it was announced that "this very liberal donation, as stated by the donor, has been made in view of the high character of the work the Hospital and the Medical School are doing in medical instruction and research, including the training of nurses."

It goes without saying that the concluding phrase "including the training of nurses" did not escape the attention of Adelaide Nutting:

"So far as I know, Mr. Rockefeller's gift is the only one ever made which has taken recognition of the *work* of the training school and of the enormous amount of teaching and supervision which is required if the duties are to be properly performed, and of the importance of such teaching. Rich gifts have been made to build homes for nurses and to provide comforts which are all very well, but no woman really enters a training school for any other purpose but to be taught and trained, and *the surroundings of the student* are what she needs more greatly than all the comforts of home (the thing I fear she sometimes enters the School to escape). She needs a quiet room to herself, libraries for reading and reference, teachers at the bedside chiefly, but also in the classroom, and the things that make the place a school. These are the necessities which occupy our present thought."

Making History

Mr. Rockefeller's tribute to the School of Nursing may have encouraged Adelaide Nutting but it did not prevent her from seeing that his gift, generous though it was, did little more than restore the Hospital to the position it had occupied prior to the disaster. There had never been much money for educational purposes then, and now there might be even less since the lion's share would be sure to go to the Hospital itself. Some means must therefore be found either of increasing the earning power of the School or of cutting down its expenses, and the outlook was not promising so far as the latter alternative was concerned. Salaries had already been reduced to a minimum by placing pupil nurses in charge of wards even when they were not fully prepared to assume such heavy responsibilities and Clara D. Noyes once gave a vivid glimpse of what such an experience meant to the pupils themselves:

"A feeling of anxiety seems to take possession of me as I face once more in retrospection the responsibilities Miss Nutting laid upon me. After a few weeks in the old operating room, Miss Sharp broke her leg—she was the head nurse—imagine my surprise to be put in charge, where I remained without losing my reason, for three months. From there, or soon after, I was sent to take charge of Ward I. It was then undivided, there being no maternity ward. I stayed about three months, perhaps longer, and I look back on it as a most valuable experience and the knowledge gained there from grappling with contagious work with almost no supervision has stood me in good stead ever since. From there, I was sent to Ward E as head nurse so you see in my last year I had nearly nine months of head nurse's work."

No one knew better than Miss Nutting that few pupils possessed the native ability and courage of Clara D. Noyes and that many of them were overwhelmed by a load that to her was a challenge and a joy. From the beginning, she had done her utmost to obtain more and better supervision in all the ward services and an entry in her journal in January 1901 shows that she had already achieved a measure of success:

"The appointment of the first supervising nurse carries into effect plans which have been made with the hope of relieving the arduous duties of the present assistants in regard to supervision and especially teaching and also with the idea of providing a more liberal training for selected nurses who show administrative ability. The present arrangement places pupil nurses in charge of the Children's Ward and Clinic and Ward E, also of Wards M and O. This territory will be under the direct daily care of two supervisory nurses who will to some extent carry on the duties of assistant superintendents. Good results are looked for from this change."

Frances Kingstone, a member of the class of 1900, is mentioned as having been appointed to supervise M and O but the name of the other supervisor does not appear although it was stated that both would "combine the teaching of certain subjects" with their supervisory duties.

Miss Nutting was determined that the ground thus gained should not be lost and that the supervisory and teaching staff must not only be retained but augmented. The only alternative was to explore ways and means by which the earning power of the School itself could be increased. The growing reputation of the medical staff was attracting private patients in ever increasing numbers and the demand for special nurses was rising proportionately. She had already warned the Trustees that "we can no longer depend on our own graduates for special duty and are obliged to call in nurses from schools where the training may not have been the same. This if continued, may bring discredit on the Hospital and the School." She began to wonder whether it might be justifiable to fill the gap by placing more pupils on special duty provided that increased enrolment kept such assignments within bounds so far as individual pupils were concerned. There were plenty of candidates but unfortunately there was no accommodation for them. The Nurses Home and the makeshift Annex were hopelessly overcrowded. There was no money for building purposes nor, under existing circumstances, much prospect of getting any. Almost in desperation, she finally made up her mind to place the following plan before the Board of Trustees:

"Attention was called in the last annual report to the large sum of money paid out annually to graduate nurses for special service in the private wards. . . . I would suggest that provision be made by which a part of this special nursing could be done by undergraduate nurses in their third year. With proper supervision they can perform the duties to the satisfaction of the patient and the experience they receive is invaluable in preparing them for private duty while the revenue derived from that source would enable us to add the urgently needed improvements and enlargements to the Training School building. The services of ten pupils, for which $21 each per week is charged to the patient should bring in an income of about $10,000 a year. Assuming the cost of maintaining each nurse at $300 per year and deducting $3,000 in maintenance we have a clear $7,000 left to appropriate to a fund for building purposes."

Much to the relief of all concerned, the School was never called upon to assume this heavy burden. In December 1905, Helen Skipwith Wilmer (Mrs. C. N. Athey) presented the sum of thirty thousand dollars to be used for the construction of an addition to the Nurses Home and to serve as a memorial to her father, Skipwith Wilmer, at one time a member of the Board of Trustees. It was announced that the Trustees "propose to erect in connection with the Nurses Home an additional building to be used as dormitories . . . to give each nurse a single room provided with a commodious closet and to place in the basement an adequate dining room and kitchen. There will also be sitting rooms on each floor for the accommodation of nurses when off duty." Mrs. Athey was a member of the class of 1905 who had, of course, been in consultation with Miss Nutting concerning the use to which the gift was to be put. A letter from Miss Nutting shows how much it meant to her: "One of my nurses just graduated has given thirty thousand dollars to build a new dormitory for the Training School, knowing how we are packed here and how I have wanted a new building. You can imagine how I am rejoicing."

The Trustees were so encouraged by this timely assistance that, prodded by the insatiable principal of the School of Nursing, they decided to build a second addition that took the form of a wing similar to that provided by the Wilmer memorial. Actual construction proceeded at the usual stately pace and the inconvenience caused by overcrowding was not immediately relieved but the positive assurance of adequate housing in the near future left Miss Nutting more time and opportunity to develop other aspects of the educational program which she had long had in mind.

Like other men and women who had been associated with the direction of the Johns Hopkins Hospital and the School of Nursing, she had a distinct sense of responsibility for the development of public health services in the community at large. At the very beginning, Johns Hopkins had declared that the School should "benefit the whole community by supplying it with a class of trained and experienced nurses" and, when the School was formally opened, Isabel Hampton had said: "a certain portion of the pupil's second year will be devoted to district nursing, among the poor in their own homes, under a competent head nurse, where it is hoped that such nurses may not only bring their sick back to health, but also leave behind them some good practical work and simple lessons in hygiene and right living, that may result in better health and happier homes." The idea that district nursing should include health teaching had already taken firm root in Boston where in 1886 the first Instructive Visiting Nursing Association was founded. Neither Isabel Hampton nor Adelaide Nutting ever gave up hope of including experience in public health nursing in the program of the School of Nursing even though the services in which it could be obtained had first to be created.

Every encouragement was given to all graduates of the School of Nursing who were willing to become pioneers in the public health services then struggling for existence. A member of the first class, Evelyn Pope (Mrs. J. W. Lord), after first serving as head nurse in the Hospital dispensary, organized the Instructive Visiting Nurse Association of Baltimore in 1896 and carried on single-handed for a year until she was succeeded by Ada Carr who resigned her position as assistant superintendent of nurses in order to develop the service still further. Later on, Mary Lent, a member of the class of 1895, took charge and also made a notable contribution.

When the "outside obstetric service" was under consideration, Dr. Hurd had said that: "It is expected that this service will eventually grow into a branch of district nursing" and it was this sort of experience that both he and Isabel Hampton had hoped to provide for the pupil nurses. During the first year that the service was in operation forty-one pupils made a total of 141 visits but by 1897 it was the old story over again: "The increased demand for pupil nurses in the maternity ward made it seem desirable to withdraw them from the outside obstetric service." Miss Nutting then seems to have refrained from assigning pupils to this service and to have concentrated her attention on building up a graduate staff. Three graduate nurses are mentioned in this connection: Anna Jammé, Mary Cloud Bean and Elizabeth Griest. A few months later, however, she commented upon a new development:

"This service remained in the hands of our graduates until June 1. Since that date graduates of other schools have been detailed for duty for a service of two months duration. Two graduates, from the Old Dominion Hospital, Richmond, and the Union Protestant Infirmary, have in turn performed this work satisfactorily. It is probable that the latter institution will make a permanent arrangement to obtain this service. This will afford training and experience in this branch of nursing to those who would otherwise be without it." This prediction turned out to be correct for in 1903, Miss Nutting noted that "the class of senior nurses from the Union Protestant infirmary attended the full course of lectures on obstetrics given by Dr. Williams and the outside obstetric work is to be carried by them."

The prevalence of tuberculosis in Baltimore had long been a source of concern to Dr. Osler and early in 1902 he tried to awaken public interest by means of an address in which he made a strong appeal to "My dear patient, long-suffering, *hopelessly inert* fellow-citizens." Three years previously, he had organized the Laennec Society of Baltimore in order to systematize and stimulate the work in tuberculosis in the hospital and to infuse in the profession and the public a knowledge of the disease. The nature of these activities, in so far as they were directly related to nursing, was later described by Miss Nutting herself:

"The first attempt in this country, so far as the writer can discover, to do special, systematic visiting of tuberculosis patients in their homes was made in Baltimore in the year 1899, not by nurses, but by women medical students, partly for purposes of education and relief, and partly for investigation. Under Dr. Osler's direction these two students followed to their homes the consumptive patients coming to the Johns Hopkins Hospital dispensary. . . . The results proved interesting, and in a brief account of the first year's efforts the suggestion was then made that if nurses could undertake this branch of work and carry it on regularly and systematically, bringing their special training to bear on some of the practical problems, very effective work could be done in this particular field. An appeal was made to friends interested in the subject to provide for a nurse for this especial purpose and two years later in November 1903 the funds were provided and a nurse finally took over the work from the medical students, beginning a regular daily system of visiting."

This nurse was Reiba Thélin, a member of the class of 1903. A year later, Mr. Henry Phipps, of Pittsburgh, gave the sum of twenty thousand dollars to the Board of Trustees of the Hospital "to increase the facilities of the out-patient department for the study and treatment of tubercular patients," thus making it possible to inaugurate a much broader program.

Yet another follow-up service was to be established in 1905, this time in connection with the orthopedic division of which Dr.

William S. Baer was the head. The ward could only accommodate fifteen children, most of whom required prolonged treatment, and it was decided to relieve this congestion by means of an out-patient clinic. Elsie Lawler has described the early stages of this project:

"About four years ago this was started by Dr. Baer and one of the graduates of the medical school of the previous year, and was held one day during the week, for two hours. The materials required consisted then of little more than a few plaster bandages and a basin, and one small room was large enough to accommodate all the patients that came. Strange to say, the assistance of a nurse at these clinics was not requested, in fact it was definitely stated that none would be needed, but as the fact was recognized that here was very useful experience to be gained, one was nevertheless provided."

In talking with the present writer, Mary B. Dixon (Mrs. Thomas Cullen) shed light on this somewhat enigmatic statement by explaining that she had offered her services on a voluntary basis in order to get the work started but that Miss Nutting had insisted that a salary of eleven dollars a week must be paid in order that "it could be entered in the books as a regular thing for which a salary had to be provided." Miss Dixon promptly returned her weekly wage to Miss Nutting who duly recorded it as "a gift from the pupils of the School toward the provision of visiting nurse service in the orthopedic clinic." This arrangement continued for several months and when Miss Dixon was obliged to withdraw, the service was taken over by the Hospital as a matter of course. The fact that Miss Dixon's father was the president of the Board of Trustees may have been a factor in the situation, and it will be remembered that this was not the first time that Adelaide Nutting and Mary Bartlett Dixon had been involved in an equally innocent and indirect approach.

All these pioneer public health nursing services developed slowly though steadily and, in point of numbers, the nursing staffs remained insufficient for several years to come. Nevertheless, Miss Nutting had accomplished what she set out to do—she had trained, guided and encouraged the exceptionally able young women who were to occupy key positions during the first difficult years and who were later to be responsible for planning the instruction of pupil nurses in the principles and practice of public health nursing.

However absorbing her other preoccupations might be, Adelaide Nutting never overlooked the importance of building up library facilities that would not be confined to technical and scientific works but which would also offer books of a wider cultural interest. As far back as 1899, she had prepared for the Paris Exposition a list of books then in use in schools of nursing in the United States. The titles have not been preserved but her summary and classification are worth examining:

Subject	*Textbooks*	*Reference*
General nursing:	11	0
Materia medica:	4	3
Surgical nursing:	5	4
Special branches of nursing:	3	0
District nursing:	2	0
Obstetric nursing:	5	3
Hygiene:	5	4
Anatomy and physiology:	7	3
Nervous and insane:	6	2
Bacteriology:	1	3
Asepsis:	0	3
Massage:	13	0
Care of children:	3	9
Dietetics:	8 (12 manuals)	13
Dictionaries:		2

Three of the textbooks in this collection, expressly intended for the use of nurses, had been written by women closely associated with the Johns Hopkins Hospital School of Nursing. These volumes were, of course, *Nursing, Its Principles and Practice*, by Isabel Hampton; *A Textbook of Materia Medica for Nurses*, by Lavinia Dock; and *A Handbook of Invalid Cookery*, by Mary Boland.

In the very early days, friends of the School had helped to establish the nucleus of a library and a bequest of four thousand dollars from the estate of Annie M. Gill also afforded some support. The next step was to encourage the nurses to use these facilities and at a meeting of the staff nurses and senior pupils, held on

December 13, 1905, Miss Nutting suggested that a society be formed for the study of the history of nursing. Its aim was defined as "the bringing into light the historical associations which have clustered around the work of men and women from the earliest times in ordered and unordered care of the sick." Reference was made to "a unique collection of rare and valuable books which would ultimately prove to be not only of immense interest and value to our own School but should also possess much wider usefulness by providing the only fairly complete library of reference accessible to nurses." This collection consisted of the source material which Adelaide Nutting and Lavinia Dock were laboriously gathering together for use in the preparation of their classic *History of Nursing*. How this incomparable work came to be written is best described by Lavinia Dock herself:

"The first intimation I had from Adelaide was in the spring of, I think, 1900. I was in Germany and had written her a full account of a visit to Kaiserswerth. She answered me briefly: 'We must have a history of nursing. Will you help me to write it?' I answered as briefly that I would and began at once to gather material in libraries and by visitations abroad.

"I do not know just when this idea took form in her mind. Of course, we know that when Teachers College was opened to nurses, Miss Nutting's course of lectures there was on the history of nursing and hospitals. I never heard those lectures, nor do I know whether they were written out in full. But when we sat down to begin our History, she had a complete and well defined skeleton of countries, time periods, leading events and sub-events, persons, and their activities down to the end of the Eighteen Nineties, and beginning with the earliest known records of ancient civilization. The only addition that I made to it was the introductory material on mutual aid. We used this skeleton in mapping out our chapters and general plan and followed it closely.

"I do not know exactly, either, just when Adelaide made her collection of Florence Nightingale's writings, including the several privately printed volumes of material intended for Parliament and the officers of the British Government, which have distinguished this collection. I remember, though, that Dr. Hurd, who was intellectual and critical, was much impressed by Adelaide's collection, and in an address that he gave at a medical meeting, he quoted at length from Miss Nightingale's report on the Crimean War, its hospitals, disasters and shortcomings in medical management and nursing.

"After our first two volumes were finished, I was in London and made a visit to Sir Edward Cook, Miss Nightingale's biographer, and he asked me how Miss Nutting had obtained these special books. I told him she had always collected books and had a special second-hand dealer in rare books in London. I do not know the dealer's name.

"You would have been surprized, perhaps, at our complete self-assurance about our History. We did not ask anyone's advice nor seek for counsel, nor need any encouragement. Of course, we spread our intention far and wide among nurses. We did not try to secure a publisher beforehand, as writers sometimes do. Miss Nutting, of course, could not spend hours in writing, with her duties and responsibilities in the hospital and school for nurses, so I, being free, could devote all my time to it. But Adelaide had her heart set on doing two special chapters, and these she did write entirely, at odd times or at night. They are the chapters on French hospitals in Canada, Spanish hospitals in Mexico, and on the Military Nursing Orders.

"She read carefully all my pages, suggested, commented, criticized, brought in more material, and finally approved. As the chapters were finished, she had them typed, and then they were passed on to Dr. Frank Smith, who was the Hospital's recognized master of good style and correct use of the English language. When all of the first two volumes were finished, we looked for a publisher. Putnam's were friendly and sympathetic, but doubtful about the cost and the returns. Dr. Hurd suggested that we make the round of the prominent publishers, but this was too slow and uncertain. Without any ado, we borrowed the money from a bank and paid the publishing costs. They were not heavy as compared with today, and the books came out and repaid the loan in a very short time.

"Adelaide was content, happy in the success of the work, and once said to me—as we heard of a wave among far countries of an interest in writing local history—'We have started something.' "

There can be no doubt that they awakened a lively interest among the members of the newly organized historical society at the Johns Hopkins Hospital Training School for Nurses. There was a discussion regarding a suitable name for the group and Miss Nutting asked to be allowed to suggest one and proceeded to read extracts from Dr. Osler's address, "Science and Immortality" which seemed to her to prove that "we ourselves have perhaps a good claim to be permitted to style ourselves 'Teresians.' " Then one of the group recalled that Dr. Osler himself had once called the little band of district nurses in Baltimore "dear disciples of St. Teresa," and the name with all that it implied was adopted with enthusiasm. The first officers were Katherine de Long as president, and Alice Fitzgerald as secretary. An early contribution to the program was a sketch, prepared by Elsie Lawler, of the work of the Christian deaconesses, Fabiola, Paula and Olympia. Miss Lawler's own comment on this literary effort was: "I found a note on my bed from Miss Nutting telling me that I had to do it."

New Horizons

FROM THE beginning, there had been a brisk demand from other institutions for the services of the graduates of the School of Nursing and by the end of 1899 no less than fifty occupied responsible positions. Not all these young women possessed special qualifications for teaching, even though they were capable administrators of nursing service, a state of affairs that was a cause of some anxiety to Adelaide Nutting. At a meeting of the American Society of Superintendents of Training Schools for Nurses, held in 1899, Isabel Hampton Robb made a strong plea for better opportunities for women who wished to prepare themselves for teaching in schools of nursing which doubtless expressed the views of all members of the Society.

"It is generally conceded by instructors in other kinds of schools that, in addition to the diploma secured, it is necessary for those who intend to teach to have a further course in a school of pedagogy or in a normal school where they may supplement the knowledge they have acquired by learning the best methods of teaching and how to apply them. Why should not this hold equally well with a woman who elects to become a teacher in a school for nurses? It is one thing to graduate as a trained nurse but quite another to enter upon the duties and responsibilities of a training school without a thorough and proper grounding in the management of such work. . . . There are already training schools for teachers established in this country, notably one just recently affiliated with Columbia University, New York."

A committee was set up forthwith and a statement of the desired objectives was submitted by Mrs. Robb to Dean James E. Russell, the head of Teachers College, Columbia University. During a second interview, at which Miss Nutting was also present, he promised to give favorable consideration to the project although the story goes that later on he ruefully admitted that he had not fully realized what he was letting the College in for when he yielded to the gentle persuasion of his quietly determined petitioners.

The new venture got under way in 1899 and took the form of a special course in "hospital economics designed to meet the needs of those directing schools of nursing in which hospital service is a predominant factor." The course was closely tied in with the department of domestic science and two courses in education were made available but it was, of course, also necessary to provide advanced instruction along professional lines:

"The College gave us much, but we also needed much that it could not give—teaching of a kind that had to be drawn from many different sources. And we were without funds. It is inspiring to recall that the expenses of that early period were almost entirely met by the contributions of nurses, chiefly heads of training schools, who paid part of the salary of the instructor in charge of our students, and of some of the lecturers. Others came in most instances at their own expense for several successive years to give instruction on hospital and training school matters."

It goes without saying that Mrs. Robb and Miss Nutting were themselves among those who spared neither time, money nor effort. Two venturesome students formed the first class and Miss Nutting recalled "coming up from Baltimore the first year to lecture solemnly to them on the history of nursing and being much impressed by their enthusiasm for the subject." It was necessary to carry on a continuing campaign for funds and a letter from Isabel Hampton Robb gratefully acknowledged a contribution from the Johns Hopkins Hospital Nurses Alumnae Association:

"I have received the notification for the Alumnae Quarterly Meeting, and I cannot, of course, be present, for which I am particularly sorry at this time, as I should have liked the opportunity of telling the Alumnae members with what great pleasure I reported to the Superintendents' Society their gift to the Hospital Economics Course. To me personally the gift meant two things—that the Johns Hopkins graduates realize their responsibility of standing for educational advancement—and that they do not intend their Alumnae, or rather *our* Alumnae, to be narrow and self-seeking in its aims; and so long as each member takes this view of her membership and her work, so long must the Johns Hopkins Hospital graduates be looked to for whatever is an inspiration to others to do likewise and to do better things."

It soon became apparent that Miss Nutting's participation in the course at Teachers College was destined to influence the policies and methods of the Johns Hopkins Hospital Training School for Nurses. The impact of new and provocative ideas, emanating from other nursing leaders, was a challenge as well as a stimulus for she had at her disposal an incomparable laboratory in which to try them out. There was seldom anything over-academic about them and it was usually possible to fit them into the administrative pattern without exciting much opposition. A certain amount of judicious indoctrination was carried on unobtrusively by granting scholarships (one of them provided by the Alumnae Association) to carefully selected members of the staff who displayed an aptitude for teaching. A subtle change took place in the terminology used in the records of the School of Nursing—pupils were sometimes referred to as student nurses—and in the title of the School itself, the word *Training* was sometimes omitted as if by accident. It all took time and infinite patience but the evolutionary process, though gradual, was unmistakable.

During the later months of 1903, Miss Nutting became involved in yet another project that took up a good deal of her time and energy. In her capacity as president of the Maryland State Association of Graduate Nurses, she guided the work of a committee which was set up to draft a Bill for the registration of nurses and to submit it for the approval of the State Legislature. In order to obtain public support for this measure, a meeting was held at the Arundel Club with Elizabeth King (Mrs. William Ellicott) in the chair. Judge Henry D. Harlan gave an address and Dr. Welch spoke on "State Registration and what it means to the Public and the Professions." Some of his contentions must have been rather a surprise to his medical colleagues:

"You have to consider exactly how to proceed to secure the State examining Board. I noticed in some of the States the law almost imperilled by efforts to secure the presence of physicians upon these examining boards. Now I am quite sure that it is not the province of the physicians to examine nurses. They have something to say in the training of the nurses; the nurse should not go forth without having come under the guidance of the physician, but your profession is a skilled profession which requires special knowledge, and a special knowledge that is possessed by the trained nurse, not by the physician. Akin as the professions of medicine and nursing are, they are still distinct professions and there is no necessity, in my opinion, and there are certain disadvantages, in the requirement that physicians should be members of the examining board."

To Miss Nutting's great satisfaction the Legislature passed the Bill "without any of those alterations or amendments which often seem slight, yet which defeat in many ways the actual purpose for which legislation has been sought." Shortly after the Bill became law, the Maryland State Association of Graduate Nurses requested Georgina Ross (at that time Miss Nutting's first assistant) "to undertake an inspection of schools and so efficiently did she fill this unofficial role that an agreement was arrived at among the hospitals of the state by which a uniform minimum of training was arranged for the junior year." This proved to be an admirable opportunity to spread the gospel of the preparatory course throughout the schools of Maryland.

Another development that arose directly out of the passage of the Bill was recorded in Miss Nutting's journal in 1905:

"The following nurses (Mary M. Thomas, Charlotte Rose, Mary A. Wallis) graduated from the Training School of the

Crippled Children's Hospital, and to meet the requirements of the Maryland law, sought a year of further training in this school. They have received careful training and instruction in medical, surgical, gynecological and obstetrical nursing, and have, in addition, had a brief course of instruction in the diet school. They have passed suitable tests and examinations and their conduct as students has been satisfactory."

The state of nervous exhaustion to which these manifold responsibilities had reduced Adelaide Nutting was reflected in letters written to her sister, who was travelling in England:

"Having thrashed around in my bed for a couple of hours in a vain effort to sleep, I got up and took a turn at the desk. These sleepless nights play the very devil with one's health, temper, ability, judgment and every other quality. I am growing positively unfit for publication under their influence. Just as I was beginning to plan for the year's meetings I took to bed and the subsequent proceedings I managed entirely from there—stenographers every morning (nice women), newspaper reporters often, and interviews with all sorts and conditions of people, to get my programme into proper shape. I got the president of the New York Board of Health down and other dignitaries up, and brought forward the question of nursing in the public schools in a splendid meeting. The reward of our efforts is that in this morning's paper, it is announced that a medical inspection and a trained nurse will begin work experimentally in some of the public schools at once. You see it is worth while to work like a galley slave."

Whenever, as on this occasion, Adelaide Nutting seemed to be taking her responsibilities too seriously, Helena Barnard was usually ready with a salutary dash of cold water:

"Let me advise you not to overdo. I think with the secretaryship of the Superintendents' Society and state registration you have assumed a good deal in addition to your other interests such as writing for the *Journal*, lecturing at Teachers College, etc., 'be moderate in all things.' That registration has been established anywhere will cause it to be adopted everywhere in this country so it will not be necessary to *pant* in order to secure it in Maryland where educational standards are well supported."

This friendly rebuke did not deter Miss Nutting from entering into everything of importance that was going on in the nursing world either at home or abroad and before long she wrote to her sister again:

"There isn't an inch of London that has not its memory for me. I spent three entire days in Westminster Abbey and prowled about the cloisters. . . . Of course, you have gone all over the Houses of Parliament and by this time you are liable to walk in there any one of these days and see a placard over a door saying: 'Nurses Committee.' A body of gentlemen from the House of Commons are bending their mighty intellects trying to find out just how dangerous it may prove to give nurses (women) an inch or two more of freedom—a chance at self-development and self-government—and that reminds me that Miss Dock is likely to be in London just about this time. You will find her views most refreshing on all the nice, correct, conventional, stereotyped hidebound English way of doing things."

One of the reasons why it was possible for Adelaide Nutting to devote so much time and energy to projects not directly related to the Johns Hopkins Hospital Training School for Nurses was that she was blest with an excellent staff. Head nurses were usually appointed for a period of one year and if they proved to be capable were "promoted" from one position to another. Among those mentioned by Miss Nutting was Elsie Lawler who served successively as head nurse, night superintendent and finally assistant superintendent of nurses. Janet Sampson and Mrs. E. M. Simpson filled similar positions in much the same order. Caroline Van Blarcom was first a supervising nurse who also taught classes in anatomy and physiology and later became second assistant superintendent. Christina Dick served as night superintendent. Katharine De Long was a head nurse in several departments and in 1906 "assumed charge of the Nurses Home with a working housekeeper to assist her." Helen Gross was for some years in charge of the operating room and Amy Miller was appointed head nurse in the dispensary in 1900. Many of these names were to become household words in the subsequent history of the School.

Thanks to these women and to others equally capable and devoted, the objectives attained during the early years were impressive: the extension of the period of training from two years to three; the expansion of the teaching program; the establishment of the preparatory course; the abolition of money allowances to pupils; the provision of scholarships; and the payment of fees to lecturers. Over and above all these, postgraduate courses were in process of development, pupils from other schools were granted certain affiliating privileges, and public health services were initiated. In one area, however, Adelaide Nutting had to admit defeat: "the introduction of the eight-hour day has proceeded much more circumspectly."

It was perhaps fortunate that, in point of numbers, the School grew rather slowly at first and that its leaders thus had the opportunity of knowing each staff nurse and even each pupil nurse personally. In the prevailing circumstances, it was necessary for these young women to assume heavy responsibility but they could be, and they were, given sympathetic guidance while they were learning to tackle it. All too often, they were overworked but they took a stubborn pride in remaining on duty until the long day and the longer night were over and the appointed task accomplished. Discipline was always strict and sometimes harsh but there was a rough justice about it and there were compensations for this and other hardships.

They knew that they had the high privilege of working with and for eminent physicians and surgeons who not only taught and guided them but who treated them with consideration and respect. They were afforded cultural facilities that were not available in many contemporary schools. Social circles in Baltimore, noted for their exclusiveness, were open to them. They were encouraged to read widely and to write on professional subjects. Their own Alumnae Association served as a practice ground for effective participation in the activities of international, national and state organizations. Here, in a bracing atmosphere of debate, they had the exhilarating experience of being close to those who were in command. Above all else, they cherished the reputation they themselves had won for giving nursing care so intelligent and skilled that other nurses, the country over, strove to emulate it. Ably directed, wisely guided, well disciplined, they laid the foundations of a School that was to set a new pattern for the education of nurses both at home and abroad. In a word, they were making history—and they knew it.

The Painting of a Portrait

A LETTER written to her family by Adelaide Nutting in the late autumn of 1905 contained a somewhat enigmatic statement:

"I am anxious to put in a splendid year of work—on the home-stretch you know, and after that you must prepare to have me on your hands. I'll do the family mending and earn my salt and that's all I shall need really. But I must make my exit from this scene with the lights up and the bands playing."

Evidently she had decided that it was time for a change but had not yet made up her mind regarding her future course of action. As early as 1900, Dean Russell had urged her to take charge of a division in Teachers College, but she had declined the invitation although the door was kept open by an enquiry in a personal letter: "May we ask you again?" In 1906, they did ask her again and she was offered and accepted the chair of Institutional Management. Her resignation was placed in the hands of the Board of Trustees in April, 1906, to take effect a year from that date.

To say that this announcement came as a painful shock to both the Hospital and the School of Nursing is to put it mildly but the news was welcomed by many of her professional associates and especially by the leaders of the nursing organizations. A message from an old friend must have pleased and heartened her—Lavinia Dock was sure that she had taken the right turning:

"So you have decided! Well, I certainly am terribly sorry to see you leave the J.H.H. I always wanted you to be there continually to shine and enjoy the fruits of your labors—yet this thing is so special that I could not advise or wish you not to take it."

Although Miss Nutting was not to relinquish her duties for another year, the graduating exercises held on May 24, 1906, were in some sense a farewell. In a masterly fashion, she traced the amazing expansion of nursing service during the fifteen years which had elapsed since she herself had been a member of the first class to graduate from the Johns Hopkins Hospital Training School for Nurses:

"Fifteen years ago the thirty-five training schools in this country furnished little in the way of opportunity for institutional work and District Nursing was in its infancy, it had indeed begun its work in but two of our cities. The latest records show about 1500 hospitals and the thirty-five training schools we had in the year 1890 are now numbered at 867. The two or three District Nursing Associations have grown to two hundred and twenty, occupying between five and six hundred nurses."

She went on to speak of the new demands made upon the skill and knowledge of nurses by the advances in medicine, surgery, neurology and psychiatry, and of the growing sensitiveness of the public mind to social and health conditions, especially in the field of tuberculosis. All this was by way of background and then she turned to her main thesis: "We have as a rough estimate perhaps 300 schools where there is some appreciation of the meaning of the word 'nursing,' of the significance of a training school, and the moral obligations which its establishment involves, and in them many new and interesting developments of our work are taking place. . . . Instructors of nursing are now a recognized feature of some of our best schools." In some, but not in all, for she went on to make a plea that every one of the 22,000 pupil nurses then enrolled "should be from the time she enters the school, until the day she leaves it, under the training and guidance of the most able, skillful and highly trained nurse instructors which we can produce, just as truly as they should be under the influence and inspiration of women of intellect, of education and culture, and of the noblest personal character."

By way of conclusion, Adelaide Nutting made a strong plea for "a new system and a new method of government" in schools of nursing:

"The matter, as one considers it in all its phases seems to point to the necessity of placing the training school on the basis of other educational institutions. In the effort to give our pupils first the preparatory teaching which has become an absolute necessity and later the complete and rounded course of training and experience which is due them, and which the community needs of them, it has become quite clear that the work of training schools in the education of nurses calls for a new system and a new method of government. Controlled by the needs of the hospital, training schools must stop at a certain point far short of their highest efficiency. Hospitals are founded primarily for the care of the sick. Invaluable centres for educational purposes they have become, but to carry out in its entirety an educational system is beyond the possibility and the province of the hospital. It has gone as far as it can well go in this direction, and the training school for nurses must turn back to the community and ask if it has no duty toward it. The public profits richly by the hospital training school, and, as has been shown, the need for the services of the nurse as an important factor in the whole life of the community, seems to be asserting itself as we have pressed her into one new avenue of work after another often for which there has been no conscious attempt at preparation on her part. To make the best and the most of our training schools the community must be as willing to give for them as for a medical school and not leave the hospital to do it all. The small hospitals struggling pitifully, ineffectually, with a problem of education quite beyond their grasp, are in urgent need of nursing schools founded on a separate and independent basis in which the course of study and training will be complete, each hospital contributing what it fairly can as a field for teaching and receiving of the student, what she must necessarily give in obtaining her practical training and experience. The formation of such a school is the next step forward in the education of nurses."

As a token of affection and loyalty, the Alumnae Association and the pupils of the School of Nursing immediately signified their intention of presenting a portrait of Adelaide Nutting to the Board of Trustees "so that she might be kept in remembrance as she had lived and worked among them." Cecilia Beaux was chosen as the artist and arrangements were made for the sittings to take place at her home at Gloucester, Massachusetts. This experience was vividly described by Adelaide Nutting in successive letters to her sister:

"I ought to have kept a journal from the very first day I came here. I came at the request of our nurses to sit for a portrait which they had arranged with Cecilia Beaux to paint and arrived here Tuesday, June 19th at 11 a.m. This little hotel had been recommended by Miss Beaux as a quiet little old house on a hill at the edge of the moor, kept by some sisters named Renton. I was told before coming that Rudyard Kipling had stayed here while writing his 'Captains Courageous,' and was happy later to find that I had his room. It seemed to bring him a little more sharply into one's life, to be in the room where he certainly thought and probably worked.

"As soon as I was settled comfortably I called up Miss Beaux, and made an appointment to go and see her the next morning. I walked about that lovely little curve of shore to a point where in among a tangle of trees and shrubs I found her cottage and studio which she has just finished building. The whole thing is so attractive that it ought to be described and yet I don't see how I can do it any sort of justice.

"The house is of plaster rough cast and one winds through an almost hidden path straight to the door. There is no obvious approach. No invitation to enter—yet once you find your way through the gate and the thicket you are at the door and almost it seems, inside. The windows are French. On entering the house one steps into a small room, in no sense a hall, one door at the right leads into the drawing room, another into a second small room from which the stairway leads in so quiet and inconspicuous a way that I forget where it is. From the drawing room one steps down into a small cloister so partitioned across that one can always be sheltered from the wind in some nook, or find the sun if sunshine is needed. A flagged sort of pavement a little above the ground faces the harbour on the southwest and takes the place that a verandah would ordinarily take. It is roofless, surrounded by shrubbery with one or two trees at the end and a pretty path losing itself shortly in the tangle. A place for quiet breakfasts and early tea, green about, water beyond and heaven above. Nothing pretentious—the absolute reverse in fact—of seclusion and remoteness perfectly open and free to those who really got within, but no hint given that you could do so easily. Someone here, Mrs. Stagg I think, tells me that Miss Beaux told her architect she wanted the house to look like the house of a working woman. She was not concerned about the expense so really did not care what cost he put into the materials, but the general effect was to be that. I do not think she has succeeded in carrying out her idea.

"I must not forget the fence, since it is her own design and built she tells me largely with her own hands. It consists of barrel staves woven in and out among posts placed pretty close together. The effect is thus in a way rustic but not too rustic.

"I have not been over the house but intend to do so before leaving to get the plan in mind. The above impressions did not come all at once but have been gathered at various times and in various ways.

"To return—in accordance with instructions I went the morning after arrival at about eleven o'clock to see Miss Beaux and, as she said through the telephone the day before, 'go through the preliminaries.' Miss Beaux was in her studio but came up to the house as soon as the maid told her I was there. As she entered the room, I saw a woman of a little over medium height, apparently about forty years of age, probably a little more—blue gray eyes not widely opened—rather a large mouth—a face longer than ordinary—a good heavy chin and jaw—a pleasant friendly smile, excellent teeth and, as she spoke, such a soft low sweet voice, with absolutely no resonance in it. As she looked at me, I met a keen level glance, which seemed to be doing a lot of things, rejecting and accepting and debating all in a moment. I am sure she was disappointed then and there in her subject. After a few moments of talk I found she had expected me to come in the things I was to be painted in instead of the nice clean shirt waist and businesslike garb I had worn. She would therefore do nothing that day, but we walked down to the studio and she talked about various matters in a very charming and entertaining way.

"Speaking of her sitters, she said that she had recently painted Bishop Grier and knowing him as a man of tremendous convictions and full of burning fiery zeal, it was interesting to see the expressions into which he fell after standing for a while. Sometimes he would look like an old pussy cat and sometimes like a petulant old woman, seldom like the man he was.

"She asked about the uniform I had promised the pupils to wear and I told her it was of soft black silk with a narrow white collar and cuffs, black girdle and a small white skull cap, saying I thought it would be pretty severe. She thought not, adding that she had always wanted to paint someone in that kind of cap and garb, and thought it ought to do well.

"She talked a little then about herself and told me of her early training by her grandmother and aunts in habits of frugality and simplicity and industry, adding that she was sure that this careful home training had much to do with her success later. She spoke then and often later with the deepest affection and gratitude of her grandmother and her aunts, talking a little about her quiet and retired life in West Philadelphia which she frankly avowed she always hated and meant to get out of as soon as possible. On a later day she described the place to me as 'hopeless,' saying that apart from her own family who lived in a semi-detached house with garden, she had no companionship. Such neighbourhood children as there were her people would not let her know beyond the merest acquaintanceship.

"The following morning I went to the studio in my uniform, carrying my cap, and an hour was spent in deciding upon the right pose, light, etc. A small platform about one foot high was wheeled out and, in a sort of arm chair placed upon it, I sat in every conceivable attitude, Miss Beaux meanwhile studying me through a small piece of paper which she had torn to resemble a frame, two by three inches. Then I stood for a while, first on one side of the room and then on the other, turning this way and that against a golden brown background and finally against the gray linen background made by the curtains of the large French windows. This seemed to satisfy something in the mind and eye of the artist and was finally decided upon. Still there were unsettled details. Miss Beaux rolled up a small sheaf of paper and placed it in my hands, asking me to hold it. Of course it did not do. Then she asked if there were no papers or something that I was used to carrying in my hand and laughingly I mentioned the little red leather notebook, which she quickly decided to be the very thing needed especially after hearing that I seldom made rounds without it so that it was as familiar to my pupils as any part of my uniform. While this process was going on Miss Beaux talked little except to give me the necessary instructions. When she got me before the grey curtain turning as though to walk away from her but looking back, she began to seem satisfied and said softly 'Yes, that's pretty nice,' once or twice over. With some slight alterations she finally settled on this asking me to fold my arms a little, or rather, cross my hands, saying that although she only intended to do a bust, she might take in the hands.

"She arranged for me to come to her studio every morning from 10 to 12.30 and talked to me about her cottage which she had only finished the year before and evidently was very proud of. The two next days were occupied in sketching me in and, by the artist, I presume, in trying to find out what I had in me. She talked almost continuously, either asking me about my work and commenting upon anything which attracted her attention or telling me some little thing about herself. Her soft sweet unresonant voice, her gay good humour, and fresh spontaneous outbursts of laughter made her a constant delight.

"She told me a good deal about her family, and of how she was not allowed to go to Paris until she was grown up and beyond the age when most students go—how as a young girl she showed no special talent, did nothing remarkable, just went on in the usual way, always doing her best to do good honest work."

At this point, the correspondence was interrupted and was not resumed until August 10 by which time Miss Nutting had arrived at Saint Johns, Newfoundland.

"I had to drop this while making arrangements to transfer myself from Gloucester to Newfoundland and since coming here have been unable to write and certain to have lost much that I had clearly in mind before leaving Gloucester. I cannot hope now to follow the days in any consecutive way but must simply gather together the fragments of conversation and impressions of the entire time as best I can. She talked one morning about this time of some sitters, speaking particularly of Mrs. Theodore Roosevelt, whom she had not long ago painted. She spoke of her as a woman of marked simplicity of character and of much nobility. She repeated what one has always heard of Mr. Roosevelt, calling him the most absolutely straightforward and direct human being she had ever seen or could imagine. She spoke of his language as almost brutally plain and frank and told of a day at Oyster Bay when she was sitting with Mrs. Roosevelt, and he came in with Secretary Taft and one or two other men, saying as he entered: 'That she-ass of all she-asses, Mrs. T. S. L.!' She mentioned other instances which I have forgotten, and spoke of Mr. Cleveland as having similar directness and absolute truthfulness and a way of giving you his whole attention in speaking or listening. She spoke with wholehearted admiration of these men, and of this particular quality of sincerity of speech, pronounced and striking honesty and clarity of mind and purpose. She spoke of Mr. Roosevelt with the utmost warmth, saying he was one of those big splendid heroic creatures she always found herself wanting to 'cherish'—and to explain the extraordinary use of this word, she went on to add: 'just as one would cherish and try to care for and preserve in perfection a beautiful flower—or a great Newfoundland dog.'

"On this and other occasions the thing which seemed to shine forth vividly was her great love of truth and honesty as the most to be desired of human qualities."

It would not be extravagant to suggest that these letters are, in themselves, a vivid portrait of an artist by an artist. The beauty of the landscape and the grace and serenity of the home are blended with sensitive skill into a rich background for the strong and vital figure of Cecilia Beaux herself. The two women were kindred spirits and became close friends and when a few months later Cecilia Beaux suffered a family bereavement, she wrote to thank Adelaide Nutting for her sympathy:

"At last, dear Miss Nutting, my appreciation of all your letters can get to you. Would you were here in the quiet afternoon sunshine in the west cloister where I am alone. Too much surges up to speak. I am so glad she saw you and you her. I am thankful for every touch of sight and hand. There was so little of the voice we love heard between her and my new friends—the ones who are to be my friends for the rest of the time. It was sudden at the last. Just after sunset on the eve of the last day of summer. What a time to die! . . . There was nothing but love and beauty—near and about her. How this little house has lived already—it seems as though it must show on the walls. Tears, agony, exaltations, mortality—a few short moments of ecstasy and many hours of labor and striving.

"Your portrait solemnises every one who sees it. And people are moved to say wonderful things and to understand it. Those were living hours. Mary at the piano—you and I tending the sacrifice! Dear Adelaide, write me again when you can.

Faithfully yours
Cecilia

The portrait was first placed on display at the Corcoran Art Galleries in Washington as part of an exhibition of the work of American artists and was considered by the critics to compare favorably with other notable paintings that also happened to be of special interest to the citizens of Baltimore:

"The *clou* of the display, without any possible question, is John S. Sargent's enormous canvas of Doctors Welch, Osler, Halsted and Kelly, grouped about a table behind which is a large globe. It is John S. Sargent at his very best, and it is quite beyond his 'The Misses Hunter.' The picture was painted as a commission from Miss Garrett for the Johns Hopkins University of Baltimore. With this are four other canvases by Mr. Sargent, his admirable and masterly Miss Thomas, president of Bryn Mawr College; a portrait of the donor, Miss Garrett; his quick sketch of William Thorne, and a most lifelike rendering of the late John Hay. No one stands up beside Sargent in this display for he is in a class by himself. But Miss Beaux crowds him a little all the same, for in her 'Miss Nutting,' the portrait of a nurse for the

Johns Hopkins school for nurses, she shows quite the best performance we have to record for her. Its simplicity, directness and feminine charm are not to be mistaken, while technically it leaves absolutely nothing to be desired."

Later on, the portrait was shown again, this time in Boston, and elicited an even more acute and penetrating critical comment:

"The portrait of a nurse by Cecilia Beaux is one of the most remarkable characterizations of a type that has come from the brush of this exceptionally talented painter. It is a type which many persons know, and which unites the *sauviter in modo* with *fortiter in re*. A useful and estimable personage, strong of will and very capable. The head is painted with extraordinary certitude, candor and comprehension."

The portrait was presented to the Board of Trustees at a simple ceremony and was accepted by its president, Judge Henry D. Harlan. The presentation address had been prepared by one of Miss Nutting's classmates, Mrs. W. S. Thayer (Susan C. Read) and in her unavoidable absence, was read by yet another classmate, Georgia Nevins. Among the other old friends was Elizabeth King (Mrs. William M. Ellicott), who seems to have expressed what was in the mind of each and every one of them:

". . . This I know, that, great as have been her powers of administration, these alone could not have given the permanent and enduring qualities to Miss Nutting's career, had not her heart as well as her brain been put into her work. Faithfulness, sympathy, loyalty and unselfishness, which have made her the best of friends, have given the final excellence to her years of active work in Baltimore.

"And now, we would be unworthy to be her friends, if, in wishing her Godspeed, we did not say we are glad to have her go—glad that in the height of her matured powers, she is entering upon a new sphere of work where her creative genius can mould into enduring form the experience she has gained here; glad that a great intellectual center has done her the honor to create a new department, in which her active mind can solve new problems and, in academic leisure, work out the experience of past years. We are glad to have her go, but we are human after all, and in the bottom of our hearts, we will be most glad when from time to time, she comes home to us again."

It was at this time that Adelaide Nutting began the long journey which was to lead her into a new world. The education of nurses had already reached and passed a critical turning point although it would be more than thirty years before she could look back upon the steep ascent and see it in its true perspective: "Surveying the course of events during the years in which we have been struggling with our educational problems, one is tempted to wonder if the decisive moment in our educational progress may not have come unseen and unrecognized on the day when the education of nurses passed out beyond the hospital and into the university, into an institution which did not need or desire to make use of the services of students, the day when Isabel Hampton with the support of the Society prevailed upon the Dean of Teachers College to open the doors of that department of Columbia University to graduate nurses."

Genius Loci

In 1905, the School of Medicine, the Hospital and the School of Nursing alike sustained a grievous loss when Dr. William Osler decided to accept an appointment as the Regius Professor of Medicine at Oxford University. In the School of Nursing, he had been guide, philosopher and friend from the very beginning and to Adelaide Nutting, as to successive generations of Hopkins nurses: "it had been a grand thing for a young nurse to accompany Dr. Osler daily in his rounds for years, to stand beside him at the bedside, to share in his teaching to his students and to gather something of his philosophy of life." It may well be that she was aware that he more than anyone else had woven the spell of which Henry James [1] had written in *The American Scene:*

"The natural pitch of Baltimore, the pictorial, so to speak, as well as the social, struck me, once a certain contact established, as that of disinterested sensibility, the passion of which her University is the highest and clearest example. There was on the splendid Sunday, in particular, a warm soft fusion of aspects, a *con*fusion in fact, while I now gather it in—which seems to defy, though all unconsciously, the sharper edge of discrimination and

[1] Henry James, *The American Scene*, London, Chapman and Hall, 1907

to offer itself insistently as a general wash of brave Southern shade of which the North knows nothing.

"Even a morning hour or two at the great University hospital —for one's experience of the higher tone, one's irrepressible pursuit of charm, in America, has, to its great enrichment, these odd sequences—even the beginning of the day did nothing to obtrude the ugly or overemphasize the real; it simply contributed, under some perversion that I can neither explain nor defend, to the general grace of the picture. Why should the great clear Hospital, with its endless chambers of woe, its whole air of *most* directly and advisedly facing, as the hospitals of the world go, the question of the immensities of pain—why should such an impression actually have turned, under the spell, to fine poetry, to some more shining view of the conditions, the high beauty of applied science?

"The conditions positively, as I think of them after the interval, make the poetry—the large art, above all, by which in a place bristling with its terrible tale, everything was made to seem fair, and fairest even while it most intimately concurred in the work. In short if the Hospital was fundamentally Universitarian—as of the domain of the great Medical Faculty—so it partook for me, in its own way, of the University glamour, and so the tempered morning, and the shaded splendor, and the passive rows, the grim human alignments that became in their cool vistas, delicate symphonies in white, and, more than anything else, the pair of gallant young Doctors who ruled, for me, so gently, the whole still concert, abide with me collectively, as agents of the higher tone.

"No example could speak more of that enlargement of function, for constituting some picture of life, that many an American element or object, many an institution, has to be felt as practising—usually with high success."

Although the literary style of Henry James does not make easy reading, it is evident that the *genius loci*—the spirit of the place—had kindled his imagination. He may or may not have known that the man who had done so much to create and to cherish that spirit had just given up his work in the Hospital and the Medical School.

There was, of course, another side to the shield. The nursing service usually pursued the even tenor of its way, but whenever a difference of opinion arose it seemed to one observer (Dr. W. S. Thayer) that Dr. Osler "flatly refused to waste time in futile controversy and discussion, and it was hard if not impossible to persuade him to enter into any controversy with nurse or superintendent. . . . There were abuses which he preferred to endure rather than to risk unpleasant discussion and he advised capitulation because of the threats of the nursing authorities." This eagerness for peace at any price is perhaps explained by a remark said to have been made by Dr. Osler himself: "I long ago made up my mind that the only way to deal with a woman is never to take her seriously—say nothing, and go your own way."

A comment by Dr. Hurd sheds another light on Dr. Osler's attitude toward the School of Nursing:

"He had a warm friendship for Miss Hampton, the organizer of the School and its first principal, and also for Miss Nutting, her successor. He gave much assistance in advice and in teaching and was warmly interested in its success. He gave two graduation addresses, one entitled 'Nurse and Patient' and the other 'Doctor and Nurse.' He was appreciative of the work of nurses and touched lightly and gracefully upon the mutual relations of the nurse to her co-worker, the doctor, and the object of her care, the patient. There was, however, a suggestion of an attitude of reserve toward nurses as a class, as may be inferred by the quotations which preceded these addresses when published. One for instance had this significant motto from the Psalms of David: 'I said I will take heed to my ways that I offend not with my tongue. I will keep my mouth as it were with a bridle.' "

Sometimes, there was what Dr. Hurd calls "a light-hearted irresponsibility" in Dr. Osler's relationships with the pupil nurses. This took the form of a series of practical jokes that occasionally bore a little heavily on the innocent victims, especially when no retaliation was possible. On a busy morning, it might be rather exasperating to discover that soda water had been squirted into the freshly filled inkwells on the head nurse's desk, or that the carefully arranged medications had been jumbled into an unsightly little heap. But, after all, these minor aberrations were nothing more than spots on the sun.

The extent to which Dr. Osler approved of the aims of nursing education as set forth by the American Society of Superintendents of Training Schools for Nurses is open to question and appears to have baffled Dr. Hurd: "Osler in fact seemed always helpful and at the same time he had an air of detachment as one who was endeavoring to see in what way the movement of the education of nurses would ultimately lead. In the end, I am sure that he learned to understand and appreciate the work of the Training School and felt its great importance to the physician and to the advance of the science of medicine."

Neither Isabel Hampton nor Adelaide Nutting leaned very heavily on the support of Dr. Osler in organized efforts to improve professional standards and it was always to Dr. Welch that they turned for help in movements such as the establishment of the Army Nurse Corps or the state registration of nurses. Nevertheless, they knew full well that Dr. Osler was more than generous in his appreciation of the value of good nursing care and that he had implicit faith in the efficacy of his favorite prescription—rest and skilled nursing. It is possible that the intellectual compulsions that were forcing nurses to seek new light may have been alien to the spirit of William Osler, but it is certain that no physician ever penetrated more deeply into the heart of nursing or came so near to its very soul.

In more ways than one, the years from 1905 to 1907 proved to be a turning point in the history of the Johns Hopkins Hospital and the School of Nursing. Change was in the air. Financial problems no longer gave the Trustees cause for anxiety and there was talk of new departments and fine new buildings in which to house them. It was evident that both the Hospital and the School were entering upon a period of expansion—in fact, a new era. Just seven years later, at a ceremony marking the twenty-fifth anniversary of the School, Adelaide Nutting, by this time professor of nursing and health at Teachers College, Columbia University, had this to say:

"The glow of this first enthusiasm was as yet undimmed when The Johns Hopkins Hospital Training School opened its doors. Not only was it to lead women into a new and absorbing field of work, but at this time, it should be remembered, there were hardly any other fields of work open to them. Teaching was practically the only profession in which women were occupied in any appreciable numbers. The whole movement for the education of women was indeed in its early years, and some of the colleges of which we are now so justly proud were then just beginning to make their influence felt. Bryn Mawr was in its infancy. Barnard was just being founded, Radcliffe was as yet a dream. The time was a favorable one for the further development of this new work for women which was soon to be rooted in the vital necessities of life, and which had made so strong an appeal.

"The city of Baltimore, with its old world tranquillity, its scholarly atmosphere, its far-famed hospitality to the stranger and to some of his ideas, had many unique institutions, educational, artistic and philanthropic, but among them there had not as yet appeared a training school for nurses. The field in this city for this new branch of women's education was wide and untouched; the time and the place were propitious. And further, this school was established in connection with a great new hospital, which had become famous in a sense, even before its doors were opened. To its planning, many years of special study and arduous labor had been devoted, and it stood as an embodiment of the best thought and skill of the time in architectural form and structure, in internal arrangement, in hygienic provisions. As a part of the noble University which had become preeminent throughout the intellectual world, it was to be a center for advanced scientific teaching and for sound methods of work. Moreover, the training school was not to be a merely necessary factor in hospital administration, but was an institution as definitely provided for by the will of the founder as was the medical school. His directions read: 'I desire you to establish'—not *in*, but *in connection with*, the hospital, a 'Training School for Nurses.' The school was, therefore, to stand on a strong foundation."

Miss Nutting went on to refer with gratitude to the staunch support given to the School by the Board of Trustees, especially by its first president, Francis T. King, and to the unfailing interest of Daniel Coit Gilman, the first president of the Johns Hopkins University. Nor was the generous co-operation of the medical staff overlooked: "The members of that first little group of students, of whom the speaker was one, like to remember their introduction to the mysteries of the human body came through Dr. Councilman; that theories of infection and immunity were presented by Dr. Welch and later by Dr. Flexner with a simplicity and clarity that reached even their 'terminal facilities'; that certain aspects of medical diseases were made known to them by Dr. Osler, coupled perhaps with sundry exhortations of a strictly personal nature. Some of them still treasure their notebooks; all of them treasure their memories."

Another builder of the School, who usually managed to remain in the background, was on this occasion singled out for special mention:

"There was one other in those early days, a woman of rare character and qualities, who as assistant and teacher filled a large space in the school for several years. Independent, fearless, loyal, Lavinia Dock exercised unconsciously an influence which was both strong and enduring, and few connected with that early life had more to do in the last analysis with shaping ideals and giving direction to future activities than this beloved teacher. A student and a thinker with a mind of a peculiarly fresh and original cast, with ideas clear-cut and logical and considerably in advance of the time, there were few of the problems of the training school or hospital, or of the professional life of nurses, to which she could not give illuminating thought. She had an extraordinary way of driving directly to the heart of a matter, pulling out the essential facts in the situation, and showing us the right way to think about them and then to deal with them. Her sense of justice was keen, but her sympathies were well-nigh boundless. It has been her chosen task to write of the lives and deeds of nurses in many fields, and she has written the history of this training school with such characteristic self-effacement that no trace of her own years of rare work with us can be discovered. It is important that her share in the upbuilding of our school should be well understood."

The far-reaching influence that the School so early exercised over nursing education in general was mentioned with a detachment that did not wholly conceal a distinct sense of pride and satisfaction:

"The school did much to break down the 'splendid isolation,' that heritage of cloistered and military ideals, which had hitherto been built up about hospital training schools. It created conspicuous traditions of hospitality, and marked courtesy was shown to all visitors from other schools. Every opportunity was granted them for study of methods worked out here which might be helpful elsewhere. Every effort was made to establish cordial relationships and to sweep away a narrow and exclusive attitude in training school administration. The heads of this school constantly studied progress made in other training schools, and in other branches of education."

It can safely be asserted that the heads of the School did a good deal more than study these matters,—they ardently debated them. The swift intuitive thinking of Isabel Hampton would be challenged by the cool and critical logic of Adelaide Nutting, and Lavinia Dock, a catalytic agent if ever there was one, would set both to rights before all three joined forces to circumvent whatever opposition threatened to block their plans for the advancement of the School.

Dr. John Billings had been right when he had told the Trustees: "It should be remembered that our buildings and machinery are simply tools and instruments, and that the real Hospital, the moving and animating soul of the institution, which is to do its work and determine its character, consists of the brains to be put in it. Whether it shall be a truly great Hospital and a charity such as was intended by its founder, is not a matter solely of arrangement and plan of buildings, it depends upon not more than half-a-dozen men and one or two women. The most difficult thing in forming this Hospital is to find the proper and suitable persons to be the soul and motive power of the institution."

Well, the men and the women were found—and as Adelaide Nutting remarked, the time and the place were propitious. Everything was new. There were no outworn traditions to uproot, nor hampering precedents to overcome. By great good fortune, the interdependence of the Hospital, the School of Medicine and the School of Nursing was mutually acknowledged from the beginning. While each sought to fulfill its own destiny, they kept in close touch and went forward together.

And yet, when all is said and done, the *genius loci*—the subtle influence that pervaded the whole enterprise—remains intangible. It was as tranquil and serene as the climate that Captain John Smith of Virginia had thought so pleasant when first he explored the shores of the Tidewater and found that in this fruitful and delightsome land: "the colde is extreame sharpe, but here the Proverbe is true, that no extreame long continueth."

Part Two: 1907-1949

Another Era Begins

THE YEAR 1907! Theodore Roosevelt was president of the United States. Universal suffrage for women was still a belabored issue. The public health movement had emerged from the era of sanitation to the era of public education; the third and present era —the era aiming to bestow on every individual the gift of a healthy mind and body—had not yet arrived. Coeducation had long since passed the experimental stage; prejudice against it had largely disappeared. College education for women was still in the great period of expansion. By 1906 there were 129 women's colleges and 335 universities, colleges, and technological schools open to women as well as to men; in these institutions 50,000 women were enrolled.

In the city of Baltimore little change was wrought during the early years of the new century. The city quickly recovered from the great fire of 1904, and the business district, the area swept by the conflagration, was entirely rebuilt by 1907. But outside the business section the face of Baltimore was not noticeably altered: the cobblestone streets were still there; the lamplighters going forth at twilight and dawn; the rows upon rows of red brick houses with their much scrubbed white steps, shining brass rails and gleaming doorknobs. Old Baltimore Town, now Baltimore City, friendly, leisurely, conservative Baltimore, held to old memories, old fashions, and old ways.

Nevertheless, Baltimore by its works had achieved distinction long before 1907. It had pioneered in the successful use of vaccination in the summer of 1800; nine years later it established a Vaccine Institute for "the better extension of the blessings of vaccination." The first issue of that journalistic institution in Baltimore, the *Sunpapers*, appeared in 1837; the Maryland Historical Society was incorporated in 1845. During the second half of the nineteenth century, the Peabody Institute was dedicated and the Enoch Pratt Free Library opened to the public. The Woman's College of Baltimore, later renamed Goucher College, was established during this period, as were also the University and the Hospital founded by Johns Hopkins.

By 1907 the Johns Hopkins University was thirty-one years old; quarters were still on Howard and Little Ross streets. By 1907 official action had been taken by the University to admit women to graduate courses, "provided there is no objection on the part of the instructor concerned." At the same time it was emphasized that there was no intention of admitting women to undergraduate classes.

By 1907 the Johns Hopkins Hospital and its Training School for Nurses [1] were eighteen years of age; the Johns Hopkins University School of Medicine a bare fourteen. The president of the University was Dr. Ira Remsen. Dr. Henry M. Hurd was superintendent of the Hospital, and Dr. William H. Howell, dean of the School of Medicine. In the Training School for Nurses, a great leader, M. Adelaide Nutting, was called away and another era begun.

Georgina Caird Ross, 1894, succeeded Miss Nutting. Miss Ross, a Canadian by birth, had been educated in the High School at Belleville, Ontario, Canada. She entered the Johns Hopkins Hospital Training School for Nurses at the age of twenty-five in 1892

[1] The School is referred to as the "Training School" in the Bylaws of the Hospital adopted October 8, 1889. The first official document found in which it is designated as "School of Nursing" is the 1935–1936 *Circular of Information.*

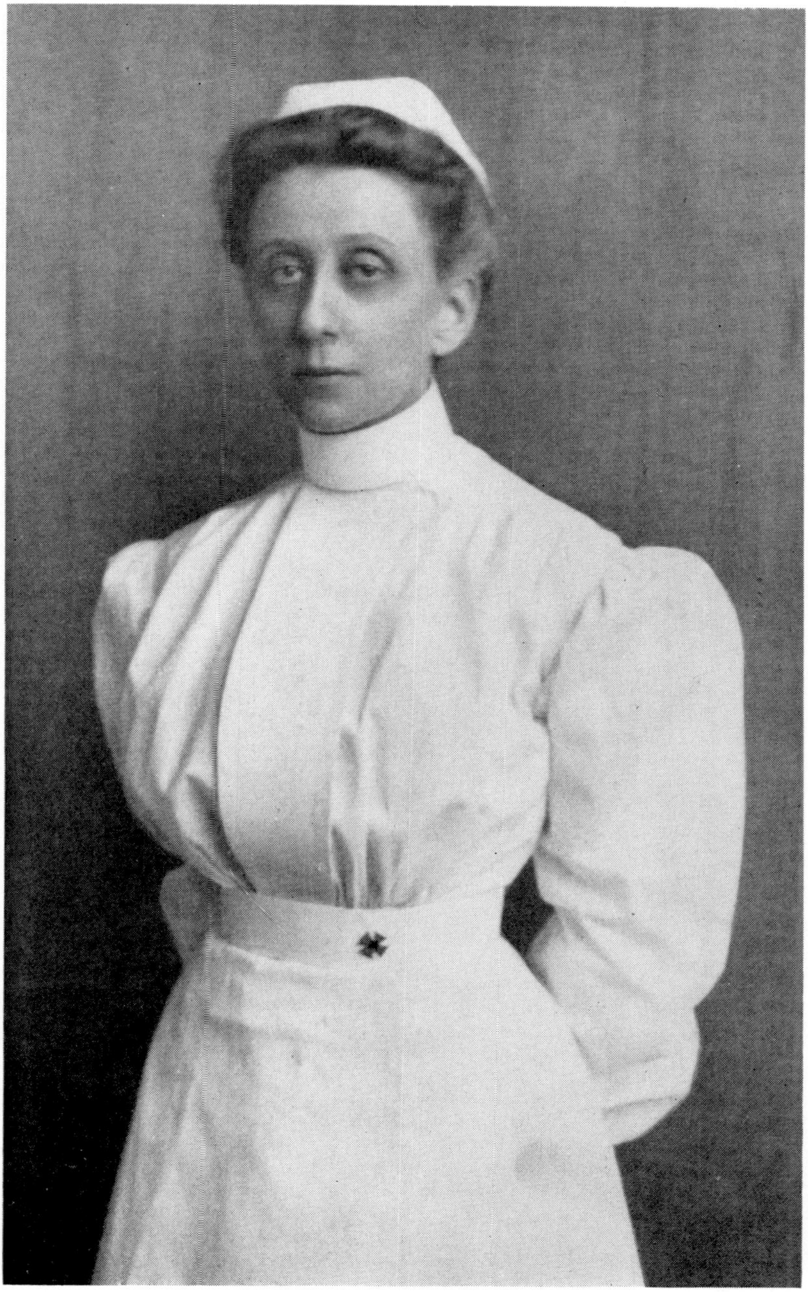

GEORGINA C. ROSS
Acting Superintendent of Nurses and Acting Principal of the Training School, 1907–1908
Superintendent of Nurses and Principal of the Training School, 1908–1910

and was graduated in 1894. Prior to her entrance, Miss Ross' experience must have been much like that of other young women of her day: she taught in Sunday School and shared the household duties of her sister with whom she lived.

After completing her nursing course, Miss Ross was head nurse in different wards of the Hospital for a time. In the autumn of 1896 a new position, second assistant, was created because of "the considerable increase in the work of teaching and supervision which the longer course necessitated." Miss Ross was appointed to the new post. She remained as assistant for two years and then resigned in order to have a much-needed rest. After the six-month preparatory course was established, Miss Ross returned to direct that program and also to assume charge of the Nurses' Home. In 1907 she was first assistant to Miss Nutting and upon Miss Nutting's departure, May 1 of that year, she became acting superintendent of nurses and acting principal of the School. In his report for the year ending January 31, 1909, Dr. Hurd announced that "At the beginning of the year Miss Ross, who had been serving as acting superintendent of nurses for a year, was appointed superintendent of the Training School."

Miss Ross had been associated almost continuously with the School in one capacity or another since 1892: first as pupil, then as teacher and assistant administrator. The same year that Miss Nutting became head of the School, she became head of a ward. It was under the tutelage of Miss Nutting that Miss Ross gained her experience; she was a devoted and competent disciple. Her incumbency as head of the School was short—less than three years—but during that time she carried on faithfully the work already begun and inaugurated some important new policies. Miss Nutting, in her annual report for the year 1906, had noted an "unusual amount of illness among the nurses during the year" and "the difficulty which a good many of our pupils find in getting through their third year." Miss Nutting then went on to say, "I have thought of asking if the vacation at the end of the second year might not be lengthened to four weeks instead of three." Miss Ross carried forward the idea and in her first monthly report, May 14, 1907, she suggested "the advisability of giving a full month of vacation this year and each succeeding year to pupils at the end of their second year." Promptly the Board of Trustees agreed to the suggestion. But the Board did not lose sight of the question of hospital nursing economics and the effect the longer vacation might have upon it. The full month vacation was to be granted to students at the end of their second year, "provided that no extra nurses have to be employed during their absence; that is, such vacation is to be given without causing increased expense to the Hospital." Actually the length of the increased vacation was four weeks. One year later Miss Ross proposed that the same vacation be provided for pupils at the end of their first year. The proposal was not acted upon favorably, and it was not until 1920 that two four-week vacations were given during the three-year course.

Another innovation in the early part of Miss Ross' regime was the appointment of a full-time instructor. In a letter to Elsie M. Lawler, dated February 17, 1925, Miss Nutting wrote, "As to the providing of a full-time instructor, I am practically certain that we led the way in that respect by appointing Miss Carr in that capacity in the winter of 1907–1908." This was indeed a happy appointment. Ada M. Carr, 1893, was a talented teacher and also a talented writer. She possessed a quiet charm and a quiet sense of humor that revealed itself now and then in smiling, twinkling eyes. Miss Carr is remembered by those who were so fortunate as to be in her classes as an outstanding and inspiring teacher.

Throughout the United States the transfer of a student from one nursing school to another was frowned upon, even though the student had good and sufficient reason. Moreover, it raised the debatable issue of granting credit in time and subject matter, an issue freighted with problems forty years ago when the enactment of state nursing laws was just beginning, and records of students were rarely available or descriptions of courses which they had covered. But as long ago as 1907 the May report of the School notes that Edith Macdonald transferred from the New York Hospital Training School to the Johns Hopkins School after being in training eight months. Miss Macdonald made the transfer because the New York School changed its course from three to two years after she had been admitted. At Hopkins she achieved a high general average in the preparatory department examinations, whereupon Miss Ross recommended that Miss Macdonald be given a time credit of six months. The Board of Trustees approved the recommendation.

In itself the incident hardly warrants mention. Historically it is important, not only in the annals of the Johns Hopkins School but in the development of nursing education generally in this country, since it represented a departure from a punitive and negative to a constructive and positive policy, based on sound educational principle. It recognized the right of the individual after she had begun her training to exercise choice of the school from which she finally received her diploma in nursing. In 1911 Mary M. Riddle declared in her presidential address before the American Society of Superintendents of Training Schools for Nurses, "It being considered an offence against their high calling . . . my plea now is against the old custom of a wholesale ostracising of those who resign from one school and try to enter another. Let them be at least heard."

On February 1, 1910, Miss Ross resigned because of ill health. In reporting her resignation, Dr. Hurd said, ". . . Miss Ross served faithfully in many capacities. . . . She devoted herself assiduously to her work and her failure in health was much deplored by all connected with the Hospital." The capacity in which Miss Ross seems best to be remembered is that of instructor. She must have been one of those individuals singularly endowed with the gift of teaching. She was a perfectionist in the art of nursing; she not only could tell how a procedure should be done, but could herself perform it with precision. Her associates recall her as a highly capable nurse with keen powers of observation, and her students, as an outstanding and understanding teacher.

Through Hospital Growth, War, and Epidemic

On March 15, 1910, Elsie Mildred Lawler returned to Baltimore to begin a regime that was to extend over thirty years. For a brief period she served as acting superintendent of nurses and acting principal of the School of Nursing; she soon received full official appointment to the position.

Miss Lawler was born in Whitby, Ontario, Canada, the third child and eldest daughter in a family of seven. She attended the Whitby Collegiate Institute and matriculated for Toronto University; she also attended the Ontario Ladies' College for Music and Drawing. Six months after she entered the University she was compelled to withdraw because of the death of her father.

Miss Lawler's application to the Johns Hopkins Hospital School of Nursing is dated October 3, 1896. She was then in her twenty-third year. To the question concerning her previous nursing experiences, Miss Lawler replied, "I have never been a nurse except at home and as I have helped nurse four younger sisters and brothers, I think I have had considerable experience." The Lawler physician who had known the family for many years wrote, "She is in every way well-suited to undertake the work of a nurse, being well-educated, sound of body and mind, of an even cheerful disposition, a widow's daughter, one of a large family, and not afraid to work." Her qualifications must have been entirely satisfactory, for one month after submitting her application she was admitted to the School. As a student Miss Lawler made a good record; she won two scholarships and was graduated in 1899.

Miss Lawler spent her first seven years as graduate nurse at Johns Hopkins Hospital. She was successively head nurse, night superintendent, and assistant to the superintendent of nurses, holding the latter position for five years. In the three years intervening between the time she left Hopkins and the time she returned, she was assistant superintendent of nurses at the Toronto General Hospital, Toronto, Ontario; superintendent of the hospital and training school, Memorial Hospital, Niagara Falls, New York; engaged for a short period in private nursing; and superintendent of nurses, Tuberculosis League Hospital in Pittsburgh, Pennsylvania. Miss Lawler came back to Hopkins in 1910 to begin thirty years of arduous labor during a period that was to see momentous changes in nursing education and to suffer a world war.

The decade between 1910 and 1920 marks the beginning of the great expansion period of the Johns Hopkins Hospital and, concurrently, the School of Nursing. The work on the new buildings had barely begun when the Hospital lost its superintendent and the School, a friend. Dr. Hurd was leaving Johns Hopkins.

Dr. Henry Mills Hurd, appointed administrative head of the Hospital, June 1889, resigned May 1911. He had witnessed the birth of the School and, it can be truly said, helped to nourish its growth for more than twenty years. Dr. Hurd was convinced of the necessity of endowment for nursing education; as early as 1906 he stated this conviction and on many subsequent occasions.[1] He was equally emphatic in his statements that nursing was a profession, and he expressed himself as believing that the education of nurses had a rightful place in the university. Not only was Dr. Hurd an able administrator; he was a writer and a scholar and "a

[1] Henry M. Hurd, "Shall Training Schools for Nurses be Endowed?" *American Journal of Nursing*, 6:843–54, Sept. 1906

man of noble and elevated character." [2] In the April 1911 *Johns Hopkins Nurses Alumnae Magazine*, Miss Nutting wrote:

"Nor can we, as nurses, forget how constantly he upheld those educational and professional standards which we are everywhere struggling to maintain. In these days of controversy it means much that the scholarly head of a great institution should . . . emphasize publicly in speech and in writings, his sympathy with our ideals. Had he been less in sympathy, the history of our beloved Training School might have been written very differently."

Dr. Hurd was succeeded by Dr. Winford H. Smith, who had been graduated from the Johns Hopkins University School of Medicine in 1903. Miss Lawler returned to Hopkins in 1910, Dr. Smith in 1911; Miss Lawler left the School in the fall of 1940, Dr. Smith left the Hospital in the spring of 1946. Their personal and professional relationship over the years was built upon the solid rock of mutual understanding and respect.

In the first twenty years of its life little physical change occurred in the Hospital—buildings or grounds. The two-story building for colored patients, Wards M and O, which later became part of the Woman's Clinic, was erected soon after the Hospital opened. Most of the buildings still lined the north side of the grounds, with the Administration Building and the two private patient wards facing west on Broadway. On the south side were the Nurses' Home and the laundry, the laundry at the extreme southeast and the Nurses' Home well toward the west. This arrangement of buildings left a broad sweep of grounds, with velvety lawns, clumps of green shrubbery, and stalwart, spreading trees. Many of the trees had been planted by the Trustees themselves, in 1883, before the opening of the Hospital. Others had, doubtless, weathered the years long before the Johns Hopkins Hospital was there.

Between 1910 and 1920 four new buildings were erected. The Harriet Lane Home for Invalid Children admitted its first patient

[2] Letter dated June 7, 1889, from James B. Angell, then president of the University of Michigan, to President Gilman. Published in *The Johns Hopkins Hospital and The Johns Hopkins University School of Medicine* by Alan M. Chesney, Vol. 1, 1943, p. 127.

in November 1912; the Henry Phipps Psychiatric Clinic in April 1913. With the erection of the Harriet Lane and Phipps Clinic, both located on the south side of the grounds, the wide and pleasing lawn was gone forever. In 1913 the Charles L. Marburg Building for private patients was also completed. The James Buchanan Brady Urological Institute was opened in January 1915.

Miss Lawler was fortunate in her choice of assistants who were to organize and administer the nursing in the new departments. Amy E. MacMahon, 1903, was appointed to direct the nursing in the Harriet Lane Home for Invalid Children; Effie J. Taylor, 1907, to direct the nursing in the Phipps Psychiatric Clinic; and Elizabeth A. Thomas (Mrs. Frank R. Kent), 1908, the nursing in the Brady Institute. In her formal reports, Miss Lawler spoke with appreciation of the work of these three women—their interest, their tirelessness, and their leadership in the face of the many problems that accompany organization of a new department.

With the opening of the new buildings, the daily average number of inpatients increased from 274 in 1911 to 424 in 1915. Other services in the Hospital, such as operating room, expanded accordingly. During the same period, the total outpatient visits jumped from 71,000 to 131,000.

Expansion of the facilities in a hospital is inevitably accompanied by increase in normal functions. The first and foremost function of a hospital is the care of sick human beings, and as the burden of this care is to a large degree one of nursing, more nurses are needed as the hospital expands. In the early years of the century the accepted way in America to increase the nursing personnel was to increase the number of student nurses. The idea of the graduate nurse for bedside nursing in the hospital barely was born. This is not the place to trace the slow but sure recognition of the graduate general staff nurse as essential for carrying out a nursing education program and for insuring a consistently good quality of nursing to patients. Suffice it to say that this doctrine was new and practically untried when the Johns Hopkins Hospital began to enlarge in the years between 1912 and 1915. Then the natural thing for a hospital to do to meet its increased nursing needs was to admit more students. During the year ending January 31, 1911, 202 students were enrolled in the School; during the year ending January 31, 1916, 284. These numbers did not include affiliating and postgraduate nursing students.

The Harriet Lane Home and the Phipps Psychiatric Clinic, the first two of the four new buildings, began admitting patients within less than six months of each other. Even though the School was larger by that time than ever before, it was still not large enough to assign student nurses to Phipps. Miss Lawler, in her report at Commencement Exercises in May 1913, sounded the note that was to be heard again and again as the Hospital grew and grew and as other events made inroads on the nursing personnel. She referred to the opening of the Harriet Lane Home and then when she came to the Phipps Clinic she said, "As yet it has not been possible to assign any pupils to this department, as our School . . . could not grow rapidly enough to meet all these new demands."

The Hospital was now confronted with a new situation—not enough pupils to nurse the patients—and a new solution had to be found. The solution took the form of employing eight graduate nurses for "regular duty" in Phipps Clinic. But the employment of graduates to give bedside care to patients made slow headway, and it was not until the Thirties that the use of this important group became more widespread in the Hospital.

With the new departments in operation, it became possible for the School to broaden its program of clinical experience. In February 1913, Miss Lawler reported, "the opening of this building [Harriet Lane] enables us to provide for our students very desirable training which we have up to this time not been able to supply." In a subsequent report Miss Lawler announced, "Each student will spend four or five months there receiving systematic bedside instruction with special attention to the question of diet and feeding." When the contagious wards in the Harriet Lane were opened several years later, student experience in this department included the care of patients "with scarlet fever, diphtheria, and measles."

By the autumn of 1913 it was possible to assign students to the Phipps Psychiatric Clinic for a two-month experience. At first the medical group were opposed to having student nurses, because of their short assignment, in this department. Later they welcomed them. The value of training in the care of psychiatric patients soon became evident. The following year Miss Lawler noted in her commencement address, "It is remarkable to observe the change in attitude displayed by the pupils after this short experience in the care of the mentally ill."

While urological patients had been admitted to the Hospital before the building of the Brady Institute, the opening of this new 60-bed department centralized the administration of the urological service. Students now received experience in urological nursing under more favorable instructional conditions.

In this period of growth in nursing service, in size of the School, and in training offered, the School faced administrative and instructional difficulties, perhaps inevitable during rapid expansion. The stress of the nursing service interfered with curriculum plans for experience and instruction in the wards, and classroom teaching also suffered from the fact that the increase in student body had not been matched by a corresponding increase in teaching staff.

Nevertheless, it seems likely that viewed in the contemporary scene the School now offered its students an uncommonly rich clinical experience. In 1913, national statistics available on hospital facilities were largely limited to the hospital as a whole, and the regular assembling of nursing school data by the national nursing organizations had not yet begun.[3] Evidence exists, however, indicating generally curriculum leanness in both pediatric and psychiatric experience in nursing schools of that period. In 1910 there were more than eleven hundred schools of nursing. The great majority of these schools were conducted by hospitals having a daily average of less than one hundred patients; many by hospitals with less than fifty patients; and an astonishing number by institutions of fewer than twenty-five patients. Some thirty-five years later an analysis of the clinical facilities in 1,047 hospitals operating nursing schools disclosed that 163 of these hospitals

[3] Two reports, giving statistics on schools of nursing, by M. Adelaide Nutting, had been published prior to 1913 by the United States Bureau of Education: one, "The Education and Professional Position of Nurses," incorporated in the *Report of the Commissioner of Education*, Vol. 1, for the year ending June 30, 1906; the other, *Educational Status of Nursing*, published as a bulletin in 1912.

had no children's service; that in the remaining institutions the fewest patients were on the pediatric service; and that not until the hospitals reached a daily average of 150 patients, might one expect to find as many as twelve pediatric patients. It is reasonable to suppose that the distribution of patients in 1910 was fairly similar to the distribution in 1944, and that the fewest patients were then, as later, on the pediatric service. Under the circumstances there must have been a paucity of clinical pediatric facilities that could not be overcome by affiliations with either general or special hospitals. Speaking before a session of the American Society of Superintendents of Training Schools for Nurses in 1909, M. Helena McMillan, superintendent of nurses at the Presbyterian Hospital, Chicago, Illinois, declared, "There is one more kind of nursing, just as important as any taken up today, and that is the care of sick children. Some schools of this country have no provision for teaching pupils anything about the care of the sick child." And one year later one reads in the proceedings of the same Society the following pronouncement by another leader in nursing education, expressing another point of view, ". . . I have come to think that in the general hospital we must give the medical, surgical, and obstetrical experience and not try to add the eye and ear, nervous and mental, children's work . . . I believe that we can only recommend that the schools affiliate with such departments so as to give optional or elective courses to the students in the third year, if they have an inclination toward any of these specialties. . . ." Obviously, at that period there were two schools of thought with respect to pediatric nursing as a curriculum requirement.

In psychiatric nursing there appeared to be even less opportunity, less concerted thought, and less disposition to include that experience in the curriculum. Sara E. Parsons, chairman of the Committee on the Nursing of the Nervous and Insane, submitted a report to the parent body, the American Society of Superintendents of Training Schools for Nurses, in 1910. One member of the committee thought at least six months, preferably nine, should be given to nursing the nervous and insane, others thought three months sufficient, and "others felt it was out of the question to introduce it into the general curriculum." Said Miss Parsons, who was then superintendent of nurses at the Massachusetts General Hospital, "I am sorry not to be able to tell you how many hospitals incorporate this training in the three years' course, but I think there are very few."

At the Johns Hopkins Hospital, as rapidly as possible, the new 100-bed pediatric unit and the new 86-bed psychiatric clinic were utilized, like all other departments in the Hospital, as fields for clinical instruction and practice for nursing as well as for medical students.

During the time when the Hospital was beginning to expand, a world-shaking disaster descended on this earth. On August 2, 1914, Germany declared war on Russia and on France the following day [4] and, according to the *Evening Sun*, "Baltimore immediately felt its far-reaching effects." Funds were sought for U.S. nationals in Europe and "Baltimore looked to her innocents abroad. . . . Cardinal Gibbons asked Catholics to pray for peace. In the synagogues, in the Protestant churches the hum of prayer rose. . . . Johns Hopkins Hospital leaders lamented. The source of their laboratory needs for scientific and medical research was Germany alone, they said. . . ." [5]

But a few years later the Johns Hopkins Hospital lamented another need, that most precious of all needs—human resources. In the early days of April 1917, the Congress of the United States, at the request of President Wilson, declared this country at war with Germany. The draining of medical and nursing personnel into military channels soon began.

In June the Johns Hopkins Hospital Unit, otherwise known as Base Hospital No. 18, left for Europe. Thirteen members of the Hospital nursing staff, all assistants and head nurses, sailed with the Unit. The same month another head nurse and a graduate staff nurse resigned to go abroad and others left at intervals during the year. The trek to war was on, and the School would lose for a time two of its ablest faculty members: Effie J. Taylor to organize the Army Nursing School at Camp Meade and Anna D. Wolf, 1915, to teach at the Training Camp for Nurses at Vassar College.

The loss of personnel not only affected the regularly employed

[4] *Evening Sun* (Baltimore), September 1, 1939

[5] *Ibid.*

nursing staff, but also the special nurses available for duty in the Hospital. The problem of meeting the demands of private patients for special nurses became increasingly acute as members of that group left civilian for military service. More students were assigned to the private wards, and when the patient's condition warranted it, a student special was provided if a graduate could not be secured. The daily census of patients continued to rise, as did also the number of patient visits to the Dispensary. The responsibility for filling these gaps fell upon the student nurses.

Other causes, than its own immediate needs, bore upon the Hospital to increase the student body. In the summer of 1917, the General Medical Board of the Council of National Defense issued a call to schools of nursing urging their expansion. M. Adelaide Nutting was chairman of the Committee on Nursing of the General Medical Board of the Council of National Defense; Pearl H. Braithwaite, 1915, assistant secretary. Miss Nutting warned: "The war might last many years" and then stated, ". . . it was justly concluded that the essential thing to do was to fill our schools . . . to the utmost and put every ounce of our energy into creating something that would be a permanent and genuine asset to nursing." That was in the spring of 1918; later that year Miss Lawler requested Dr. Smith to bring before the Trustees the proposal, received from Dean Annie W. Goodrich of the Army School of Nursing, that senior students be permitted to complete their training in the Johns Hopkins Base Hospital in France. Before the proposal could be put into effect, the war ended.

How did the Johns Hopkins Hospital School of Nursing react to the internal and external pressures for expansion? From its early days the School had had many more candidates for admission than it could accept. It had consistently maintained a high level of selection, and the 1905–1906 *Circular of Information* specifies that applicants "must show they have graduated from a High School or have received the equivalent of such a degree of education, and while this is indispensable, women of superior education and cultivation will receive preference, provided they meet the requirements in other particulars." Although for more than fifty years public high schools in the United States had provided secondary education for the great masses of people, this educational specification was, nevertheless, a bold advance for a school of nursing in 1905. At that time the great majority of training schools had not formulated entrance requirements beyond a grammar school certificate or, more vaguely, "a thorough knowledge of the simpler branches of English." [6] Some seventeen years later, out of the findings of the Goldmark Study came the pronouncement, "Completion of four years of high school should be the minimum entrance requirement." [7] Too many schools were still admitting students with one year of high school or even less.

Miss Lawler's reports during the period of hospital expansion and World War I emphasized that there was no dearth of applicants and that the applicants were of "the most desirable type." In her commencement address in May 1913, she stated that 1,230 requests for information and 184 applications for admission had been received during the year; five years later on the same occasion she could cite 2,396 requests for information and 245 applications for the previous twelve-month period. Not only were there more applicants in 1918 than in 1913, but a greater proportion must have had "superior education." Sixty-two students were admitted in 1913 and of that number 13 per cent had an academic degree and 16 per cent, one or more years of college; ninety-five students were admitted in 1918, 38 per cent of them had a degree and 30 per cent one or more years of college work. This considerable increase in the admission of women with college preparation was doubtless due, in part at least, to the efforts of the Committee on Nursing of the Council of National Defense to enlist the interest of college groups in nursing. A notable outcome of the work of that committee was the Training Camp for Nurses at Vassar College.

[6] M. Adelaide Nutting, "The Education and Professional Position of Nurses." *Report of the Commissioner of Education.* Year ending June 30, 1906. Government Printing Office, 1907, Vol. 1, pp. 155–205

[7] Committee for the Study of Nursing Education, *Nursing and Nursing Education in the United States.* New York, Macmillan Co., 1923. This study, made under the aegis of the Rockefeller Foundation, is often referred to as the "Goldmark Report." Josephine Goldmark was secretary of the sponsoring committee. The publication contains a report by the committee and a report of the survey made by Miss Goldmark and her associates.

The Vassar Training Camp, "The College Woman's Plattsburg," was a war recruiting measure under the auspices of the National Council of Defense and the American Red Cross. It brought into nursing more than four hundred graduates of more than one hundred colleges. On the distinguished faculty were Dr. Florence R. Sabin and Anna D. Wolf. Dr. Sabin, professor of histology at the Johns Hopkins University, earlier taught anatomy and physiology in the School of Nursing. Anna D. Wolf was then assistant and instructor in the School and later became its fifth director. M. Adelaide Nutting, who was chairman of the Committee on Nursing of the Council of National Defense, was a member of the General Advisory Committee for the Camp.

America needs nurses! That was the cry in 1917 as it has been in other wars since Florence Nightingale hoisted her banner in the Crimea. Vassar College heard the cry and responded. The Provisional Alumnae Council passed a resolution requesting "the Board of Trustees at Vassar College to grant the use . . . of the college plant . . . during the summer of 1918 as a training school for young women for patriotic service in whatever lines of work offer the greatest opportunities or present the greatest needs." [8]

The Vassar Trustees referred the resolution to a committee of three, of which Mrs. John Wood Blodgett was chairman, Frank R. Chambers and Frank L. Babbott, the other two members. The committee reported as follows:

"That it is the unanimous opinion of this committee that the fundamental need at the present moment for women is in the department of nursing; that the country is facing a serious shortage of professional trained women, which will become more acute as the war goes on; that if a skilled service is to be available for the care of the wounded abroad, as well as the sick at home, the necessary supply of trained nurses must be greatly increased. Our committee would therefore recommend that such buildings at Vassar as may later be designated be given over to a summer school for intensive theoretical training of hospital nurses, and limited to college graduates who shall be recruited from all the colleges

[8] *Announcement*, The Training Camp for Nurses at Vassar College (3rd ed.), 1918, p. 16

recognized by the A.C.A.[9] beginning with the graduates of 1918 and extending back ten years." [10]

The Trustees of the College approved the plan.

When apprised of the suggested summer course, the Committee on Nursing of the Council of National Defense passed the following resolution which was moved by Annie W. Goodrich and seconded by Lillian D. Wald:

"That this Committee considers the suggested offer of special preliminary summer courses at Vassar for women of college rank an important educational step both for the college and for the training schools for nurses and would gladly take up the matter and cooperate in endeavoring to work out a practicable plan of putting it into effect." [11]

The American Red Cross appropriated $75,000 from the Red Cross War Fund to finance the course. The cooperation of the National League of Nursing Education was sought and the League appointed a committee consisting of Isabel M. Stewart, Elizabeth C. Burgess, and Anne Strong to cooperate in organizing the curriculum. More than $13,000 in scholarships was contributed by organizations of Vassar College Alumnae, by Vassar Alumnae personally, or by the efforts of the Vassar Alumnae Recruiting Committee.

The Training Camp opened officially June 24, 1918 and at the convocation in Vassar Chapel, 435 women graduated from 110 colleges, assembled to begin an intensive program covering twelve weeks. Instruction was provided in those subjects usually taught in the nursing school during the first four to six months. The plan stipulated that a student who had satisfactorily completed the course should be given credit therefor and be permitted to graduate from the school of nursing she chose in two years and three months.

Thirty-four schools of nursing, approved by an Advisory Committee composed of nurses, were requested and agreed to join in

[9] Association of Collegiate Alumnae. In 1921 the A.C.A. combined with the Southern Association of College Women to form the American Association of University Women.

[10] *Announcement*, The Training Camp for Nurses at Vassar College, pp. 16–17

[11] *Ibid.*, p. 17

the plan. The list of these thirty-four was published in the *Announcement*. The *Announcement* also stated that four other schools "unable to reduce the required time of study, either because of the laws of their states or because of previous arrangements, are receiving students from The Training Camp. . . ." [12] The Johns Hopkins School was one of these four. However, upon the recommendation of Miss Lawler a time credit of three months was allowed to Alma J. Speer, 1921, and Agnes L. Barland (Mrs. E. B. McDaniel), 1921, two students from the Vassar Camp who chose Hopkins.

The Vassar Training Camp students were a mature group. They had had the benefits of a broad general education and were soundly prepared in the preclinical subjects. They doubtless brought into those schools they entered a social outlook and an appreciation of nursing as a broad human service. But the Vassar experiment was significant in other ways. True, it came out of the war and was born of an urge for patriotic service. Nevertheless, it symbolized an unmistakable trend toward recognition by colleges and universities of their responsibilities to nursing education and nursing.

The first suggestion that the Johns Hopkins Hospital School of Nursing should benefit by the educational opportunities of the Johns Hopkins University was found in the records of 1916. During the first two decades of its life, the Hopkins School was acknowledgedly a leader in this country and indeed throughout the world. With such a record and as a department in a Hospital closely related to a great University, it is hardly likely that the import of transferring the control of the School from the Hospital to the University escaped either Miss Hampton or Miss Nutting, both of whom played an important part in the establishment of courses in 1899 for graduate nurses at Teachers College, Columbia University. But during the last years of the nineteenth and the first years of the twentieth century, "nurse training" was still wrapped in its swaddling clothes and taking whatever steps it could in the traditional atmosphere of the hospital. One can only surmise that in the thinking of those best informed the time had not arrived for the Hopkins School to seek university recogni-

[12] *Ibid.*, p. 30

tion. Nevertheless, there are indications that the idea was latent in the Alumnae Association early in the history of the School; one would be hard put to it to say just when it was born. In 1916 it was expressed in a letter, soliciting contributions for an endowment for the School, sent by the Endowment Fund Committee to Alumnae Association members. Enlarging on the undeveloped areas of the School of Nursing, the committee wrote, ". . . Baltimore with its many interesting educational and social institutions, its well-developed public health work, and its great university . . . offers for study and training a rich field which would be of incalculable benefit to the students of our school of nursing." Beyond this pronouncement, the idea rested for another ten years.

With the increase in students, resulting from the expansion of the Hospital and the exigencies of war, the residential accommodations became less and less adequate. Indeed, before 1900 the School had outgrown the once spacious Nurses' Home and acquired temporarily an additional dormitory, known as the Nurses' Home Annex. This Annex was over the pharmacy and officers' dining room. In 1904 the third floor of Private Ward B was taken over for the growing number of students. When the east and west wings to the Nurses' Home were occupied in the fall of 1907, for the first time in eleven years, all students were living under one roof, and second- and third-year students enjoyed a single room.

This comfortable state of affairs did not endure. Early in 1913 the superintendent of nurses reported that "the Nurses' Home is uncomfortably crowded and it has been necessary to put two nurses in a room." Later in the year, when the private patients on Ward B were transferred to the new Marburg, the entire B building became available and provided temporary relief from the housing strain.

But the relief was brief. In 1916 two houses on Broadway were secured by the Hospital for the School and a third was rented the following year. The spreading of personnel in so many different buildings complicated the supervision of living quarters. This situation was somewhat bettered when 318 Broadway was acquired and the three other Broadway residences closed. By the early Twenties the housing question was again in the forefront, and the School was again looking for new living quarters.

The School had weathered the demands of an increased hospital census; it was still weathering the war when Baltimore was stricken with an ominous epidemic.

In 1918 the world was swept with influenza, "one of the great historic scourges of our time which . . . destroyed more human lives in a few months than did the European war in five years. . . ."[13] The "Spanish influenza," which took pandemic form, attacked all peoples, all races, all ages, and all classes—rich and poor alike. The drama of the epidemic was the swiftness with which it spread, the deadliness of its nature, and the toll it exacted, not of the young or old, but of the adolescent and the adult who had barely reached forty.

In the United States as early as March 1918, a comparatively mild form of influenza was reported at the Army Training Camps in the United States. In September, influenza-pneumonia appeared along the eastern seaboard, especially in the port of Boston. From Boston and other eastern ports it spread rapidly; within a month the entire country was engulfed.

Baltimore, a highly urbanized city of some 600,000 souls, was in the grip of the epidemic by early October. In a canvass of 34,000 persons in that city between November 20 and December 10, 1918, 7,900 cases were reported. Of these, 156 died.

For the year ending January 31, 1919, the Johns Hopkins Hospital recorded the treatment of 379 patients and fifteen deaths from "influenza epidemic." When the epidemic first exploded in Baltimore, the Hospital was well filled and, because of limited isolation facilities, unable to admit influenza patients. But soon the population within the Hospital itself felt the deadly impact of the disease and, with the exception of emergency surgical and urgent medical cases, all admissions were discontinued. Six wards were entirely filled with influenza patients, mostly nurses, medical

[13] Ministry of Health, *Report on the Pandemic of Influenza, 1918–1919* (Reports on Public Health and Medical Subjects, No. 4). London, His Majesty's Stationery Office, 1920, p. iv

students, medical staff, and other members of the Hospital family.

The number of patients and the number of personnel available to care for them varied from day to day. During the month of October, the number of ill student nurses averaged seventy-four daily or about one-third of the total student body; on November 1 there were still ninety off duty. When the epidemic broke there were no general staff nurses in the Hospital; students constituted the entire bedside nursing staff. The illness of so large a number reduced the nursing personnel to a point where help was acutely needed.

The graduates of the School who were married or for some other reason no longer engaged in nursing hurried back into the Hospital to give assistance wherever they were most needed. All classes were suspended in the School of Nursing and the School of Medicine for a time. Third- and fourth-year medical students assisted the medical staff with the care of patients, acted as orderlies, helped with the preparation of food, and made surgical supplies. A large class of preliminary students was admitted in the fall of 1918. Soon they were sent to the wards and took their posts beside the older nursing students.

Because of the desperately ill condition of many of the patients and the diminishing professional staff, the nurses and all who assisted them were confronted with an almost overwhelming task. But such is the human spirit that it rises above seemingly insurmountable obstacles, particularly in time of crisis. In May 1950, Dr. Arthur L. Bloomfield, resident physician at Hopkins during the epidemic, recalled that there were no such drugs as the "sulfas" in 1918 and that little could then be done medically for the influenza patients. "The important treatment was nursing," said Dr. Bloomfield, "and there was no deterioration in nursing—patients were kept clean, their mouths kept in good condition, and they received the proper nursing care." Of Dr. Bloomfield, Miss Lawler wrote, "So long as the School exists, we shall owe a debt of gratitude to Dr. Bloomfield for his splendid, untiring care of our sick nurses." To Miss Lawler and her faithful staff, a debt is also owed.

As the year 1918 drew to a close, so did the epidemic. There was some recurrence in February, but the disease had spent its force. In its trail it left heartbreaking events. Three of the medical staff and three medical students died. Six nurses died: two from the 1918 class, just graduated, and four students in the School, including a preliminary student. It can be truly said that each lost his life in service to humanity.

Excluding the illness caused by the influenza epidemic, the School does not appear to have suffered from an undue amount of serious sickness during the period from 1910 to 1920. Typhoid fever had not yet disappeared, although the number of students contracting this infection decreased after 1910. But the incidence of other acute infectious diseases reflected the fact that their control was still in the future. During this period the infection most prevalent was diphtheria. Fourteen pupils and two head nurses were off duty with diphtheria during an epidemic of that disease in the early months of 1911. After 1915, scarlet fever made its appearance more frequently and continued to do so throughout the next ten years.

Before 1912 the only illness record kept was the number of students *who reported off duty* with each of the then prevalent acute infections, tuberculosis, and appendicitis. After that date the total days lost through illness were recorded, but the types of illness represented in those data were not indicated. No mention was made of minor conditions such as colds and skin infections—it is likely that students having mild indispositions, more often than not, did not report off duty. In any event until the influenza struck, the loss of time was not excessive considering the size of the School, then ranging from 150 to more than 200 students. During the years between 1912 and 1918, the average number off duty daily was somewhat less than four nurses.

While student health programs—defined, planned, and implemented as such—were practically unheard of during this period, some positive health measures had been taken by the School. Vacations had been increased from three to four weeks for second-year students in 1907. In the 1909 Hospital report, it is stated that "the general health of nurses has been better for the past two years." The improvement is credited to the fact that each nurse had a single room and that special attention was given to diet.

As the School grew larger, the problem of medical attention

correspondingly grew. Among the responsibilities of the medical resident was that of caring for sick nurses. Because of his many duties in the Hospital, it was not always possible for the resident to respond promptly or to give the necessary time to the increasing health and medical needs of the School. Early in 1911, Miss Lawler requested that a physician be designated who would be in the Nurses' Home at a stated time each day. Within the year, the admitting officer was appointed as physician to the Nurses' Home.

Still there was much to be desired in the way of a health program. It was not until 1920 that first-year students, as well as second-year, were given a four-week vacation and that an illness allowance of one month was given during the three-year course. Previous to that date all time lost through illness had to be made up, a policy not conducive to reporting sickness.

Probably the most flagrant violation of the laws of health during that period was the work schedule. True, Hopkins had broken a path for the shorter day, when it introduced the eight-hour day and the ten-hour night, less than ten years after the School was organized. Then some years later, in 1920, night duty was further reduced to eight hours. These schedules still meant an official 54-hour week by day and a 56-hour week by night. The term "official" is advisedly used, because no record was kept of recurring overtime work for either day or night nurses. To the fifty-four or fifty-six hours of ward service were added from six to twelve hours of recitations, demonstrations, and lectures, bringing the total weekly scheduled hours up to sixty to sixty-eight hours. Sometime within their waking time and outside of on-duty and class hours, students were expected to write up their lectures and prepare for classes. The miracle is that they usually did, although nobody knows the effect on their health in after years of this heroic program.

Actually—it seems preposterous to state—Hopkins was still in the vanguard of schools having shorter hours. In 1920 there were twenty-five schools of nursing in Maryland having state approval. Ten of these schools reported weekly "hours on duty" from fifty-five to fifty-eight during the day. Seven others had day schedules varying from sixty to sixty-eight hours. Four schools reported a 70-hour, and one an 84-hour week at night.

The picture in Maryland was not dissimilar to the national picture.

Whether or not these hour schedules had any relation to the state's attitude on working hours for women is a matter of conjecture—probably not. Maryland did not enact labor-hour legislation for women until 1912; by that time the majority of states had laws regulating the length of women's working day. The Maryland statute provided for a ten-hour day and 60-hour week in manufacturing, mercantile, and certain other establishments; however, between 10 o'clock at night and 6 o'clock in the morning the hours were limited to eight. By January 1, 1950, one-half of the states had an eight-hour day and/or a 48-hour week for women; nine, a maximum nine-hour day and all but one of these a weekly maximum of fifty or fifty-four hours; another nine, a maximum day of ten hours and a week varying from fifty to sixty hours. The State of Maryland fell in the last classification; she had clung to her labor-hour law of 1912 for women. This brief reference to the legal working day of women in industries is not to imply that hours in schools of nursing should be regulated by law. A school of nursing is an educational institution and should function as such. One might properly presuppose, however, that the daily hour-schedule of student nurses would not exceed that of women in industry. The eight-hour night was legislated for women in certain establishments in the state in 1912; another eight years was to pass before it became operative at Hopkins. But the Johns Hopkins School of Nursing had introduced the eight-hour day for its students sixteen years before the legislators of Maryland awoke to their social responsibility of protecting the health of women in industry by labor-hour laws.

For the Johns Hopkins Hospital School of Nursing, the years between 1910 and 1920 were indeed years to remember. The School's spirit, courage, endurance, and will to do, were tried and found true, as it successively encountered hospital growth, war, and epidemic. Bright spots there were along the way, the comradeship and appreciation of one's fellowmen that spring from sharing deep human experiences. Another decade was being ushered in and with it a new kind of interest and inquiry into nursing education.

The School Looks at Itself:

Studies Are Made

To try to recapture the spirit of the Twenties is like peering into a valley where the haze is beginning to lift and the sun is breaking through. The carnage of war was over and the time was now for new effort, new action, and new hope. It was a time of revival of spirit in America.

Nursing shared in the awakening. The Twenties saw the publication of two significant studies: *Nursing and Nursing Education in the United States* [1] and the first of a series of extensive reports by the Committee on the Grading of Nursing Schools.[2] At the Johns Hopkins Hospital School of Nursing a "cherished hope" was rekindled: the hope of establishing a place for the School in the Johns Hopkins University. This aspiration must have been encouraged by Dr. Frank J. Goodnow, then president

[1] Committee for the Study of Nursing Education, *Nursing and Nursing Education in the United States*. New York, Macmillan Co., 1923

[2] The membership of the Committee on the Grading of Nursing Schools included representatives from the medical, nursing, public health, and hospital national associations; also members-at-large who were mostly educators. Elizabeth G. Fox, 1910, Gertrude E. Hodgman, 1916, and Dr. Winford H. Smith, then director of the Johns Hopkins Hospital, were members of the committee; Blanche Pfefferkorn, 1911, a consultant to the committee.

of the University. Speaking at the launching of the second campaign for an endowment of the School, Dr. Goodnow said:

"Nursing education must of necessity be preëminently practical, and this would rank nursing schools with vocational schools —but on no account should the fact that the education of nurses is practical rather than academic debar it from taking its place in the great universities. There is a place for it there.

"In recent years architecture, engineering, and other professions of which the basic principles are practical have taken their places in the universities. Nursing schools should and will have a similar place."

On the same occasion Dr. Henry M. Hurd also expressed the hope that the School of Nursing would have its place in the University.

Dr. Goodnow and Dr. Hurd made their statements in February 1921. At that time the study, *Nursing and Nursing Education in the United States*, was in progress. When the report of the study was published in 1923, it discussed the "unique" advantages of the university school of nursing; its value in furnishing "a body of leaders who have the fundamental training essential in administrators, teachers, and the like" [3] and thereby "gradually but steadily improve . . . the efficiency of every institution for the training of nurses of whatever type." [4] The committee sponsoring the study concluded, "that the development and strengthening of University Schools of Nursing of a high grade for the training of leaders is of fundamental importance in the furtherance of nursing education." [5]

When *Nursing and Nursing Education in the United States* was published, the Johns Hopkins Hospital School of Nursing actually and potentially possessed the basic essentials of a "high grade" university school. The Hospital of which it was a part was a teaching institution; the School was linked by name with a great university; the public health work in Baltimore offered fertile opportunities for the development of a public health field

[3] *Nursing and Nursing Education in the United States*, p. 26

[4] *Ibid.*, p. 26

[5] *Ibid.*, p. 26

where nurses could be trained. Moreover, the School had always attracted in considerable numbers students of good cultural and educational background, and from the beginning it had sent out leaders, not only to important posts in this country, but to Europe, Asia, India, and the furthermost corners of the globe.

The "Goldmark Report" acted as a catalyzer for some much needed reforms in nursing education. It exposed "un-school-like" practices and made clear-cut suggestions for their correction; it also stimulated affiliations with universities. The day seemed to have arrived for consideration of a university relationship for the Hopkins School of Nursing. Upon the recommendation of Elsie M. Lawler, then principal of the School, the Hospital Trustees invited Carolyn E. Gray, formerly dean of the Frances Payne Bolton School of Nursing, Western Reserve University and a participant in the Goldmark study, to survey the School and, at the same time, to explore the field in Baltimore for untapped resources in nursing education.

After six weeks of study in the late fall of 1924, Miss Gray submitted her report to the Training School Committee. Members of the committee present were Miss Lawler, Dorothy D. Filler (Mrs. E. H. McBride), 1920, Dr. Smith, Dr. Warfield T. Longcope, and Dr. J. Whitridge Williams. One part of the report dealt with plans for the revision of the curriculum.

Miss Gray proposed that the School offer two programs: a five-year program, which she outlined, and a three-year program. The five-year program provided for an affiliation with the Johns Hopkins University. It specified that the first two years be given to work in the University and the next two years to work in the Hospital. "Hospital work" refers to the portion of the program given in the School of Nursing dealing with the principles and practices of clinical nursing. During the fifth year provision was made for four months in the public health and four months in an elective field with courses given coordinately in the University; the public health program was to be developed cooperatively with the University School of Hygiene and Public Health. Upon the successful completion of the five-year program, a diploma in nursing would be granted by the Hospital and a bachelor of science degree by the University.

The second program covering three years was to be given entirely in the School of Nursing, including, however, four months of field experience in public health nursing. One of the Gray recommendations was that *all* students, those admitted to the three-year as well as those to the five-year program, should be qualified "to matriculate at [the] University and meet requirements for entrance." This recommendation accorded with the proposal that students enrolled in the three-year program should be eligible for work in the University leading to the degree.

The Training School Committee approved the five-year program, but withheld action on the recommendation that *all* students meet the matriculation requirements of the University. Both programs were submitted to the University. In November 1924, the University Advisory Committee on the Bachelor of Science Degree acted favorably on the five-year plan. With reference to the three-year program, the Advisory Committee voted to postpone action until a detailed plan was submitted.

Early in 1925 President Goodnow proposed a radical change in the educational policy of the University. The president's proposal, called the "Goodnow Plan," [6] included elimination of instruction "in most of the subjects now taught in the first years of college" and discontinuance in the future of granting the bachelor's degree. In view of these proposals, the University authorities agreed that no further action, for the present, be taken on affiliation with the School of Nursing.

The denial of university benefits was a bitter disappointment both to the School and to the Alumnae. Even though the recommendation for relationship with the University was laid on the table, for the time being at least, there were other recommendations, dealing with administrative policies, in the Gray report that urged immediate attention. The Hospital Trustees promptly appointed a new Training School Committee to consider the curriculum and reorganization of the School. This committee dealt solely with the School as a hospital school, but because it did act as a link in the chain of events leading to renewal of efforts for

[6] The "Goodnow Plan" never became wholly operative. Certain features of it were temporarily adopted, but instruction in subjects given during the first two years of college was continued.

recognition by the University, a brief account of its activities is indicated here.

The Alumnae Association from the time of its founding was keenly interested in the progress of the School. This interest was sharpened into a more positive form with the appointment of the Endowment Fund Committee. In the work of that committee the Association was using its substance and its energies to create an endowment for the School; it considered keeping abreast with developments in the School one of its important functions.

In 1925 an event occurred that spurred the Endowment Fund Committee into action—the launching of the Half-Century Campaign by the Trustees of the University and of the Hospital on the fiftieth anniversary of the University. The campaign program included two items for the School of Nursing as a department of the Hospital—one of these items was a general endowment of $500,000.[7] The Half-Century Committee through its chairman, Daniel Willard, invited the cooperation of the Alumnae Association. Before accepting the invitation the Endowment Fund Committee desired to know how the endowment would be used for the School. It was agreed to ask the Hospital Trustees through the Nurses Guild, a subdivision of the Half-Century Campaign organization, to enlarge the new Training School Committee; it was also agreed to suggest names to the Trustees for additional personnel. The personnel suggested were: Mrs. John S. Gibbs, Jr., representing the public; Dr. William H. Welch (and later Elizabeth G. Fox), representing the field of public health; M. Adelaide Nutting, Anna D. Wolf, and Carolyn E. Gray, the field of nursing education; and Amy P. Miller, 1900, representing the Alumnae Association.

As originally appointed by the Trustees the new Training School Committee consisted of three members of the Medical Board—Dr. J. Whitridge Williams, Dr. Warfield T. Longcope, and Dr. John Howland; three members of the School staff—Elsie M. Lawler, Mrs. Dorothy Filler McBride, and Loula E. Kennedy, 1903; and the director of the Hospital, Dr. Winford H. Smith. The Trustees granted the request of the Endowment Fund Com-

[7] See "The Work of the Endowment Fund Committee," pp. 347–9.

mittee and added the suggested personnel to the new School Committee. Because of Miss Nutting's absence in Europe, Isabel M. Stewart, professor of nursing education, Teachers College, Columbia University, served in her place.

At the first meeting of the enlarged Training School Committee in January 1926, a small committee was appointed "to study the question of a program" for the School. The small committee, consisting of Miss Lawler, Miss Wolf, Miss Miller, Dr. Welch, and Dr. Smith, met in February and drafted a program for the reorganization of the School, which was presented to the parent committee the following month. With some editorial revision, the Training School Committee accepted the proposed program and voted to recommend the report to the consideration of the Medical Board of the Hospital for approval and recommendation to the Board of Trustees of the Johns Hopkins Hospital.

A key recommendation of the program was the appointment of a director of the School of Nursing, an official separate and distinct in function from the superintendent of nurses. The Medical Board was not in sympathy with this proposal and recommended instead the appointment of an educational director. The Board of Trustees agreed to the change.

But the Alumnae Association was unwilling to let the matter rest there. In May 1926 it appointed a committee, with Effie J. Taylor as the able chairman, known as the Special Committee of the Alumnae Association.[8] The Special Committee requested that it be permitted to present directly the case of the School before the Board of Trustees. The request was granted and on January 27, 1928, the committee submitted to the Trustees a scholarly and exhaustive report of a twelve-month study. In its conception and execution, in its exposition of fundamental nursing education principles and practices, this report stands as a monument to the Special Committee. It dealt with those factors vitally important in the development of the School program. It considered the operation of the School in relation to the operation of the nursing service at the Johns Hopkins Hospital, and the effect the operation of one had upon the operation of the other. It looked to the future of the School of Nursing as a unit related to the Hospital,

[8] For personnel of committee, see, "The Work of the Endowment Fund Committee," p. 352.

to the School of Medicine, and to the Johns Hopkins University. Finally, the report stated unequivocally:

"To see our school a part of the Johns Hopkins University has been the ambition and hope of its alumnae. The efforts of the graduates were bent towards this end in planning to raise an endowment which would place the school on a sound financial status and enable it to make the connection. . . ."

The report ended with the recommendations:

"That the Johns Hopkins University be again asked to consider the possibility of an affiliation with the Johns Hopkins Hospital School of Nursing on the closest terms the policies of its organization will permit.

"That a committee be appointed immediately to discuss with the university a means of establishing a connection between the school of nursing and the university."

The report was received by the Board of Trustees with sympathetic interest and consideration. But medical opinion in the Hospital did not favor recognition by the University and the Hospital administration held reservations. The study of the Special Committee did not then secure, as the committee had hoped, affiliation for the School with the Johns Hopkins University. Affiliation was delayed for another seven years.

Although the report of the Alumnae Special Committee did not achieve university association for the School, it did lead to other important action. In April the Trustees appointed a Special Training School Committee to consider the curriculum of the School. On this new committee were Dr. Joseph S. Ames, president of the Johns Hopkins University, and Blanchard Randall, a University Trustee; John M. Glenn, Dr. H. Barton Jacobs, Judge Henry D. Harlan, Trustees of the Hospital; Drs. Edwards A. Park and Warfield T. Longcope of the Medical Board; Dr. William H. Welch, director of the School of Hygiene and Public Health; Dr. Winford H. Smith, director of the Hospital; Effie J. Taylor, Anna D. Wolf, and Florence M. Patterson, 1907, representing the Alumnae Association; and Elsie M. Lawler and Loula E. Kennedy, representing the School.

The newly constituted committee met in May. A subcommittee was appointed to consider the desirable education for nurses, with the understanding that the program of the School should be based on the decision of the committee. Dr. Ames, Dr. Park, Dr. Welch, Miss Taylor, and Miss Patterson were appointed to the subcommittee with Dr. Ames as chairman.

When the subcommittee met a few months later it "resolved that the first step to be taken is to establish an Advisory Board for the supervision of the Training School for Nurses . . ." and proceeded to draw up recommendations as to the Board's functions, composition, and organization. The recommendation for such an Advisory Board was duly approved and on October 7, 1930, the Board of Trustees adopted a resolution creating an Advisory Board of the School of Nursing. The resolution took the form of an additional rule to be incorporated in the *Rules and Regulations* of the Hospital. The full text of the rule is printed in the November 1930 issue of the *Johns Hopkins Nurses Alumnae Magazine*. The first two paragraphs, defining the functions and membership of the new Board, are here given.

1. There shall be an Advisory Board of the Training School for Nurses which shall meet regularly once a month during the academic year. The duty of the Advisory Board shall be to advise the Trustees of the Hospital upon all matters relating to the welfare of the Training School for Nurses. Without being confined thereto their recommendations should concern the following subjects:
   a. The purpose, scope, and form of organization of the School of Nursing.
   b. The curriculum.
   c. Appointments to the Teaching Staff.
   d. Award of diplomas.
2. The Advisory Board shall consist of eleven members as follows:
   a. Two members of the Medical Board of the Hospital and one member of the Advisory Board of the School of Hygiene and Public Health.
   b. The Director of the Johns Hopkins Hospital, the Director of the School of Nursing, and the President of the Johns Hopkins University, ex officio, and a member of the Staff of the School of Nursing.
   c. Two members at large who are interested in the School of Nursing.
   d. Two alumnae of the School of Nursing to be elected by the Alumnae Association.

While forces without the School were helping to shape its future, what was taking place within the School itself? In the School and in the Hospital, events were occurring that added to the problem of educational administration and also to that of nursing service.

The Hospital authorities in association with the authorities of the University adopted an expansion program, presented to the Hospital Trustees by Dr. Winford H. Smith in his report for the year ending January 31, 1920, "designed to round out the Hospital as an effective instrument of medical education and of medical care." The program included the erection of the Woman's Clinic for gynecologic and obstetric patients, completed in 1923; the Wilmer Ophthalmological Institute, completed in 1928; and the Carnegie Dispensary Building, in 1927. The completion of the first two structures brought the daily average number of inpatients from 453 in 1920 [9] to 602 in 1929; [10] during the same periods the opening of the new Dispensary raised the annual outpatient visits from 143,000 to 230,000.

The School of Nursing adopted the following policies in 1920. An allowance was granted of one month of illness during the three-year course. This allowance represented a fair approximation of the average illness time lost per student at that period. The vacation time was extended from seven to eight weeks. Students at the end of their first year, as well as those at the end of their second, were now to have a four-week vacation. About the same time the ten-hour night was changed to an eight-hour night and the seventy-hour week at night to a week of fifty-six hours. The adoption of these policies necessarily reduced the number of students available for nursing service in the Hospital.

The longer vacations, the illness time allowance, and the shorter night schedule unquestionably represent right procedure in an educational institution. The time must have seemed propitious for these innovations since the largest classes in the history of the School had been admitted during the previous two years. But the Hospital had also grown and continued to grow. To maintain

[9] For year ending January 21, 1921.

[10] For year ending June 30, 1930.

good standards of nursing service and a good field for educational practice presented a difficult problem to the nursing administration without additional graduates. Reading the School reports of this period, one is aware of the pressure exerted on the School to supply nursing service, not only because more patients were in the Hospital, but also because of the accelerated activity in practically every department, the complexity of new medical treatments, and the demands upon the nursing personnel by the School of Medicine. Moreover, in the Twenties a new method of equating nursing service needs and nursing personnel was developed which tended to alert both hospital and nursing administrators to nursing shortage. The old measuring rod, nurse-patient ratio, gradually began to be superseded by a more reliable and comparable index, nursing hours per patient. Miss Lawler noted in one of her reports during this time, "The question of how many hours of nursing care are required by each patient is receiving much attention now, but it is practically dependent on the number of nurses in the School." For the idea still generally prevailed that students provided the natural and *most desirable* nursing service personnel for the hospital. The persistence of this idea seems to have been partly grounded in tradition, partly in hospital economics, and strange as it may seem now, looking back over quarter of a century, partly in the preference of many nursing administrators for the student rather than the graduate staff nurse. In a study of data submitted by five hundred superintendents of nurses, 76 per cent preferred student nurses to take care of their patients.[11] The work of the Committee on the Grading of Nursing Schools, begun in 1925, started a new way of thinking on a subject that had hitherto escaped the logic of a formidable array of facts.

With a School grown to 250 students providing the major portion of the bedside nursing, vacations became increasingly difficult to arrange. In 1924 when it was necessary to have forty to fifty nurses absent almost the entire summer in order to complete vacations by the time the school term began, Miss Lawler wrote, "If the Hospital is as busy as it was last summer, I do not see how we can care for the patients without additional help," and

[11] May Ayres Burgess, *Nurses, Patients, and Pocketbooks*, New York, Committee on the Grading of Nursing Schools, 1928, p. 391

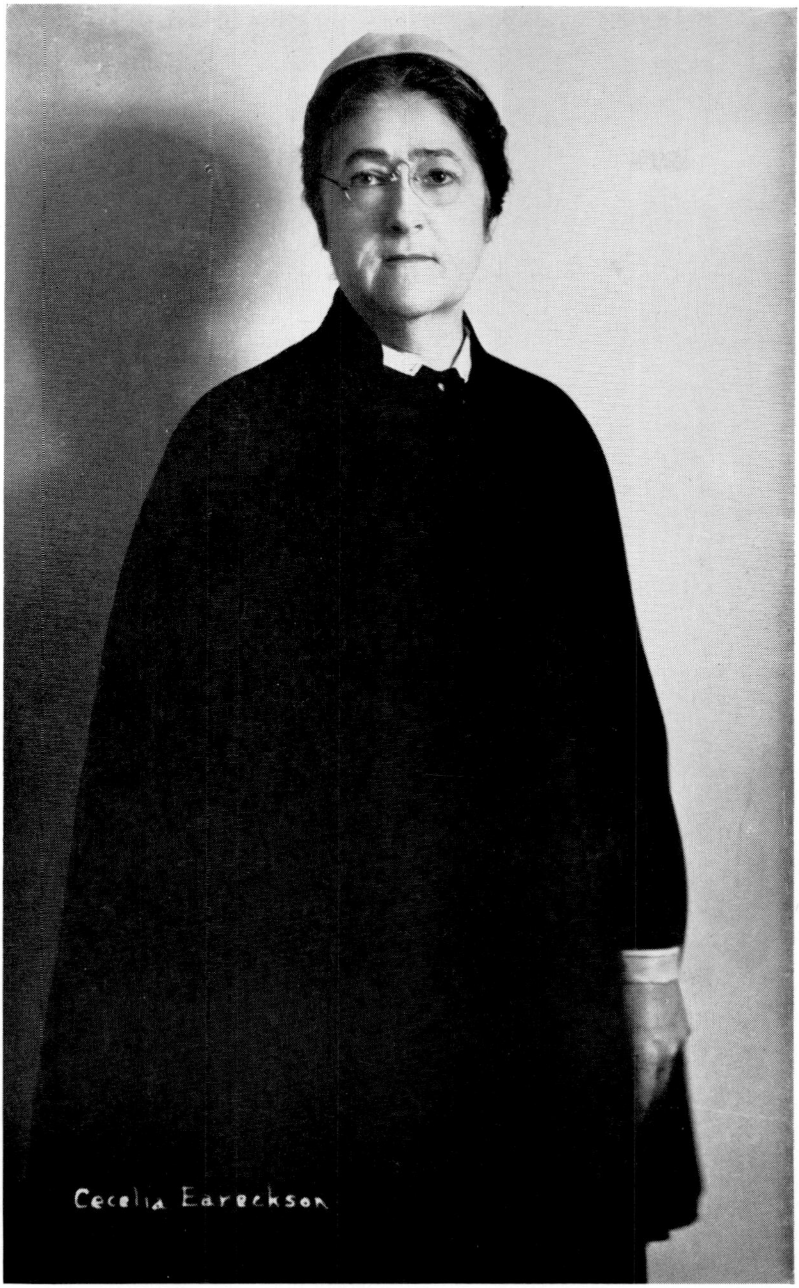

ELSIE M. LAWLER
Superintendent of Nurses and Principal of the Training School, 1910–1940

CECELIA EARECKSON

then she asked, "If the necessity arises, might we consider employing graduate nurses?" Sometime later the employment of graduate nurses must have been authorized. In the annual report of 1927, the temporary appointment of twelve graduate nurses is noted, and the next year it is recorded that thirty-one graduates were temporarily appointed for "vacation and sickness relief." Otherwise the graduate staff grew slowly and it was not until the Thirties that this group began to appreciably increase.

In 1920 the School had two full-time instructors: Amy P. Miller, director of theoretical instruction, and Hester K. Frederick, director of practical instruction. Miss Frederick resigned in 1927 to return later as assistant to Miss Lawler. Miss Miller's resignation in 1921 ended her official connection with the School.

Miss Miller had had varied experience in the public health nursing and teaching fields as well as special work at Columbia University, Harvard Medical School, and Johns Hopkins School of Medicine before she was appointed to the position of instructor at Hopkins. She began her work there when the instructor in schools of nursing was still expected to teach a wide variety of subject matter courses. Miss Miller, herself, taught a considerable number, including both nursing and biological science subjects.

Miss Miller is described by those who knew her as tall, slender, aristocratic and immaculate in appearance; as having a keen sense of humor, great human understanding, a quiet strength and serenity. She must have had unusual teaching endowment which, combined with her fine personal qualities and her efforts to add to her skills and knowledge, made her a rare teacher. Held in universal respect and affection, a quotation from a letter of a colleague soon after her death portrays Miss Miller as a teacher and a friend. Wrote this colleague, "I learned so much that was fine in the expression of her own life and in her teaching of students. The impression she made upon all of us was indelible and . . . I am sure she lives on in hundreds of students whom she taught. . . ."

Loula E. Kennedy, who succeeded Miss Miller in 1921, was to continue as teacher and counselor for the next twenty-five years. Her reports of the Department of Instruction, also referred to as the Teaching Department, are concise and specific and historically valuable in viewing the School program during that period.

Miss Kennedy analyzed course by course for subject content, for appropriateness of placement in relation to other courses, both classroom and practice, and to the program as a whole. "In the preliminary course," suggested Miss Kennedy in her report for 1923–1924, "take out *Diet in Disease* and discuss principally diet in health. Diet in disease may be given in the Junior year as soon as the student begins to take responsibility on the wards in the serving of meals, and after the courses in General Medicine and Surgery have been given. . . ." Then she asked, "What arrangements can we make to put chemistry into the Curriculum?" A course in chemistry was promptly introduced—"an excellent straight lecture course with demonstrations," covering twenty hours. Ten hours of laboratory work were soon added, and by 1928 Miss Kennedy could report a 45-hour course in that subject, "as recommended by the Curriculum of the National League of Nursing Education." About that time provision was also made for laboratory in bacteriology. Other courses introduced during the Twenties were a 15-hour course in communicable diseases, described as "a much needed course in the third year . . ."; courses in body mechanics and studies in personal adjustment for the preliminary students; one month of experience in the Social Service Department, and, with the establishment of the Wilmer Institute, nursing of patients with diseases of the eye.

The Department of Instruction was not unmindful of the health of the students. A course in physical education was proposed for the preliminary group. "This," the record reads, "would be a part only of a *definite health program* which it is most desirable to initiate . . . ," and then the report goes on to say that the program should include yearly physical examinations as well as the examination given on admission. The appointment of student advisors from the faculty was also proposed. This proposal was promptly put into effect, but from subsequent reports it appears that the advisory program was only "fairly successful," and its life was short. About the same time a "student council" was organized. The life of the council, too, was brief; by the middle Thirties it had ceased to exist. To understand these abortive efforts one must review the discipline system of the School from the time of its beginning.

Among the Nightingaliana in the historical collection of the Johns Hopkins Hospital School of Nursing is a letter from Florence Nightingale dated October 30, 1861. In this letter Miss Nightingale states tersely her belief in the absolute power of the "Matron":

"I do not see however how it would be possible, with *any Matron* whatever, not to vest 'the power of instant dismissal' with her alone. If the Nurse can appeal to anyone else, there is an end of all discipline. It is a power I have contended for always for *all* Hospital Matrons—& given it to the Military Supt. of Nurses."

Miss Nightingale's statement epitomizes the authoritarian principle which survived for many years in American schools of nursing, including the School of the Johns Hopkins Hospital. Isabel Hampton, a graduate of Bellevue, must have been reared in an atmosphere of military discipline; Lavinia L. Dock, her first assistant, stated on various occasions her categorical belief in the system. As a member of the first class Adelaide Nutting was trained in the military tradition; she regarded it as essential to the efficient conduct of the nursing service and the effective operation of the School. In 1910 Elsie M. Lawler, graduated from Hopkins in 1899, was appointed principal and continued in that office for the next thirty years. Miss Lawler, too, was the product and exponent of the rule of authority.

What were some of the evidences of military discipline at the Hopkins Training School for Nurses? How did it manifest itself in the daily life of pupils?

Essential to the system was recognition of rank. The head of the School held the highest rank, next came the assistants, then head nurses. Rank extended down through the pupils. Senior pupils were of a higher rank than intermediate, and intermediate pupils higher than junior. Lowest in the ladder were probationers. Rank established the head of the School as the sole source of authority; it also provided the means for transmitting authority and fixing responsibility in a straight line from the source.

Inherent in the recognition of rank was a well-defined pattern of behavior. One always stood in the presence of persons of superior rank; one had no social and personal relations with individuals of either higher or lower rank. Seniors were not permitted to mingle socially with intermediates, nor intermediates with juniors, upon the premise that familiarity jeopardized the acceptance of authority. Obedience to authority, unquestioning obedience, was the order of the day.

Evidence of the system was apparent in other ways. Pupils were described as "faithful, obedient, and industrious"; it was recorded that two pupils withdrew from the School "without permission," and a notation found on another student record reads "ward etiquette poor." A common form of censure was "suspension." Pupils were suspended for "misconduct," for "carelessness"—carelessness in general or carelessness resulting in a mistake in the performance of a procedure in the wards. No record was found of how the pupils spent their time during a suspended period and little of the effect of suspension upon their work or behavior.

These few illustrations are indicative of the form imposed by the system; the substance could go deeper. The early pupils seem to have accepted the form as a necessary part of training and escaped the blight of the substance upon their spirits and minds. They had been brought up to accept the authority of home, school, and church and to abide by recognized social mores; they were prepared to accept the authority of the training school. An occasional individual might privately chafe under the regulations, but overt rebellion was rare.

As the twentieth century advanced an awareness dawned at the Johns Hopkins School that external authoritarian rule was contrary to democratic principles and inimical to democratic development, individual and group. Many of the students entering Hopkins during the Twenties were college women. They had lived in a societal group where the individual was expected to exercise independent judgment and to have a moral sense of responsibility; they recognized the dangers inherent in a system of concentrated authority and its withering effects upon personal growth. One J.H.H. graduate of the Twenties has thus described her reaction to the prevalent discipline: "What I felt was a barrier which obstructed the exchange of ideas and participation in thinking."

With this backward view it is understandable why neither the student advisor nor the student council movement took root in the Twenties. The scene was not yet properly set. Another fifteen years had to pass before a counseling program, encouraging independent judgment and self-direction of students, could be introduced.

All through the Twenties two notes could be heard. One sounded the need for more clinical instruction by qualified personnel in order to realize the educational opportunities in the broadening experience. Wrote Miss Lawler in 1927:

"Since so much of the head nurse's time must be given to administration and the work of the Medical School, one of our greatest needs at this time is additional instructors who might be called teaching supervisors—nurses who could give their entire time to supervising the work of the pupil over her patients."

One of the recommendations of the Gray survey was that assistants to head nurses be appointed "in order to relieve them of some administrative duties, and make it possible for them to *teach* student nurses." Two years later the study by the subcommittee of the Training School Committee again stressed the need for more clinical instructors. In another two years the Alumnae Special Committee submitted its findings on the program of the School. Included in that committee's report were the following comments:

"That the students have not an equal opportunity to profit by the ward experience.

"That there is no apparent plan for correlating the theory and practice.

"That the resources within the Hospital are not adequately made use of for the instruction of the student nurses."

From 1925 on the annual reports of the Department of Instruction show a growing concern for the ward teaching program. Loula E. Kennedy, who prepared these reports, urgently declared in her 1925–1926 summary that applied instruction in the wards "needs to be emphasized and definite plans made to connect the classroom teaching with the care of the patient more than has been possible in the past." While clinics for student nurses had long been held in the psychiatric department, it was not until the middle Twenties that the ward teaching program included weekly clinics of one-half hour for students assigned to the medical wards. One year later it was possible to report, "Great progress has been made this year in the development of systematic 'ward rounds' [clinics] in practically all departments." The school year 1926–1927 also saw the introduction of case studies in the teaching of medical and pediatric nursing. In another year the case study method was "being applied in nearly all the departments," and seminars for seniors were begun.

Another recommendation in the Gray survey was the discontinuance of the "specialization method of student assignment" and the substitution of the case method. In the specialization or functional method, assignments are made according to activities—one nurse takes the temperatures of all patients, another gives all medicines, and so on; in the case method, each nurse is responsible for the total nursing of the patients assigned to her care. In Phipps, the psychiatric clinic, the case method system had been in effect from the time the department was opened in 1913. During the late Twenties it was introduced in Ward F, the men's medical unit. But the pressure of nursing service together with the persisting belief that more work could be accomplished with the functional method discouraged the use of the case assignment method and delayed its application throughout the Hospital for almost twenty years. It was tried out at intervals in other wards as well as F, only to fall into disuse under the weight of nursing service.

The second note in the Twenties, lack of classrooms, resounded from the early days of the School. In 1903 Miss Nutting, in no uncertain manner, stated the need of more classrooms. Ten years later the same complaint was voiced by another principal of the School: ". . . we are still without an adequate classroom. The one in the Home is entirely too small, and though it would seem with the number of lecture rooms in the Hospital now that we ought to have no difficulty, yet each lecture room seems to be in almost constant demand." Then within another ten years the cry was again heard. Wrote Miss Lawler in her annual report of 1922, "The question of classroom accommodation has been more complicated than ever, and it is only by the most careful planning that we are able to fit in our work so we may occupy the classrooms when not in use by the Medical School. . . ." Herein lay the keynote of the problem; the same classrooms were used by the School of Medicine and by the School of Nursing. Good economy predicates that such physical facilities shall not be duplicated, but the practice ceases to be economical when the same classrooms are used for different groups with conflicting class schedules. Then one group inevitably has difficulty in locating classroom space. Over many years this was the predicament of the School of Nursing, especially as its curriculum expanded during the Twenties.

One of the original motives of the Alumnae Association in seeking to raise a school endowment was to provide funds for a properly equipped teaching building. Then in 1920 when the Hospital expansion program was adopted, an item of $250,000 for a "Teaching Building for the School of Nursing" was listed as one of the "needs." With reference to this item, Dr. Winford H. Smith, director of the Hospital, said in his 1922 report, "She [Miss Lawler] also stresses the difficulties due to lack of classroom facilities which is a matter of such importance to warrant the hastening of that part of the expansion program dealing with that matter as soon as possible." It was not until November 1927, however, that the School had a centralized teaching department—not a new building, but one which served it well for almost a quarter of a century.

Soon after the Carnegie Dispensary was completed, the General Operating Rooms were moved to that building. This transfer released the entire fourth floor of the old Surgical Building. It is related that the Medical Department wanted the space for teaching, but that Dr. Smith also had designs on the vacated floor. Dr. Smith thought the Nursing Department in more urgent need of the teaching facilities than the Medical. At any rate the Trustees decided in favor of the Nursing School and the much loved old "General" was remodeled into a teaching center for the School of Nursing. When the alterations were completed, the floor provided two classrooms, a model ward with accessory rooms, "a diminutive Marburg [private] room," a pharmacy laboratory, a library with open book shelves, and instructors' offices. The amphitheatre was used for lectures and demonstrations to large groups. Nor was the new teaching unit a place merely to hold classes. Prideful care went into making it inviting and attractive. Portraits and pictures were hung on the wall, and plants at the windows gave a bit of outdoors. Now, at last the School had space and a place of its own. In the remodeled old "General" it conducted a large part of its teaching activities until the building was razed twenty-three years later.

While many difficulties disappeared with the new School center, not all of the classes could be held there. The School of Medicine had shared with the School of Nursing the use of its laboratories for instruction in anatomy, bacteriology, and chemistry.[12] The School continued to use these facilities and also lecture rooms in the Hospital for advanced classes.

Another memorable occasion of this period was the opening of Hampton House in 1926. The expansion program, previously referred to, provided an increase in the Hospital capacity of more than three hundred beds. The General Education Board in 1921 granted $3,000,000 toward the financing of the proposed expansion. At that time enlargement of the living quarters of the School was again a pressing need, and the projected increase in the Hospital facilities made additional accommodations urgent. Out of the moneys given by the General Education Board, Hampton House was built and equipped at a cost of $750,000.

Pride in its institutions is a characteristic of the City of Baltimore. On June 28, 1924, the *Sun* of Baltimore announced that a new nurses' home was planned by Hopkins and that plans for it were being prepared by Joseph Evans Sperry, architect. The new eight-story residence, facing the Hospital, was erected on property purchased on the west side of Broadway. The front of the building, on either side of the doorway, is enclosed by iron railings in keeping with instructions of Johns Hopkins in a letter,

[12] The new educational unit, located in the Main Residence and opened in 1950, includes a laboratory for anatomy and microbiology and also one for chemistry.

dated March 10, 1873, to his Trustees. "I wish," wrote Mr. Hopkins, "the large grounds surrounding the hospital buildings to be properly enclosed by iron railings. . . ." The railings enclosing Hampton House are similar in design to those surrounding the Hospital and serve as a symbol of a trust carried out a half century after the trust was bestowed.

Hampton House is built of tapestried brick with stone trim. The beauty of the exterior of the building is its simplicity, dignity, and excellent proportions. Within, the appointments match the charm of the exterior. Mrs. George Weems Williams, onetime professional decorator and wife of one of the Trustees, selected and arranged the furnishings and directed the interior decorations.

To describe minutely the new residence would cover a disproportionate amount of space in this volume. To Alumnae who have not visited Hampton House and to others who may be interested, the article by Patience Carr, 1927, in the November 1926 issue of the *Johns Hopkins Nurses Alumnae Magazine* is commended. Miss Carr, who has an eye for detail and the gift of describing happily what she sees, has left a delightful account of the new Hampton House. But let it be said here that in the original building all bedrooms were designed as single rooms; during World War II it was necessary to house temporarily two students in one room. Hot and cold water is in every room and furnishings combine attractiveness with functional comfort. A lounge and small parlors are on the first floor; a sitting room on each of the upper floors. The House also provides kitchens, laundries, a court for outdoor games and play, and a gymnasium; a roof with recreation rooms for social occasions; sun decks for gathering to review the affairs of school life, or just for relaxing and taking an idle hour in the life-giving sun.

Fittingly the new residence was named Hampton House, thus associating the beloved first principal, Isabel Hampton, with the School for all time. Her portrait, painted by Sergeant Kendall, was moved from the old Home to the new Home and hung facing the entrance to the spacious lounge on the first floor. There she stands, smiling, beautiful, and serene, that all who pass through the portals of Hampton House may know her.

When the School was organized a monthly allowance was made to students, a practice common in the better nursing schools of that day. But Isabel Hampton had wanted to abolish the allowance and to use the money instead for educational purposes. In 1896 allowances were discontinued. Then in 1902, the School announced in the *Circular* a "caution money" charge of $10 to cover the cost of "possible breakage and damage to hospital appliances," and the following year an entrance fee of $50 was begun for instruction during the preparatory period. The aptly descriptive term, "caution money," derives from the Johns Hopkins University practice of requiring "a fifty-dollar caution money deposit" from a candidate for a higher degree to insure his fulfillment of publication regulations for dissertations. In 1921 the School abolished the caution money deposit, and raised to $100 the instructional fee.

About this time, too, a change was made in the age requirement for admission. Since 1903–1904 the *Circular* of the School had stated, "Applicants must not be under twenty-two years of age. . . ." In the 1922 *Circular* this statement was revised to read, "Applicants must not be under twenty years of age. . . ."

At the close of 1922, the School lost Effie Jane Taylor, then associate principal. Although Miss Taylor continued to serve the School in other ways, her departure at that time ended her official connection with the School of Nursing.

Effie J. Taylor entered the Johns Hopkins Hospital School of Nursing in the spring of 1904. Her correspondence for admission shows that she clearly foresaw the importance to her future in selecting a good school and the social and spiritual values which a nursing career offered. In her letter of application she wrote:

"I am very desirous of taking the training and for several reasons. In the first place because I believe that with such a training I shall become a more useful and capable woman and will be better fitted to occupy the position and to do the work in life for which I was intended. I do not know of any training which if taken with the right motive will so broaden or develop a girl's character . . . I wish to become the very best nurse that I have the ability to become and will not try to get into an inferior school. . . ."

Miss Taylor was born in Hamilton, Ontario, Canada. She was graduated from the Hamilton Collegiate Institute which qualified her to enter a university. Her formal education did not end with her graduation from the Institute; she received a diploma in English, elocution, and physical culture from the Wesleyan Ladies' College and also from time to time took university extension courses. Wrote the principal of Hamilton Collegiate Institute in certifying Miss Taylor's educational qualifications for entering the School, ". . . and [she] possesses at the present time an education far in advance of the average young lady."

At Hopkins Miss Taylor must have continued her good scholastic record for she received two scholarships, one in her junior and one in her intermediate year. Her official connection with the School, as a graduate, began in 1907 and continued in various capacities for the next fifteen years. During that period she was granted one leave of absence for study at Teachers College, New York, and another to organize the Army School of Nursing at Camp Meade, Maryland, during World War I.

As the first nursing head of the Henry Phipps Psychiatric Clinic, Miss Taylor organized the nursing service in the new department. She held that position until 1920 when the office of associate superintendent of nurses was created, with Miss Taylor as its first incumbent. Probably her most signal contribution to the Johns Hopkins Hospital was her work in Phipps Clinic.

Effie J. Taylor knew good nursing and was a good nurse herself. She had an unflagging zest for work, combined with educational vision; she was always willing to compromise, but never to sacrifice principle. Endowed with a warm personality and a broadly humane spirit, Miss Taylor was ever ready to help the young head nurse and the uncertain student. She gave unsparingly of herself during difficult and critical years. After she left the School, Miss Taylor had many honors, but perhaps none which she treasured more than the esteem and the affection in which she was held by those who had been associated with her at Hopkins, both graduates and students.

How much of the new hope and the new effort of the third decade of this century was translated into reality at the Johns Hopkins School of Nursing? Some new bright paths were broken, but not all of the trails explored led to the hills of promise. Three considered studies were made and out of these studies came the Advisory Board of the School of Nursing. The curriculum was broadened, both in the classroom and practice areas, and a beginning was made in a clinical instructional program. And the School could now rejoice in a new, much-needed teaching center and a fine new residence.

The hoped-for relationship with the Johns Hopkins University did not materialize. This was indeed a disappointment. The Johns Hopkins Hospital School of Nursing had from its beginning been a leader; other schools were to forge the university movement in the history of nursing education.

Mileposts and the End of Three Decades of Service

In the United States and in the world at large, the years between 1930 and 1940 were turbulent years. The high tide of hope that pervaded the Twenties for better things to come, faded out toward the end of the decade in a rising wave of gloom and apprehension. In October 1929 the stock market crashed, and Americans soon sensed that hard times were ahead. As the year 1929 made its exit and 1930 came upon the scene, the great depression was on. On corner after corner stood the apple salesman, a depressing symbol of rising unemployment.

By 1932 there were in the United States eight million unemployed men and women, and many of those who were employed already had had or were facing wage cuts. Out of this bleak situation emerged the five-day week, a share-the-work movement in business and industry to cut down unemployment. In spite of governmental and private efforts to provide relief and to restore a balanced national economy, businesses continued to collapse and banks continued to fail. In the first days of March 1933 came the bank crisis, and on March 5 the Government ordered a four-day nation-wide bank holiday—a festive name for a grim event. Still, a new president had been inaugurated, and hope surged through the country. But despite the New Deal, recovery was wavering and slow. Frank R. Kent wrote in the *Sun* of Baltimore on January 2, 1940:

"While it is true that in 1939 there has been a considerable business expansion, more employment, more goods produced, and large profits made, no informed person holds that a real recovery has been made. The fact remains that we are still in the great American Depression which began ten years ago in the fall of 1929."

Hospitals and nurses, with other groups, felt the grip of the depression. In families impoverished by the loss of savings, as well as the loss of regular income, the incidence of illness took an upward trend. The average patient census in hospitals in 1940 exceeded the average census in 1930 by 265,000. Although the largest proportion of the increase occurred in publicly supported institutions, the census in voluntary hospitals had also risen. In the meantime the income of voluntary hospitals had fallen off distressingly, partly because of decline of income from patients and partly because of decline of gifts and contributions. It was inevitable that public hospitals, too, should feel the pinch of the economic disaster. Said President Glenn Frank of the University of Wisconsin, addressing the American Hospital Association in September 1933, "We have had a bank holiday, but no hospital holiday" and then went on to say that hospitals had weathered the depression with financial deficits but they had no service deficits.

Before 1930 the profession of nursing had become increasingly aware of overproduction in its ranks. The unemployment tragedy which hundreds of nurses suffered during the early Thirties cannot be attributed primarily to the depression, although it undoubtedly precipitated and exaggerated the crisis. Private duty nurses soon found themselves unemployed in appallingly large numbers; the demand for their services depended upon a group of patients whose ability to pay shrunk greatly during the lean depression period. Many nurses were dropped in the public health and industrial fields. In institutions the opportunities to absorb unemployed nurses were extremely limited; in some hospitals four hours of service were exchanged for meals.

The measures adopted to relieve the unemployment pall in nursing were similar to those adopted in industry and business. Salaries were cut in hospitals and public health agencies. The depression years saw the eight-hour day for private nurses with the accompanying decrease in fees gradually take hold—a share-the-work movement for the nurses, and for the patients, three nurses in twenty-fours hours at approximately the same rate as two. In 1930 a comparatively small number of hospitals operating nursing schools made use of general staff nurses. The bitter days of the early Thirties brought home to hospitals and to others concerned the inequities of a system which produced large numbers of graduates and provided employment for relatively few; they also changed the attitude of many nurses who, before the depression, were unwilling to accept the position of general staff nurse.

Such was the economic status of this country in 1930, and with short periods of abatement it continued throughout the decade. How did it affect educational institutions? Schools, colleges, and libraries were compelled to curtail their activities because of insufficient funds. Schools of nursing are, by and large, self-supporting agencies; if the hospitals conducting them were unable to increase their budgets, the schools, at least, could continue their existing programs without major curtailment. Salaries of the school staff were cut, as were the salaries of all other hospital personnel. But, since the financial base upon which schools of nursing rest derives so largely from service rendered by the schools through their students, it is not likely that they were affected by the depression to the same extent and in the same way as were other educational institutions.

In spite of the depression, or perhaps because of it, the trend to determine causes of financial and social phenomena, begun soon after World War I, continued into the Thirties. The machinery for several important studies, national in scope, had been established before 1930. The five-year program of the Committee on the Costs of Medical Care [1] was adopted in February 1928; the final report of the committee, in October 1932. In the autumn of 1929, President Hoover asked a group of scientists "to examine into the feasibility of a national survey of social trends in the

[1] Elizabeth G. Fox was a member of the Committee on the Costs of Medical Care.

United States," [2] and in December of that year the President appointed a committee to undertake such a project. Another important committee appointed in 1929 by President Hoover was an organizing committee for the White House Conference on Child Health and Protection.[3]

The pronouncements of these committees, emerging from economic, social, and medical studies were of cardinal significance to nursing. They indicated a penetrating insight into the current status of nursing education. The President's Research Committee on Social Trends viewed rather dismally the trend in nursing education. "Nursing education," said the committee, "has grown rapidly in volume, but there has been only slight improvement in quality." [4] The Committee on the Costs of Medical Care recommended "that nursing education be thoroughly remoulded to provide well-educated and well-qualified registered nurses." [5]

All three committees substantially agreed on the vital part of the nurse in a national health and welfare program. In *Recent Social Trends* it is stated, "The importance of the public health nurse cannot well be overestimated. William H. Welch has said, 'America has made two unique contributions to medicine—the Panama Canal and the public health nurse.' " [6] The White House Conference affirmed "the nurse should . . . always be a health teacher. . . . In fact the meaning of nursing is fundamentally health supervision." [7]

About the same time as the work of the above named three committees was in progress, a fourth committee, the Committee on the Grading of Nursing Schools, launched a nation-wide

[2] Report of the President's Research Committee on Social Trends, *Recent Social Trends in the United States.* New York, McGraw-Hill Book Co., 1934, p. v

[3] Alta E. Dines, 1914, and Chelly Wasserberg, 1916, served on the Subcommittee on Obstetric Teaching and Education of Nursing and Trained Attendants.

[4] *Recent Social Trends in the United States,* p. 1067

[5] Final Report of the Committee on the Costs of Medical Care, *Medical Care for the American People.* Chicago, University of Chicago Press, 1932, p. 138

[6] *Recent Social Trends in the United States,* p. 1090

[7] White House Conference on Child Health and Protection, *Hospitals and Child Health: Hospitals and Dispensaries, Convalescent Care, Medical Social Service.* New York, Century Co., 1932, p. 219

study. The Grading Committee adopted a program in 1926; its final publication appeared in 1934. The committee collected more facts about nursing, by the questionnaire method, than had ever been collected before; these facts dealt with supply and demand, nursing economics, educational and administrative characteristics of nursing schools, and the activities performed by nurses. The Grading Committee never actually graded schools of nursing, as might be inferred from its name. It did, however, supply every school with highly informative reports, showing the place the particular school occupied among other participating schools in each significant characteristic.[8]

It was clear from the Grading Committee reports that few schools, if any, had a flawless record; it was also clear that even if a school had a good standing in a particular item as compared with other schools, that fact did not necessarily predicate desirable practice. In the Second Grading, for example, in all schools of nursing only 20 per cent of the nurse faculty members had some college preparation, 51 per cent, four years of high school, and 29 per cent had less than four years of high school work. At the Hopkins School 46 per cent of the nurse faculty members had some college preparation and the other 54 per cent, four years of high school.[9] While Hopkins had a favorable record in its nurse faculty preparation as compared with all other nursing schools in the study, it had an unfavorable record as compared with other types of professional schools.

The Johns Hopkins School had a 56-hour week at night for the students, and in that respect it was better than 64 per cent of all schools whose weekly night schedules ranged from fifty-seven to

[8] It is of interest to note that M. Adelaide Nutting, as chairman of the Committee on Education of the American Society of Superintendents of Training Schools for Nurses, included in her 1911 report to the Society the statement, "They [the committee] believe that . . . a close, careful and exhaustive study is now needed on the whole question of the education of the nurse, inclusive of the fields of professional work which she occupies . . . The Committee therefore recommends that this Society request the Carnegie Foundation for the Advancement of Teaching to make such a study."

[9] Committee on the Grading of Nursing Schools, *The Second Grading of Nursing Schools*, p. 25. (All data for the Second Grading were collected during 1932.)

eighty-four or more hours.[10] Thus, in terms of practice in the majority of nursing schools, the Hopkins night schedule seemed reasonable enough; in terms of sound educational principle, it was conspicuously unreasonable.

However, there were aspects of the Hopkins program that were good not only in relation to other schools but were good in relation to good nursing education. In some of the services, though not in all, the length of the clinical assignment closely corresponded to that recommended by the National League of Nursing Education. In the majority of schools there was a wider divergence from the League's recommendations in practically all services. In the psychiatric department, Hopkins students received approximately sixty days of nursing experience, the same as recommended by the League. In all reporting schools, three-fourths of the students had nine days or less in the care of psychiatric patients.[11]

The initial and major contribution of the Grading Committee to nursing education was not the reports to particular schools, but the findings on all schools all over the country and the general poverty disclosed of their educational programs. It was plainly evident that whatever broad national benefits would stem from the work of the committee must come out of the action of individual schools to upgrade their own programs.

It would be difficult to assay the extent to which the Johns Hopkins Hospital School of Nursing was affected by the depression, by the reports of the Committee on the Grading of Nursing Schools, and the pronouncements of other national health and educational committees. Members of the administration and of the Alumnae Association were associated with the various national committee activities and informed on their findings. Certain it is that important changes were achieved in the School between 1930 and 1940.

A highly significant event in 1930 was the organization of the Advisory Board of the School of Nursing. By the creation of this Board the Hospital Trustees recognized an official group whose sole function was deliberation of the School as an educational en-

[10] *Ibid.*, p. 45
[11] *Ibid.*, pp. 73–101

tity. From the beginning the Advisory Board maintained a distinguished personnel. The first members were: Dr. Joseph S. Ames, president of the Johns Hopkins University, Elsie M. Lawler, director of the School, and Dr. Winford H. Smith, director of the Hospital (ex officio members); Dr. J. Whitridge Williams and Dr. Edwards A. Park, representing the Medical Board of the Hospital; Dr. Wade Hampton Frost, representing the Advisory Board of the Johns Hopkins University School of Hygiene and Public Health; Effie J. Taylor and Clara D. Noyes,[12] 1896, representing the Johns Hopkins Hospital Nurses' Alumnae Association; Mrs. John S. Gibbs, Jr., and Dr. Esther L. Richards, members-at-large; Hester K. Frederick, member of the School staff. Dr. Joseph S. Ames was elected the first chairman of the Advisory Board and Hester K. Frederick, the first secretary. In 1938 an amendment to the *Rules and Regulations* of the Hospital provided for membership on the Advisory Board of a member of the Hospital Trustees.

The first meeting of the Advisory Board was held on December 18, 1930. At this meeting, the Board authorized the chairman to appoint two committees: one, "to consider the purpose, scope and function of this school for nurses" and another, "to consider the curriculum." Effie J. Taylor was appointed chairman of the committee to consider the purpose, scope, and function of the School. Two months later Miss Taylor submitted a report. As chairman she had written to more than two dozen individuals, outstanding in their special fields and including nursing, medical, and public health educators, and asked their opinions on the "function and scope of a high-class school of nursing." Miss Taylor summarized the replies she received in ten statements, each of which lent to the concept that a school of nursing should be primarily educational, that it should have the essential facilities and financial resources, and that it should plan its curriculum on changing community needs. M. Adelaide Nutting wrote in reply to the inquiry she received:

[12] Other Alumnae who have been members of the Advisory Board are K. Virginia Betzold, 1933, Gertrude H. Bowling, 1915, Alta E. Dines, Virginia M. Dunbar, 1923, Loula E. Kennedy, Mrs. Dorothy Filler McBride, Lucile Petry, 1927, Elizabeth C. Phillips, 1927, and Anna D. Wolf.

"I believe that a school is a place for instruction and that a school of nursing is a place for instruction in nursing. It has to my mind no other legitimate functions. . . . If, in the performance of its duties, something outside and beyond its educational purpose and aim is accomplished, this is in reality a by-product of education and should be regarded and treated as such, no matter what its value from any other standpoint."

The Advisory Board, in appointing the two committees, one to consider the function of the School and the other the curriculum, announced its intention to start anew. This action should assure, first, a common definition of function for its membership and, secondly, such reconstruction of the curriculum as essential to bring it into harmony with the accepted function. The function of a nursing school, reported the chairman of the committee to consider function, is primarily educational. This definition, completely interpreted, would ultimately affect not only curriculum content but also the conditions under which the curriculum operated: adequacy of faculty, weekly hour schedules, and character of the nursing service where students learn to nurse.

Elsie M. Lawler, then director of the School, was appointed chairman of the committee to consider the curriculum. The committee was instructed to interpret the term "curriculum" in its broadest sense, involving both the theory and practice of nursing. Miss Lawler, in the next ten years, brought before the Advisory Board a list of recommendations, some of which were adopted and some of which were modified or delayed. She and her associates, particularly Hester K. Frederick and Loula E. Kennedy, initiated a series of studies in support of the recommendations submitted. Revision of the curriculum had already begun; Miss Kennedy, as director of theoretical instruction, had prepared during the Twenties convincing reports, analyzing the separate courses and setting forth the needs of a program directed primarily toward education.

The changes in the curriculum between 1930 and 1940 were characterized chiefly by consolidation of courses and refinement and expansion of subject matter. During this period, the curriculum prepared and published by the National League of Nursing Education was thoroughly revised. There is no doubt that some of the changes at Hopkins were influenced by the philosophy set forth by the League Curriculum Committee; there is also evidence that the Hopkins School made its own evaluations and, after reasonable deliberation, accepted, modified, or rejected the national proposals as they were suitable to the Hopkins program. This was exactly what the League Committee hoped that schools would do. The committee states in the revised *Curriculum Guide*, "It is not intended that these recommendations be accepted uncritically and applied *in toto* to every situation. The assumption is that each school will have its own curriculum committee and will work out its own curriculum using the best advice and materials available." [13]

Early in the Thirties the course in materia medica was thoroughly overhauled. In the 1904–1905 *Circular*, it is stated that "Instruction in the properties and uses of drugs is given mainly in the Hospital Pharmacy under the direction of the Pharmacist." This instruction included the actual preparation of "solutions, tinctures, liniments, ointments, powders, etc." The graduates who were in the School during the first twenty-five years of this century will remember the pharmacist, Jacob L. Walz, who taught them the proper proportions of the proper ingredients of the various preparations. Mr. Walz possessed an all-seeing eye and an uncanny ability in detecting the slightest mistake whether he stood at the side of the erring student or whether he stood off at some distant point in the pharmacy. He must have been amused by the enthusiasm over the preparation of a jar of cold cream. It was Mr. Walz' responsibility to see to it that his young and eager charges became "familiar with the practical handling of all drugs in daily use in the Hospital." What a far cry it seems to that time when familiarity with all drugs in daily use in the Hospital could be achieved!

While the pharmacy program was modified during the Twenties, it was not until 1933 that the course in materia medica was reorganized, with less emphasis on the compounding of pharmaceutical preparations and more on the action of drugs, their ad-

[13] Committee on Curriculum, National League of Nursing Education, *A Curriculum Guide for Schools of Nursing*. New York, National League of Nursing Education, 1937, p. 10

ministration, and the importance of observing and reporting their effects. The course in dosage and solutions, according to the 1932–1933 Report of the Department of Instruction, "now represents a course in pure mathematics." All students had to learn to deal accurately with fractions.

Reorganization of the dietetic program began between 1930 and 1940. A major weakness in the dietetic course was the lack of an instructor who gave her full time to supervising and helping the student interpret and correlate her dietetic classroom instruction with her dietetic experience. The supervision then given was provided by a staff member of the Hospital dietetic department; it was but one of her many responsibilities.

In 1938 the Advisory Board approved the appointment of Katherine Rose Nelson as supervisor and instructor in nutrition and dietetics. Miss Nelson was a well-qualified dietitian by training and experience; she was also a graduate of the Johns Hopkins School of Nursing. Her appointment as a full-time member on the faculty of the Nursing School brought a new emphasis on the nutritional factors in the nursing care of patients.

One of the chief curriculum developments during the Twenties was the strengthening of the science courses, with particular reference to laboratory work. The bacteriology course then provided for ten laboratory hours; the instructor requested that the laboratory hours be increased to twenty. In 1938 this request was approved with instruction in bacteriology now covering forty-five hours of which twenty-four were devoted to laboratory.

There is no phase of the curriculum in which the plan of education has explored more often new directions than that covered during the early months in the School, known variously as the probationary, the preparatory, the preliminary, and the preclinical period. In the spring of 1933, according to a report of the Department of Instruction, "A very successful experiment was tried this year of sending the preliminary student . . . on the wards for periods of observation early in their course. . . . The three periods determined on were as varied as possible and included (1) early morning activities (2) late afternoon activities (3) Sunday morning 9–1. . . ." The next year the observation periods were extended to include a half-day in the Dispensary following a new patient and an afternoon with a social worker visiting the homes of patients. It was evident in the reports prepared by the students and in the conferences with their instructors that these preliminary observations of bed patients in the Hospital, of ambulatory patients in the Dispensary, and of patients in their own homes stimulated an early appreciation of the relationship between social conditions and health.

Public health nursing, practice as well as theory, was introduced into the curriculum at Hopkins in 1933. While the incidents which led up to this course are fully described in the special study, "Nursing the Community," any reference to curriculum development during the Thirties would be highly incomplete without mention of this significant event and its invigorating influence on the entire program. At that time college graduates were granted a six-month time credit. The incorporation of public health experience necessitated a special planning of the programs of such students. This planning presented certain problems, and in 1934 time credit was discontinued.

While the curriculum changes so far described in this chapter have been concerned largely with classroom teaching, the program of instruction and supervision in the clinical departments was slowly forging ahead. The crying need to vitalize and expand the clinical program was the appointment of instructional personnel with the sole function of planning and developing the opportunities in the fields of practice and of tying together learning in the classroom with doing in the actual nursing situation. Miss Lawler had repeatedly stated this need; the reports of the Department of Instruction reiterated it again and again. Late in 1933 Mrs. John S. Gibbs, Jr., announced that the Women's Auxiliary Board of the Hospital had appropriated the salaries of two full-time ward instructors for one year; the appropriation was continued by the Women's Board for four years when it was taken over by the Hospital Trustees. The first two appointees to the position were Anna T. Beckwith, 1928, assigned to Osler Clinic, the medical service, and Dorothy E. Blackman, 1929, to Halsted Clinic, the surgical division.

After 1933 the appointment of instructors who gave all or the major part of their time to student supervision was gradually extended to all departments in the Hospital, both during the day and during the night. The title of this official was later changed to "instructor and supervisor," thus expressing the philosophy of the School that clinical faculty should share in the supervision of nursing service.

The Instructors' Meetings had been inaugurated in 1928. The discussions in the instructor group must have stimulated and nourished the growth of the new clinical teaching efforts. One year after the appointment of the first ward instructors, the report of the Department of Instruction noted, "We have progressed considerably in our program of ward instruction." Not all was smooth sailing; difficulties loomed in the way, especially in the medical and surgical departments where assignments were less definitely blocked than in the "specialty" departments, such as ophthalmological and psychiatric. One other lament was heard: weekly ward rounds were not regularly held and they required "a good deal of persistent attention" in making arrangements and seeing to it that they were kept up. Nevertheless there was evidence of solid achievement. During the school year 1935–1936, clinical teaching programs were outlined for seven different services. About that same time Virginia H. Walker, 1929, then ward instructor in Halsted Clinic, wrote, "The ultimate object of our entire program in nursing is to secure the maximum amount of mental and physical comfort for each individual patient." Miss Walker then proceeded to tell how the clinical teaching program not only helped the student to gain confidence and acquire skills, but also safeguarded the physical care of the patient and contributed to his peace of mind.

With the changes in the curriculum, expansion of subject matter and increase in instruction by more than three hundred hours, it was inevitable that the worrisome question of student hours should again be on the agenda. Students were still on a 54-hour week of practice during the day and a 56-hour week during the night.

In 1934 Miss Lawler reported a thorough study of hours had been made by herself and her staff. It was the opinion of the group that a 48-hour week *exclusive of classes* could be introduced for all students by adding to the nursing staff seventeen workers, four general staff nurses and thirteen ward helpers. While the shorter hour schedule was not then granted, it was approved in principle by the Board of Trustees. Four years later the Trustees authorized a 48-hour practice week. It was not possible, however, to put the schedule fully into effect, especially during the summer months, because of the continued need of the Hospital for student service. Nevertheless the School was not without hope that eventually student hours would more nearly accord with sound principles of education.

Student hours, the employment of general staff nurses, and hospital economics are inextricably tied together. As the Thirties began the country was sinking into the morass of a devastating depression. The Johns Hopkins Hospital inescapably felt the economic tightening; a reduction in student hours had to be offset by an addition of *paid* nursing personnel and the Hospital, patently, at the beginning of the decade, was unwilling to undertake the added expenditure. Moreover, the idea of the general staff nurse had still to take hold in Baltimore along with the country as a whole. In 1932, 63 per cent of all hospitals with state approved nursing schools did *not* employ any general staff nurses; by 1937 this per cent had dropped to 10.[14] The Johns Hopkins Hospital employed thirty-seven general staff nurses in 1930; in 1940 it employed 188.

Not only were general staff nurses added to the nursing service personnel, but by 1940 the nonprofessional workers consisted of six ward clerks (the ward clerk was introduced in 1931), forty ward helpers, and forty-two attendants, the attendants being assigned to Phipps Psychiatric Clinic. In the meantime the Osler Clinic for medical patients and the Halsted Clinic for surgical were completed and occupied. The completion of these two buildings added to the Hospital capacity about 170 beds. The increase in hospital accommodations counteracted somewhat the personnel gains. Nevertheless the staffing of the nursing service reached a new degree of stability, which greatly facilitated the program of the School.

A schedule of long hours of practice to which are added class hours and hours of study inevitably predisposes to fatigue and

[14] *American Journal of Nursing*, 38:186–87, Feb. 1938

lowered resistance. Apparently the 54-hour day and 56-hour night together with some other weak links in the health program exacted their toll in the years between 1930 and 1933. The illness days recorded for the year ending June 30, 1930, were 2,087; for the year ending June 30, 1933, 4,127, the largest number for any one year during the Thirties. The illness days included those lost by students and also those lost by graduates. The number of graduates who were ill during either year was small in proportion to the number of students. Student illness, doubtless, constituted the bulk of the time lost.

The high incidence of sickness caused considerable worry in the School. More intensive and more frequent medical examinations were instituted and especial emphasis was placed on the teaching of personal hygiene. For many years the infirmary for sick nurses was located on the first floor of the old Nurses' Home. After the remodeling and converting of old Wards D and E into the Thayer Memorial Clinic for semiprivate patients, the infirmary was transferred to the first floor of the Thayer Clinic. That was in January 1934. Mary S. Purcell, 1919, was appointed supervisor of Thayer, in which capacity she was responsible for the administration of the infirmary. This arrangement must have proven highly satisfactory for later Miss Lawler wrote, "To have . . . a part of Thayer 1, where sick nurses can be under Miss Purcell's watchful eye, has been a great blessing."

Because of the concern of the School and of the medical group responsible for the care of sick nurses and with the transference of the infirmary to the Thayer Clinic, a number of important changes were gradually made in the health program. By 1938 a broad medical care plan had been adopted. The plan included procedures of diagnostic significance and was directed toward prophylaxis and the early detection of infection. The scrutiny of the health program continued through the Forties. The School owes a debt of gratitude to the chiefs of staffs and their associates for the tireless and skillful care given to student and graduate nurses. When the health services for all personnel in the Hospital and the University were coordinated under one administration in 1948, the same excellence of medical attention was provided for the School of Nursing.

An account of the activities of the School between the years 1930 and 1940 would be incomplete without some mention of the library, even though the steps in its development are traced in the special library study. After much tilling of the ground the library was reorganized; the reference books which had been housed in the Teaching Department on the top floor of the old surgical building were transferred to the School library, now remodeled and enlarged, in the old Nurses' Home. The development of the library as an actively functional unit of the School was well on its way.

At the beginning of this chapter, reference is made to certain nation-wide studies, dealing with nursing and related medical and social fields. Spurred on by the national groups and the disclosures of their research, nursing schools undertook to blueprint their own educational and administrative performance and to compare what they were doing with what was being done in other schools and with the recommendations of the national groups. At Johns Hopkins the teaching and administrative staff made a number of well-considered studies, some of which originated in the Advisory Board, to improve the structure of the School and nursing service and to support with facts its recommendations. Among the studies made were those which dealt with head nurse duties, staffing requirements of the different departments, prenursing education as related to achievement, student withdrawals, curriculum, teaching load of instructors, nursing education costs, illness, and library needs. The School also sought the services of experts in the fields of general and nursing education for appraisal of its curriculum. In the preliminary study of the National League of Nursing Education leading to the League accreditation program, Hopkins was one of the fifty nursing schools included; it was also one of the first schools granted accreditation by that organization.

The long-sought relationship with the Johns Hopkins University was accomplished in 1935. When the Advisory Board of the School of Nursing was created in 1930, Dr. Joseph S. Ames, president of the Johns Hopkins University, was elected chairman. He was, therefore, in a position to keep informed on the current of educational affairs in the School of Nursing.

In 1934 Dr. Ames, as president of the University, was approached by the Advisory Board concerning the attitude of the University toward allowing academic credit for work in the School. Dr. Ames requested the Committee on Advanced Standing on the Bachelor of Science Degree to survey the School of Nursing in order to determine whether its program merited university credit. The report of the committee included the statement:

"The investigations of the Committee led to the conclusion that the administration of the School is efficient, the instruction competent, the facilities adequate, the students in the main earnest and attentive, and the personnel of the student body of high quality. The teaching methods also compare favorably with those in ordinary college instruction."

The result of the survey was an arrangement made early in 1935 whereby graduates of the School of Nursing, who could submit evidence of two years of college work, including certain prescribed subjects prior to their entrance to the School, were eligible as candidates for the bachelor of science degree granted by the University through its College for Teachers. The arrangement also required that at least thirty points of credit should be obtained in work taken at the Johns Hopkins University. In effect this meant that the University evaluated the program pursued during the three years in the School of Nursing as the equivalent of thirty points of undergraduate work under university auspices.

The School had now established a form of official relationship with the University. This was a step forward and an important step, since it signified recognition by the University of the program of the School in academic terms. Relatively few of the graduates, however, took advantage of the affiliation, doubtless because they could secure more credit for their nursing course in other high-ranking universities, and also because they could matriculate for programs in nursing offered by these universities for graduate nurses.

Of Miss Lawler's assistants who helped the School reach new mileposts during the Thirties, and before, none served more loyally or more steadfastly than Hester King Frederick. When Miss Frederick retired in 1941, she had devoted twenty-one of her twenty-nine years of professional activity to the School of Nursing and the nursing service of the Johns Hopkins Hospital. She was director of practical instruction and taught principles and practice of nursing for eight years; later she was assistant to Miss Lawler for ten years.

Hester Frederick was one of those fortunate individuals who possess not one but several well-developed abilities. She was an able and resourceful administrator; she was an instructor of charm and magnetism thoroughly absorbed in the subject she taught, the Principles and Practice of Nursing. According to those who knew her the welfare of the patient was always a foremost consideration, and it might have been that her devotion to the teaching of nursing was linked with her ever-present concern for the patient.

There was no "gray" in Miss Frederick's character or personality; she was all "black" or all "white." She was patient, she was also impatient. Her impatience was always short-lived; it was like a summer storm, soon blown out by its own intensity, the sun and the blue skies quickly breaking through the clouds. That her patience was more enduring is reflected in the memories of her students. They remember that she was approachable, that she was exacting and expected much of them, that they liked her and admired her, even though their liking and admiration were tinctured with awe and fear. They are grateful to her for what she taught them and the ideals she gave them.

Miss Frederick was a beautiful girl and a handsome woman. She had a sense of humor that was refreshing and contagious, a spirit that was gay and lively. Her outside interests were many, and it may be that the many facets of her personality and character grew out of the richness of her life.

As the year 1939 drew to a close the departure of Elsie M. Lawler, head of the School, approached. The School had just passed the half-century mark; Miss Lawler had been its head for thirty of the fifty-one years of its existence. In March 1910 Miss Lawler began a regime that ended in November 1940.

In 1910 little change had been made in the original hospital structure; by 1940, new buildings had been erected and new clinics had replaced practically all of the old wards, and those which still stood had been remodeled. In 1910 the daily average number of patients was less than 300. In 1940 it had reached 750. Literally Miss Lawler saw the Hospital rebuilt.

Miss Lawler saw other things. She saw World War I and she lived through the 1918 influenza epidemic and during both events gave unsparingly of herself. She saw the remodeling of the "Old General" operating room into a much-needed teaching center; she saw Hampton House, a dignified and beautiful residence for the School, arise on Broadway.

Miss Lawler loved Johns Hopkins—the Hospital, the School, the Hopkins traditions. Her profound regard and pride for all that Hopkins stood for seemed to have grown a part of her. Honors came to Miss Lawler in recognition of her years of devoted service. The Johns Hopkins Hospital Nurses' Alumnae Association celebrated her twenty-fifth anniversary as principal of the School at a dinner at the Hotel Belvedere. On this occasion the Board of Trustees and the Director of the Hospital presented to Miss Lawler a silver bowl and tray, and the Alumnae Association, a diamond bar pin. In February of the same year, 1935, the Johns Hopkins University conferred on Miss Lawler the honorary degree of master of arts in recognition of twenty-five years of "outstanding work as a nurse, teacher and administrator." The Alumnae Association established the Elsie M. Lawler Scholarship Aid Fund in 1948, initiated by the class of 1928. The auditorium of the new Educational Unit in the Main Residence (old Nurses' Home) was dedicated to Miss Lawler.[15] This tribute after ten years of retirement must have given her special pleasure. Miss Lawler's portrait, the gift of the 1925 class and the Alumnae Association, hangs in the entrance hall of the Main Residence.

When Miss Lawler retired in 1940, 2,209 nurses had been graduated from the Johns Hopkins Hospital School of Nursing. By her own record she signed the diplomas of 1,796, and "helped to start out that many women to lives of usefulness." Although Miss Lawler's students generally regarded her with awe, a host

[15] This is epilogue as the history ends with the year 1949. The dedication took place May 1951.

of them admired and respected her and held her in affection. She endeared herself to them by her kindliness, her sympathy, and her practical counsel and help, especially in times of personal distress. In her annual reports Miss Lawler testified to the support and loyalty and assistance she received from her staff. To earn the affection, admiration, respect, and loyalty of one's students and associates, is surely one of the greatest rewards that can come to an official in high office.

A New Architect Designs

By the end of 1939 Europe was again embroiled in conflict; by the end of 1941 the United States had joined the battle. In America with the outbreak of European hostilities, private as well as governmental agencies aligned their forces. The mobilization of both material and human resources was quickened after Pearl Harbor. The watchword of the nation was "defense."

The organized nursing profession clearly saw its responsibilities early in the war. In July 1940 the Nursing Council on National Defense was inaugurated. Its membership included representatives from the national nursing organizations, the federal nursing agencies, and the American Red Cross Nursing Service. Early in 1942 the Council changed its name to the National Nursing Council for War Service, and, as the war continued, considerably broadened its membership representation. At the close of hostilities the Council deleted "for War Service" from its title and became the National Nursing Council.

As early as 1944, the Council sponsored a postwar planning committee, known as the National Nursing Planning Committee.[1]

[1] Marjorie B. Davis, 1925, was appointed secretary of the National Nursing Planning Committee. Members of the committee included Virginia M. Dunbar, Lucile Petry, Ruth G. Taylor, 1924, and Anna D. Wolf.

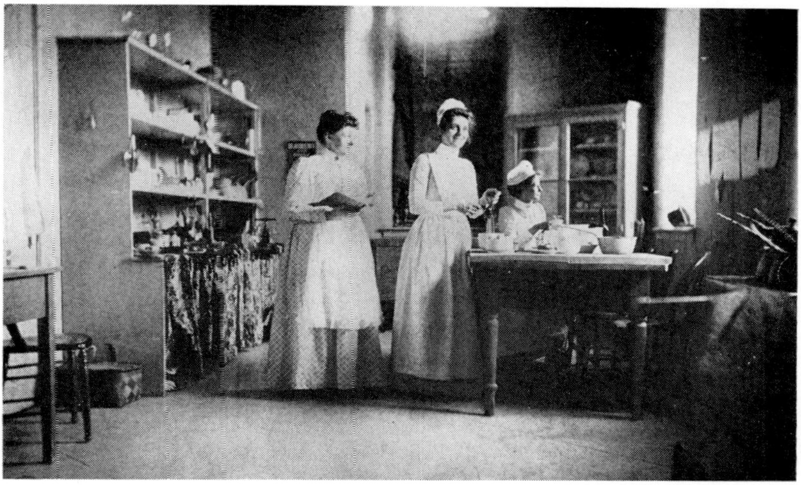

The Diet School, 1890

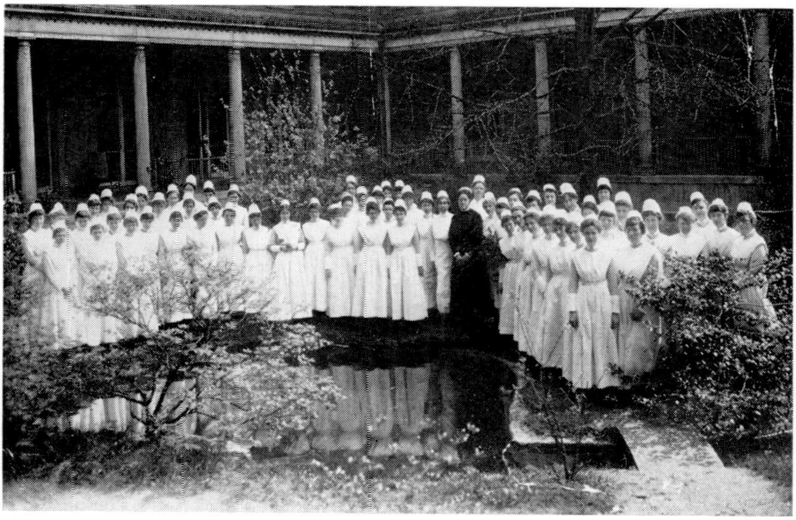

Graduating Class, 1920

When, in 1948, the work of the Planning Committee was completed, the National Nursing Council considered its obligations fulfilled and, having made recommendations for implementing the studies concluded under its sponsorship, passed a resolution to go out of existence.

The activities of the Council, before and during the war and for several years thereafter, affected importantly programs in schools of nursing. It stimulated through field services the accelerated curriculum, which later became the basis for the program required by the United States Cadet Nurse Corps. The Council affirmed and reaffirmed the necessity of increasing the number of superior young women in schools of nursing whose graduates would qualify for enrolment in the American Red Cross Nursing Service and, also, add to the ranks of hospital and other civilian nursing personnel. To accomplish this objective the Council coordinated its efforts with the efforts of the national nursing organizations, the American Hospital Association, the nursing units of the United States Public Health Service, and the Subcommittee on Nursing of the Health and Medical Committee, Office of Defense Health and Welfare Services. For an equitable civilian distribution of nurses and to insure the maximum number with the armed forces, the Council also worked closely with the Nursing Division in the Procurement and Assignment Service, Placement Bureau, War Manpower Commission, and the nursing consultant in the Medical Division of the Office of Civilian Defense.

In the wake of the war and during the years between 1940 and 1950, momentous changes—political, social, and economic—were to sweep the globe. In this country before the outbreak of hostilities, there had been a growing manifestation of the federal government's concern in the economic betterment of the population, in health measures, and in education, professional as well as general. The Social Security Act of 1935 authorized the use of federal funds for the training of public health workers, including public health nurses. In 1940 the Committee on Educational Policies and Resources of the Nursing Council on National Defense presented the needs in nursing to the United States Office of Education, and, as a result, the Training for Nurses (National Defense) Act was passed by the Congress in July 1941. Under this Act the sum of $1,200,000 was originally appropriated for increasing enrolment in basic nursing schools, for refresher courses, and for postgraduate education in special fields—all devices intended to strengthen nursing resources. The Congress placed the administration of the program under the United States Public Health Service. Within the next two years, twelve thousand additional students were admitted to basic nursing schools.

But that was not enough. The United States had entered the war after the enactment of the Training for Nurses Act, and with its entrance, the drain upon civilian nursing personnel rapidly gained momentum. Seventy-six thousand nurses had volunteered for military duty by the end of 1944, although not all of them were equipped to stand the rigors of the service. In 1940 there were 940 nurses in the Army Nurse Corps; by 1944 there were approximately 50,000. The Army was now asking for 10,000 more nurses, the Navy, 4,000.[2] The urgency of a plan that would bring much larger numbers of students into nursing schools was crystal-clear as the year 1943 began. Out of this urgency came the Bolton Bill, enacted into law in June 1943, and the establishment of the United States Cadet Nurse Corps. The Division of Nurse Education of the United States Public Health Service, with Lucile Petry as director, was created to administer the Bolton Act program. The Division worked closely with the National Nursing Council for War Service. The major program for student recruitment was administered by the Council. During the year 1943–1944 (July 1, 1943 to June 30, 1944), 65,500 students were admitted to schools of nursing, an increase of more than 27,000 over the number admitted during the calendar year 1940.

Other events occurred during the Forties which undoubtedly influenced the development of hospital nursing service and of nursing education. The Hospital Survey and Construction Act

[2] President Roosevelt informed the Congress in January 1945 that "volunteering has not produced the number of nurses required" for the armed forces and urged that provision be made for drafting nurses. A few months later Germany unconditionally surrendered. The "Draft Bill" was not enacted into law.

was passed by the Congress in 1946. This Act provided for large appropriations for hospital construction. The work of the Commission on Hospital Care, resulting in the publication, *Hospital Care in the United States*,[3] stressed the inadequacy of the nation's hospital facilities. More hospital beds presuppose more nursing personnel and an available source from which the personnel can be obtained.

The American Red Cross Volunteer Nurse's Aide Corps originated during the first World War. After the outbreak of the second world conflagration the Corps was revived. During the summer of 1941, the American Red Cross and the Office of Civilian Defense announced as their goal the training of one hundred thousand Nurse's Aides within the year. The Nursing Council on National Defense cooperated to the fullest extent in the endeavor as an official measure for supplementing professional nursing service.

The Volunteer Nurse's Aide program provided for formal instruction, supervised practice in a hospital, and a certain amount of voluntary service under supervision upon completion of the program. As the war progressed and the shortages of professional nurses became more and more acute, the Nurse's Aides gave valuable service in assisting the professional nursing staff in hard-pressed civilian hospitals.

A major event during the Forties bearing directly and importantly on nursing and nursing education was the Brown Study. In 1945 the National Nursing Planning Committee outlined a plan to reconvert wartime to peacetime nursing activities. One of the principal proposals set forth in the plan was a study of selected aspects of nursing education: organization, administration, control, and sources of financial support. Esther Lucile Brown, Ph.D., director, Department of Studies in the Professions, Russell Sage Foundation, undertook the project.[4] Dr. Brown prepared a

[3] Commission on Hospital Care, *Hospital Care in the United States*. New York, Commonwealth Fund, 1947

[4] The Professional Advisory Committee to the study included Virginia M. Dunbar, Lucile Petry, Anna D. Wolf, and Blanche Pfefferkorn, ex officio.

report for the National Nursing Council, sponsor of the study, under the title, *Nursing for the Future*.[5]

Nursing for the Future gives few lines to looking backward, but many to looking toward the future. A major thesis is positive health, and, as a corollary, the statement that health agencies, including hospitals, are on the increase and that the obligation of every health agency is to see to it that patients and patients' families are given health instruction, as such instruction is indicated. Another contention is the need of recognition of several strata of nursing personnel; of a supplementary force of nursing workers, trained to perform functions not requiring skilled nursing service.

Nursing for the Future reviews the current educational status and wide differences in existent schools of nursing. It classifies hospital schools as "Socially Undesirable Schools," those that should be closed immediately; "Relatively Good Schools," those with uncertain future; and "Distinguished Hospital Schools," those which Dr. Brown is convinced and so recommends, should be placed under university control. The author has probed deeply into her subject; she has submitted reasonable and realistic argument in support of her recommendations.

Such was the climate of the Nineteen Forties in which schools of nursing carried on: a climate of intense effort to meet the day by day urgencies arising out of the war and the problems which follow with war termination. Some schools survived better than others, some performed better than others, but there can be little doubt that all did their duty as best they could. What account did the Johns Hopkins Hospital School of Nursing give of itself during this critical period?

As the Forties began, the School at Hopkins had a new architect to design its broad pattern. Anna Dryden Wolf was appointed director of the School of Nursing and the nursing service, the Johns Hopkins Hospital, November 1, 1940.

Miss Wolf, a graduate of the Johns Hopkins School of Nursing, was the daughter of missionaries. She was born in Guntur, Madras

[5] Esther L. Brown, *Nursing for the Future*. New York, Russell Sage Foundation, 1948

Presidency, South India. Her father was head of the American Evangelical Lutheran Mission College, a school for Hindu boys in Guntur; her mother, a former school teacher, organized the first school for Mohammedan women in that community. Her sister, Dr. Eleanor Wolf Stewart, graduated from the Johns Hopkins University School of Medicine, was a medical missionary in India for six years. Miss Wolf herself gave evidence of social interests from her college days; during vacation each year she engaged in some form of social work.

Brought to America in her third year, a large part of Miss Wolf's life was spent in Maryland. She attended private school, later went to Goucher College in Baltimore where she received a bachelor of arts degree. In 1912 she entered the Johns Hopkins Hospital School of Nursing and was awarded two Trustee scholarships, one as an intermediate and one as a senior student. Upon graduation from Hopkins and with the aid of the Trustee scholarship received as a senior, she matriculated at Teachers College, Columbia University for a master's degree.

Miss Wolf held positions of distinction before coming to the Johns Hopkins Hospital as director of the School of Nursing. Her first appointment at Hopkins was to the position of instructor and assistant superintendent of nurses, a good apprenticeship for important work she was soon to assume. She was one of an outstanding group of young nurse educators selected to teach at the Vassar Training Camp for Nurses in the summer of 1918. Her appointment as superintendent of nurses at the Peking Union Medical College, Peking, China, extended from 1919 to 1925. There she reorganized the nursing service, organized a school of nursing for women students, and laid the foundation for the university nursing program which was later established. Upon her return to this country, she reoriented herself to American nursing and spent another year at Teachers College, Columbia University. Then, in 1926, she was appointed associate professor of nursing and director of nursing at the University Clinics, the University of Chicago, where she organized an all-graduate nursing service assisted by a staff of supplementary workers; she also developed at that university courses in teaching and administration in schools of nursing.

When the New York Hospital and the New York Hospital School of Nursing moved into their stately new quarters on the East River, Miss Wolf was appointed director of the school and the nursing service. In that capacity it was her task to effect a reorganization which involved the consolidation of the activities and personnel of four different hospitals, an outpatient clinic, and a newly established psychiatric institution. From New York she returned to Baltimore and to her own School. Miss Wolf brought to Hopkins a rich background of education, general and professional, and a record of educational organization and administration, international in scope and internationally recognized.

One of the first acts of the new administration was to bring before the School Advisory Board the matter of faculty organization and responsibilities. Less than three months after taking office, the director reported that organization of the faculty was under consideration and, two months later, she presented recommendations concerning the personnel to constitute the faculty and the functions to be delegated to that body. Out of these recommendations came a well-knit faculty with specifically defined functions. Bylaws were drafted and by October 1941, the faculty was organized as prescribed by these bylaws. This was a highly significant step in the total growth of the School. It established official recognition for the faculty *as a group* responsible for the initiation of the educational policies of the School; it provided by this recognition a means for keeping the faculty members informed and for the sharing of members in the progressive development of the School; and, finally, it gave to the faculty status and responsibilities similar to those given to faculties in institutions of higher education.

About the same time the faculty was organized, the students were given the opportunity to form a student organization. Apparently the time and the setting were now right for their active participation in the affairs of the School. They at once set about drafting a constitution and bylaws for an association, to be known as the Student Association of the Johns Hopkins Hospital School of Nursing. With the organization of the Association an official channel was created for a cooperative working relationship between the students and the faculty.

In the preamble to the constitution and bylaws the students declared they desired "to assume individually and collectively responsibility for the conduct of students in their hospital life, and thus to promote loyalty and self-control. . . ." They adopted an honor code; they published *The Dome*, the student handbook to guide students and to inform them what they might expect of the School and what, in turn, the School might expect of them; they carried on other social and School activities. During the war they took an active part in the student recruitment program. With the organization of the Student Association, the School grew up to adult stature.

An immediate problem confronting the faculty was the recruitment of students, so important in the national defense effort with the increasing absorption of graduate nurse personnel into the armed forces. Then Pearl Harbor was bombed. Immediately national and state recruitment measures were accelerated and schools of nursing everywhere redoubled their efforts. Well they knew that now the country was at war the depletion of their graduate nurse staffs would become increasingly acute. The National Nursing Council for War Service, after analyzing nursing needs, suggested that hospital nurses were one of the groups that could be released most readily from civilian service. Directives would soon be issued by the Procurement and Assignment Service, War Manpower Commission, specifying the amount of professional nursing service allowed to patients in hospitals. Surgeon General Thomas Parran emphatically stated, "Nursing is a strategic defense skill of which we have a serious shortage."

Two hospital units were organized at Hopkins on request of the Surgeon General of the Army: General Hospital No. 18 and General Hospital No. 118. Sixty nurses from the Johns Hopkins staff went overseas with the two units in the spring of 1942, of these twenty-three were in teaching positions. By June 1943 another seventy-one had joined the Army and Navy.

The Johns Hopkins Hospital School of Nursing had launched a vigorous and widespread recruitment program during the latter part of 1941. Sixty-three students entered the School in February 1942, the largest spring class admitted to that date. The total admissions for the year 1942 were 195 as against 101 during 1941 and 82 during 1940. The 1941 campaign had paid well.

The establishment in 1943 of the United States Cadet Nurse Corps gave a tremendous impetus to national recruitment. The extent to which Hopkins cooperated with the Corps program is indicated by the fact that by February 1945, 404 of the 465 students enrolled in the School were also enrolled in the Cadet Nurse Corps. Admissions increased, though not appreciably; during 1943, 202 students were admitted; during 1944, 214. It seems probable that the approximate maximum admissions had been reached during 1942 as a result of the excellent and intensive work on recruitment by the School itself and the program of the National Nursing Council for War Service.

The military and civilian exigencies which forced student nurse recruitment to the limit inevitably tended to react on admission requirements. In good schools of nursing and in the nursing profession at large, it was recognized that numbers alone would not suffice, that quality of recruits was of equal importance to meet either the emergency created by a terrible war or the health and hospital needs that follow war. While principles should not be conceded, flexible admission procedures, wisely administered, were essential for securing quantitative goals without sacrificing basic qualitative standards. For the war period, at least, formal rulings should be reconsidered.

During 1941 and 1942 at the Johns Hopkins School of Nursing, the general education of the newly admitted students did not differ markedly from the education of students admitted prior to that time. One hundred and one students were admitted in 1941; of this number 36 per cent had baccalaureate degrees and 49 per cent from one to three years of college. In 1942, 195 students entered the School; 40 per cent had degrees and 44 per cent one or more years of college. During the 1943–1944 national campaign, these proportions tended to shift, and a larger per cent was admitted whose education did not extend beyond high school.

Until this country entered the war the minimum age requirement for admission was twenty. The 1942–1943 School bulletin stated, "Because of the need for a larger number of well qualified nurses due to the war, exceptions to this general policy may be made." At the same time the School adopted a policy designed to provide one other admission instrument for judging the suitability of a candidate with questionable credentials. The faculty recommended to the Advisory Board of the School and the Board approved the recommendation, "that psychological and aptitude tests, as offered by the Psychological Corporation . . . be required of those applicants . . . whose credentials leave us in doubt as to their eligibility or suitability for nursing."

As a part of the national defense and recruitment effort, five summer preclinical programs were offered by cooperating schools of nursing; during 1941, 1942, and 1945 at Bryn Mawr College, Bryn Mawr, Pennsylvania, and during 1943 and 1944 at Goucher College in Baltimore. The program at Bryn Mawr was patterned after the program at the Training Camp for Nurses at Vassar College and was the brain-child of Mrs. Thomas Raeburn White, an alumna of Bryn Mawr and also of the Vassar Training Camp. The American Red Cross sponsored the Bryn Mawr plan and generously subsidized it the first year.

The educational requirement for admission to the program at Bryn Mawr was two or more years of acceptable college work; at Goucher, high school graduation. The Johns Hopkins Hospital School of Nursing had the largest number of students in each of the summer courses. The School also lent faculty members to participate in the teaching at both colleges: at Bryn Mawr, K. Virginia Betzold, Frances U. Reiter, 1931, Della Lang (Mrs. Chester J. Bramhall), 1944, Elizabeth Gould, Katherine K. Sanford, Eleanor A. Hall, Barbara L. Tate, Mrs. Anne D. Joslin, and Senior Cadet Lucille Wright; at Goucher College, Miss Sanford, Miss Hall, Olga Andruskiw, Wilhelmina Stafford, Elizabeth Moser, 1926, and S. Evelyn Moore, 1943. Jessie B. Black (Mrs. G. J. McVicar), 1930, was dean of both Goucher summer programs.

The National Nursing Council for War Service considered the recruitment of college women into nursing a highly important phase of its program.[6] All during the Forties, colleges and uni-

[6] In response to a request from the Council the following members from

versities were graduating annually between seventy and one hundred thousand women, and it was important that the opportunities in professional nursing for a socially useful and personally satisfying career be brought before this group. It was equally important that college graduates enter schools of nursing whose educational standards were high and whose administrative policies conformed generally to those operating in colleges. Otherwise nursing would neither attract nor hold the college woman.

At Hopkins early in 1944 the Advisory Board of the School of Nursing and the Trustees of the Hospital concurred with and approved the recommendation of the faculty that a baccalaureate degree from an institution of higher education, accredited by a national or regional association, be made the educational requirement for admission. Historically this action reflected the philosophy of the School since its beginning—the selection of applicants with superior qualifications as fundamental to the conduct of a sound, a broad, and an effective program in nursing education. At that time the Trustees also favorably considered the transfer of the School from the control of the Hospital to the control of the University, and this change in admission requirements represented one step toward the accomplishment of this transfer. The director of the School, Anna D. Wolf, believed that nursing could render its most beneficent service nourished in the atmosphere of a university. It was in the order of things that Miss Wolf should strive to have the School made an organic part of the Johns Hopkins University, coordinating its activities with the Johns Hopkins Hospital.

In the autumn of 1946 the Special Committee for the Consideration of a University School of Nursing was appointed with Dr. Francis F. Schwentker as chairman. Other members of the committee were Dr. Alan M. Chesney, representing the School of Medicine of the Johns Hopkins University; Dr. Ernest L. Stebbins, the University School of Hygiene and Public Health; Dr.

---

the Hopkins School faculty were temporarily released to assist with the program: Mrs. Jessie Black McVicar, Leona V. Bowman (Mrs. P. B. Day), 1939, Alice N. Burton, 1940, Harriet Baker (Mrs. A. L. Woodruff), 1939, Harriett J. Stech (Mrs. R. D. Sloan), 1942. Other members of the faculty, not graduates of the School, also released to assist with the program were Martha Johnson and Mrs. Eloise Rallings Lewis.

Charles R. Austrian, the Johns Hopkins Hospital Medical Board; and Dr. Russell A. Nelson, the Hospital administration. The faculty of the Johns Hopkins Hospital School of Nursing was represented by Anne M. Hahn (Mrs. A. I. Lindblad), 1929, Martha Johnson, Mildred Struve, 1926, and Anna D. Wolf.

One year later, in October 1947, the Special Committee submitted its report. A major recommendation was the amplification of the already existing relationship between the Johns Hopkins Hospital School of Nursing and the University. Out of this recommendation came the decision of the University to establish a new degree, the bachelor of science in nursing, to be awarded through the medium of McCoy College [7] to candidates who had completed at least two years of approved college work in an accredited institution of higher learning and passed successfully the prescribed program of study covering thirty-two months at the Johns Hopkins Hospital School of Nursing. Provision was made at the same time that graduates who did not have two years of college work before admission would receive, after making up their deficiencies, the full senior college credit of sixty points for their program in nursing. Soon after the new arrangement became effective, the University also awarded to students graduating from the School and holding either their bachelor of science or bachelor of arts degree, the new degree of bachelor of science in nursing. For the administration of the new plan, committees with representatives of the University, the Hospital, and the School of Nursing, were appointed to recommend basic policies satisfactory to each of the institutions concerned.

The action of the University in the new arrangement bears scrutiny. In 1935 the University allowed to candidates with two years of approved college work a credit of thirty points for the 36-month nursing course at the Johns Hopkins School of Nursing and required the completion of at least thirty academic credits at the Johns Hopkins University before awarding the degree. The degree then awarded was the bachelor of science. In 1947 the University allowed to candidates with two years of acceptable

[7] McCoy College of the Johns Hopkins University was established in 1947 "by the consolidation of units of the University that had provided similar educational opportunities for nearly forty years."

college preparation a credit of sixty points for the 32-month program of the School and did not require that any work be taken within the doors of the Johns Hopkins University. The degree now awarded was a newly established degree, the bachelor of science in nursing, and was conferred only upon graduates of the Johns Hopkins Hospital School of Nursing.

Dean Francis H. Horn of McCoy College called the agreement "an unorthodox academic wedlock," and then went on to say:

"Hopkins nurses may well take satisfaction in this unique academic union. It is recognition by the University, first, that a sound program of nursing education is the equivalent of upper division college work, and second, that the superior achievement of the Johns Hopkins School of Nursing justifies this departure from the customary type of cooperative program in nursing education."[8]

An echo of pride must ring in the heart of every nurse graduated from Hopkins as she reads the words of Dean Horn. But the fact remains that the School did *not* become a collegiate school of nursing and it was still denied the educational stature and privileges predicated to schools with university status. It was still a hospital school but could rightfully claim to be one of those "distinguished hospital schools" which are defined by Dr. Esther L. Brown as having had "a long and distinguished history in providing much of the potential leadership of the profession. . . ."[9] For such schools Dr. Brown recommended "that provision should be made within the university for the continuing [of their] undiminished contribution. . . ."[10]

With the adoption of the baccalaureate degree for admission early in 1944, the School immediately reviewed its recruitment program. Since recruitment was now aimed at college graduates only, some new recruitment devices were introduced in order to reach more directly the college group and to rouse their interest in nursing as a career. The School *Circular of Information*

[8] Francis H. Horn, "Unorthodox Academic Wedlock," *Johns Hopkins Nurses Alumnae Magazine*, 47:37–39, Apr. 1948

[9] *Nursing for the Future*, pp. 127–28

[10] *Ibid.*, p. 132

was revised and sent to all colleges and universities accredited by regional and national associations. The students in the School organized a program to establish contact with their own colleges; they also participated in radio programs, told what they found interesting and challenging in nursing, and discussed what an applicant should look for in the choice of a school. Colleges requested representatives to present nursing as a career to their student body and the special advantages offered by the Johns Hopkins School. In compliance with these requests, arrangements were made for speakers, faculty and Alumnae, to visit a number of colleges throughout the country.

Fifty-six students with baccalaureate degrees entered the School in the fall of 1944; in the spring of 1945, another twenty-five. While the number admitted during the school year 1944–1945 was considerably smaller than the number admitted during each of the three prior years, it still approximated the admissions during 1939 and 1940. Considering a new trail was being explored, the results must have been regarded as encouraging.

Within a few months after the admission of the spring class, Germany surrendered, and by September Japan acknowledged defeat. The termination of hostilities brought to an end a period of unexampled, nation-wide expansion in schools of nursing. At Hopkins the total number of students in the School more than doubled the total number before war recruitment began. Unquestionably, many of the applicants admitted during the war were motivated by a genuine interest in nursing. Many others were moved by a patriotic urge to perform a service which their country needed greatly in a time of peril; with the coming of peace the urge was no longer present. During the war a traditional policy in schools of nursing, nonacceptance of married candidates, was generally reversed, and married applicants were admitted. Now that the world-wide battle was over, husbands and betrothed soldiers were returning home. Doubtless many of the married applicants cancelled their appointments, as did also many of those who were engaged. It is also likely that many potential candidates, either married or engaged to returning veterans, never submitted their applications.

In any event, even though the national and state nursing associations, the American Hospital Association, and individual schools kept up unflagging recruitment in 1946, the flow of students into nursing schools sharply diminished. One year after hostilities ceased, schools of nursing were polled by the American Hospital Association on the number of students they had appointed to their 1946 fall class; 953 schools reported the appointment of 60 per cent of the desired number.

At the Johns Hopkins Hospital not only did the national decline affect admissions, but, without doubt, one other cause entered into it. A school of nursing and a hospital were no longer synonymous to the public; there were hospital schools of nursing and there were university schools of nursing. Women with college education were aware of the significance of the university stamp upon their future professional career. This fact was soon thrust upon Hopkins, even with its half-century of prestige.

Whatever the cause or combination of causes, admissions dropped alarmingly at Hopkins in 1946 and 1947. Before Pearl Harbor, the School considered the admission of one class yearly because of the limited number of applications for the spring group. Then because of defense pressures and war activities three classes were admitted each year from 1941 through 1945. Although great effort continued to recruit a February group, the results were disappointing and would neither appreciably increase admissions nor justify the expense and work of repeating the preclinical program. After 1945 one class only was admitted in the fall of each year.

With the demobilization of military nurses, it was thought that hospitals would be able to bring their graduate nurse staffs to approximate peacetime strength. Early in 1946 the director of the School reported the approval of the Board of Trustees to increase the amount of patient nursing care as graduate nurses became available. In June of that same year new personnel policies for graduate nurses became effective, providing for higher salary scales and other benefits not previously granted. In 1948, a 44-hour weekly schedule for day and a 40-hour schedule for evening and night services were established for graduate nurses. Other favorable personnel practices were adopted in 1949.

To strengthen further the nursing service, the Hospital trained and employed large numbers of nurses' aides. In the fall of 1947, 123 trained nurses' aides were employed, with unfilled positions for a considerable number more. The Red Cross Volunteer Nurse's Aide group still contributed a certain amount of service. It was hoped that these measures—more time to nurse patients, training auxiliary workers to perform duties not requiring professional nursing skills, better personnel policies—would attract and hold qualified workers and stabilize the nursing service.

But shortages persisted. A certain restlessness prevailed among nurses returning from the war. Many were uncertain as to what they wanted to do and a considerable number took advantage of the G.I. Bill of Rights. Many of those who had been employed in hospitals were unwilling to go back into those institutions because of conditions of work, personnel policies, and exclusion at that time, of hospital workers from Social Security benefits. Moreover, demand continued to exceed supply in every nursing field.

In November 1940 there were 188 regularly employed nurses on the general staff at Hopkins; in December 1947, ninety-nine. To somewhat offset this depletion, a number of graduate nurses were employed by the day. Shortages, by no means, were confined to the general staff group. They included administrative officers, instructors, supervisors, and head nurses.

During the war when hospitals were being drained of their graduate nurses for the military, it was expected that student nurses would step into the breach. But the acute nursing emergency did not end with the end of hostilities, and senior students continued to fill the gaps left by unfilled positions. In the spring of 1946, three seniors at Johns Hopkins were given assistant instructor and supervisor assignments, ten, head nurse, and 159, assistant head nurse and general staff assignments. The strained nursing service and the large number of student substitutes, of necessity, affected the administration of the curriculum.

What was happening in the Hospital during this lean time of nursing personnel? Since 1940 the daily average number of patients had been gradually increasing. For the year ending June 30, 1941, the daily average was 756; for that same period in 1947, it was 827. To maintain even adequate nursing, a corresponding increase in nursing personnel was essential. The Johns Hopkins Hospital prided itself upon the quality of nursing it traditionally gave its patients. Now, because of inability to secure personnel it was seriously handicapped in carrying out that tradition.

By the end of 1947 the situation at Hopkins had become grave. Well did the executive committee of the faculty know that a critical emergency existed; that prompt action was urgent because of inability to secure graduate nurses and auxiliary workers, reduced student enrolment, and the growing hospital census. Before submitting recommendations, the executive committee was of the opinion that both the Advisory Board and the faculty should hear the report of the Special Committee for Consideration of a University School of Nursing, appointed in the autumn of 1946.

The Special Committee reported in October 1947. The recommendations of the committee included the re-establishment of the minimum educational requirement for admission during the war, high school graduation. Two months later the executive committee of the School recommended to the Advisory Board that "the diploma of the school be granted to matriculants with less than two years of college work upon the satisfactory completion of a 36-month program. . . ." The Advisory Board was favorable to this action, and voted to recommend it to the Board of Trustees which body approved it. Another recommendation made by the faculty was that all applicants with less than two years of college be required to take at their own expense the battery of tests given by the Prenursing and Guidance Test Service of the National League of Nursing Education. Applicants with two or more years of college would also be requested to take the tests when, in the opinion of the Admissions Committee, additional information was indicated to determine their suitability for nursing. In 1942, because of the war urgency for students, *only* candidates with questionable credentials, irrespective of their educational background, were required to take psychological and aptitude tests; now these tests were required of *all* students who had *less than two years of college.*

A curriculum is created out of the experience and vision of those who design it. It does not operate in a vacuum; it progresses and regresses, expands and contracts according to many environmental factors, both within and without the institution it represents. This is true of all curricula. It is particularly true of curricula in schools of nursing. For the nursing curriculum is affected not only by budget allowance, by quality of faculty and of students, by essential facilities, but by two other conditions which bear traditionally upon it: the responsibility of the school for nursing service in the hospital and—war. The Johns Hopkins School, like some twelve hundred other nursing schools, carried on its curriculum from 1940 to 1950 during a war and a postwar period when the Hospital leaned heavily on the School for nursing personnel. To maintain a balanced educational structure called for imagination and ingenuity, to adjust educational needs to Hospital and war demands.

Early in 1941, Miss Wolf reported to the Advisory Board that the annual review of the School program had been begun. About the same time the policy was adopted of granting a six-month exemption to college graduates who maintained a general rating of "B" during their first eighteen months in the School. The exemption was optional since some students might prefer to complete the three-year program required for registration in some states.

Before another annual review was due the United States had entered the war. The tempo of nursing school programs was soon attuned to critical wartime needs. At Hopkins in the spring of 1942, the curriculum was accelerated so that *all* students secured the full theoretical content and the minimum nursing practice within thirty months.[11] This arrangement released students dur-

[11] The National League of Nursing Education issued recommendations concerning curriculum adjustment in September 1942. One recommendation specified: "That schools offering the three-year curriculum plan to complete within thirty months all organized instruction and clinical experience in at least the four major services, medicine, surgery, obstetrics, and pediatrics, leaving six months free for supervised practice wherever needed in the hospital. This arrangement would also make it possible should a plan be worked out in co-operation with Army and Navy hospitals for students who choose to go into military service to have such

ing their last six months for elected or assigned supervised practice where their services were most needed within the Hospital, or for a military affiliation, should such an affiliation be established. As a further war measure and until rescinded by the Advisory Board, the time allowance policy was broadened. Students with a baccalaureate degree maintaining a "C" instead of a "B" average were eligible for a six-month exemption; students with two or three years of college work maintaining a "C" average, for an exemption of four months.

The acceleration of the program involved faculty reconsideration of the content of courses with special reference to elimination of repetition and inclusion of essentials only. Many classes and lectures were repeated for a better correlation of theory and practice, and clinical instruction was stressed. By the time the United States Cadet Nurse Corps was established, the accelerated curriculum had been in operation for more than a year. The School program was then well-organized to expand its opportunities, especially those in the public health nursing field, offered during the supervised practice or senior cadet period.

When the educational requirement for admission was changed to baccalaureate degree in the spring of 1944, the Advisory Board of the School authorized a special committee to examine the curriculum and to determine whether it would satisfy graduate standards of education. Professor Lowell J. Reed, director of the Johns Hopkins University School of Hygiene and Public Health, was appointed chairman of the committee. Other members were: Dr. Warfield M. Firor and Dr. Russell A. Nelson from the faculty of the Johns Hopkins University School of Medicine; K. Virginia Betzold, Dr. Katherine K. Sanford, Mildred Struve, and Anna D. Wolf from the faculty of the School of Nursing.

The Special Committee on the Curriculum began its work by a detailed study of the program of the School. After comparing the *Curriculum Guide for Schools of Nursing* of the National League of Nursing Education, the curricula of the Yale University, the Frances Payne Bolton, and the Johns Hopkins Hospital

an affiliation during this six months; or later if the need becomes more acute, students might be released to enter military service at the end of the thirty months." See *American Journal of Nursing,* 42:1182, Oct. 1942.

schools of nursing and also examining course outlines of the School and other pertinent materials, the committee decided that its task consisted of two parts: (1) recommendations for the curriculum for the class to be admitted in October 1944; (2) recommendations for the curriculum to be established as soon as possible after the war.

With some modifications the Special Committee recommended the 30-month curriculum as outlined in the 1944–1945 *Circular* for the classes admitted during the war. For the postwar program the committee submitted a 32-month curriculum. Students who desired a 36-month program to comply with registration requirement in one or more states could elect an additional four months.

The clinical portion of the postwar curriculum consisted of two clinical units for students registered for the 32-month program and a third unit for those desiring a three-year course. Clinical Unit 1 covered sixty-four weeks; Clinical Unit 2, forty. Clinical Unit 1 was planned upon the premise that sequence of assignment in clinical nursing is *not* all-important, "provided basic preclinical instruction is inclusive, instruction in the clinical subjects is correlated with practice, and adequate guidance is given the student as she participates in patient care." [12] In accord with this premise the postwar curriculum proposed that at the completion of the preclinical period the class be divided into four groups, each group to be assigned a 16-week practice unit. Group 1 would be assigned to four weeks of psychiatric nursing, followed by twelve weeks of medical; Group 2, to eight weeks of surgical nursing, then to eight weeks of operating room; Group 3, to sixteen weeks of pediatric nursing, which provided for observation of the well child and sequence of experience in the care of prematures and infants, in the play activities program, in the care of children, and in the outpatient department; Group 4 would be assigned to obstetric and gynecological nursing with experience sequence in the care of prenatal mothers, the delivery room, the care of the newborn, postpartum mothers, gynecological inpatients and outpatients. As a group completed a 16-week unit it would be assigned to another unit. By the end of sixty-four

[12] K. Virginia Betzold, "Our New Curriculum," *Johns Hopkins Nurses Alumnae Magazine*, 46:51–52, Apr. 1947

weeks all four groups would have rotated through the four blocks of practice with a program of instruction, changed sufficiently for each group, to be built upon previous learnings. Nutrition in health and illness would be given as part of each clinical assignment, and emphasis placed on the social and psychological aspects of nursing.

Clinical Unit 2 followed a more orthodox pattern. It included eight weeks of psychiatric and eight weeks of public health nursing; four weeks each of urological, ophthalmological, communicable disease, medical, and surgical nursing; and also four weeks in the nursing care of medical and surgical patients in the outpatient department.

Clinical Unit 3, designed for those students wishing to complete a three-year program, provided an elective of sixteen weeks in any one of the clinical fields or in public health.

The plan of Clinical Unit 1 was frankly an experiment with a new pattern in nursing education, contrary to traditional practice. From this experiment it appeared that neither the type of patient nor the sequence of experience, but the nature of instruction, carefully selected and carefully interrelated, and its correlation with practice, were the key factors for successful student learning and growth.

The Board of Trustees approved in 1945 the postwar curriculum recommended by the Special Committee. With the class admitted in September 1946, the implementation of this program began.

A reconsideration of the curriculum was again in order when, late in 1947, the minimum educational requirement for admission reverted to graduation from high school. As a result two programs were offered. One extended over thirty-six months for students with less than two years of college work. The second program provided for a 32-month course and was offered to students with two or more years of acceptable college work. It was this second program for which the Johns Hopkins University agreed to grant sixty senior college credits and to award upon its successful completion the degree of bachelor of science in nursing.

The changes made in the 1948 curricula were largely concerned with the preclinical subjects. The clinical portion of the program was not at that time revised. The following year certain changes were made in service assignments in Clinical Units 1 and 2. The basic philosophy underlying the clinical program remained the same.

In May 1946 the faculty voted that the case method assignment of patients be instituted. For the successful operation of the new educational program it was essential that a student be assigned to a group of patients for whose complete care she was responsible. Plainly the student who saw the patient only when she took his temperature or gave him a hypodermic injection could know little about the man, no matter what she knew about the disease.

While revisions were being made in the general curriculum design, other important curriculum developments were occurring. An innovation in 1946 in the pediatric area, was the inauguration of the "Play Activities Program," subsidized by the Women's Auxiliary Board. Organized and directed by the Pediatric Nursing Department, this program provided not only service to children but also a practice field for the education of nurses.

To mention the play activities program is to recall Helen Mary Schnetzer. Miss Schnetzer was graduated from St. Vincent's Hospital School of Nursing in New York City. When she came to Hopkins as assistant director and head of pediatric nursing in the Harriet Lane Home for Invalid Children in 1943, she had already served six years at the New York Hospital as head nurse, instructor and supervisor of pediatric nursing.

Helen Schnetzer was endowed with an overflow of kindness, understanding, and confidence in human beings and a profound desire to give service. Combined with these qualities were great teaching talent, a fine precision in writing, exceptional insight into the nursing needs of children, and the ability to translate that insight into a working program. It was she who organized and directed the program of play activities, later named "The Helen Schnetzer Play Activities Program." When Miss Schnetzer's career, so full of useful and brilliant promise, ended in 1949 at the age of forty-four, her death was truly a loss to the children and students whose lives she might have touched.

Another event which affected significantly the curriculum was the return to the School in 1947 of Harriet Kennelly (Mrs. W.

T. B. Mitchell), 1917. Mrs. Mitchell was appointed assistant director, instructor of social psychology, mental hygiene, and psychosomatic nursing. Following her graduation from Hopkins and studies at Northwestern University and later McGill University where she secured the degree of doctor of philosophy, Mrs. Mitchell held a number of important positions in the field of mental hygiene. She was exceptionally well-qualified for her post at the Hopkins School of Nursing.

When Mrs. Mitchell began her work in the School she participated in the direction of the four-week psychiatric assignment which preceded medical practice in Clinical Unit 1. As she experimented with that block of instruction and practice, she became convinced that more extensive social science should be included in the preclinical term so that students having their first experience in clinical nursing would have an understanding of the social and psychological aspects of nursing. As a result of this experimentation, a course of seventy-five hours in social psychology was added to the preclinical program. This course and an inservice program for faculty and staff, given by Mrs. Mitchell, stimulated and influenced the application of the psychosomatic concept to clinical nursing. Students became more acutely aware that nursing consists of several essential ingredients—the social, the psychological, and the physical—and that neglect of any one of these might have tragic results for the patient.

Mrs. Mitchell's responsibilities also included counseling of students. The first appointee to the position of counselor to students was Loula E. Kennedy. Officially Miss Kennedy began her work as counselor in 1943; actually she had served in that capacity throughout the twenty years she had been director of instruction.

Miss Kennedy retired in 1946. Then for several years the director of the School and two other faculty members assumed the major responsibility for counseling activities.

In 1948 important changes were made in the counseling program. These changes grew out of a plan, initiated in 1935, which provided for a psychological examination of first-year students and a conference of one-half hour. This program was first administered by Dr. Esther Loring Richards, associate professor of psychiatry in the Johns Hopkins University School of Medicine and lecturer in the School of Nursing; after January 1936 by Dr. Rachel Gundry, instructor in psychiatry in the School of Medicine. Dr. Richards continued to serve as consultant to students with personality and psychiatric problems until 1942. By 1948 Dr. Gundry was unable to carry further the program because of the burden of her own work. Thereafter all students were scheduled for a one-hour conference early in their preclinical term with Mrs. Mitchell.

Mrs. Mitchell outlined a counseling plan based upon the premise that practically every student has counseling needs at some time during her course. These needs she classified administratively into four major areas: educational, physical health, emotional health, and social and recreational. The plan emphasized that such counseling divisions were purely arbitrary and largely for administrative efficiency.

The director of the School was the coordinator of all counseling services. While the entire faculty participated to some extent in counseling, inasmuch as student guidance is implicit in every learning experience, especially qualified members assumed the major responsibility in each of the four areas. In the educational area the associate director had the major role. She interpreted policies of the School to the student and assisted her with matters pertaining to the educational program; she arranged for special tutoring, for financial assistance when needed, and for opportunities for work for pay when desired. She discussed study following graduation and opportunities in the nursing field. It was also the responsibility of this counselor to consider with the student any personal difficulty and advise her of special aids and services relevant to her problem.

In the area of physical health the supervisor of the health service was the major counselor. She was head of the semiprivate patient division where the Nurses' Infirmary was located, and where physical examinations and health recommendations were made and health records filed. The health counselor early became acquainted with the health status of the individual student, and was able to give well-considered advice on problems of physical illness and health throughout the course.

Mrs. Mitchell who had outlined the new counseling program

became counselor in the emotional health area. Her responsibilities were primarily preventive. The one-hour conference which she had with each member of the preclinical group enabled her to become acquainted with the student as a person. She provided opportunities to discuss, in a confidential relationship, any special problems of adjustment; gave personal guidance to the student with regard to any immediate problem she might be experiencing; and initiated and developed a friendly relationship. The student's state of emotional health and growth was of paramount importance to this counselor.

In the social and recreational area the residence director had been acting as counselor since 1944. Her functions were more sharply defined in the new plan of counseling. It was stressed that the residence director operated in a double capacity: as counselor to the individual and as counselor to the group. Generally speaking, the guidance she gave was extracurricular in character. She advised and assisted in matters pertaining to the student's life and comfort in the School residence and at the recreational cottage in Sherwood Forest; she assisted with plans for social events and helped organize groups of various kinds—choral, hobby, and so on; she made available to students information about the rich and varied community resources for entertainment and recreation.

Great emphasis was placed, in the implementation of the program, upon the fact that effective counseling required the closest cooperation and discreet exchange of significant information between the four administrative areas; that "the individual student functions as a unity" and that constructive guidance must be built upon the treatment of the student as *a whole person.* "Individual growth and maturity cannot be forced. It can only be encouraged and guided. The student grows and matures most wholesomely under school conditions that enable her to learn self-direction, self-discipline, independent judgment, and the assumption of responsibility for self and others through experiences intelligently designed to progressively promote such learnings." [13] Upon this concept the new counseling program of the School was developed. The objectives and activities of the Student Association, which

[13] From unpublished material by Mrs. Harriet Kennelly Mitchell.

by 1948 had operated for seven years, facilitated student understanding and cooperation with the program.

Other noteworthy changes during the Forties concerned reorganization of the central administrative offices, hour schedules, vacations, fees, and the introduction of an orientation period. In the reorganization of the central administrative offices, two non-nurse workers were employed early in the Forties as registrar and assistant registrar, positions previously held by two nurse office assistants. After 1941 the hour schedule was consistently given in terms which included *both class and practice*. Late in 1942 a 52-hour week, with one day each week free from practice, was approved for students during the clinical period. A few months later, in 1943, the 48-hour week became effective for first-year students; by the end of 1946, for all students. Early in 1947 the Board of Trustees acted favorably on the recommendation of the faculty that the class of 1949 and succeeding classes be scheduled not more than forty-four hours of classwork and practice each week. Vacation time was extended to ten weeks for students taking the 32-month program, to twelve weeks for students taking the 36-month course.

No change had been made in tuition fees since 1921, but some charges, such as those for books, had been added to student expenses. In 1941 a health fee and the cost of all uniforms were charged to students. Two years later a tuition fee of $50 for the second term of the first year was established. In 1947 tuition fees for the entire program were increased to $400, total expenses to approximately $580.

While the School had provision through loan funds and scholarships for financial aid to students, the moneys so available were necessarily limited. To help students further, rates of pay were adopted early in the Forties for certain student services, such as typing, library, or tutoring of other students. Of special interest was the service described as "work experience." Work experience referred to controlled extension of practice over that specified for curriculum requirements. Students who had maintained a certain level of achievement and a good health record were permitted to work ten hours more each week than their regular schedule, either on clinical services where they were currently assigned or on services where they already had had practice.

A four-day orientation period was inaugurated late in the Forties as part of the total program. During this period there were no classes; registration, health examinations, pretests, and other preliminary activities were conducted. On the first day a parent conference was held. Miss Wolf and other members of the faculty met the parents, explained to them the general plan of the School program, took them on a tour of the lecture rooms, laboratories, and library, and entertained them at afternoon tea and an evening reception. The reception followed a general convocation ceremony, begun in 1941, to bring together and to welcome the new class and to award the diploma to senior students who had completed their program since the May commencement or were in the last month of their course of study.

During the Forties the loss of instructors and supervisors wrought havoc with the administration of the curriculum. According to the oft-quoted dictum, attributed to Mark Hopkins, a school consists of a log with a student at one end and a teacher at the other. Figuratively, if not literally, especially during the war years, in schools of nursing the teacher end of the log was without a teacher. Early in the war, twenty-three teaching members of the Hopkins School faculty left to go overseas with the Hopkins Hospital units. The migration had begun.

Not only was there loss of nurse instructors but also of physicians who lectured on the medical aspects of the curriculum. The School soon realized that the depletion of the medical staff might require a change in the teaching plan, with less dependence on instruction by physicians and more on instruction by nurses.

While the nurse instructors at Hopkins assumed greater responsibility for incorporating in their teaching of clinical subjects those aspects usually given by the medical staff, instruction in the science courses was transferred from nurse members of the faculty to other professional groups. In 1941 the biological and physical sciences were taught by nurse instructors; in 1942 by members of the faculties of the Johns Hopkins University School of Medicine and the School of Hygiene and Public Health. Then in 1943 the appointment of a highly qualified instructor of sciences, Katherine K. Sanford, Ph.D., neither a nurse nor a physician, stabilized instruction in the science area for the duration.

The instructional difficulties of the School were not only concerned with securing qualified instructors to replace those entering the armed services, but also with increasing the number of teachers to keep pace with the increasing enrolment. Within three years, between 1941 and 1944, student enrolment had practically doubled. Three new appointees in three newly created positions took office in September 1944: Margaret F. Grainger, 1930, as coordinator of medical and surgical nursing; Carrington F. Owen, 1937, as instructor of obstetric nursing; and Ruth L. Greenfield, 1941, as instructor of surgical nursing of children. A few months later the Board of Trustees approved additional instructors in other departments of the Hospital where students were assigned. About the same time a survey of the programs in obstetric and pediatric nursing by Ruth Doran, 1924, a representative of the United States Children's Bureau, resulted in a subsidy by the Bureau for an assistant director in charge of the obstetric program and an instructor and supervisor in the care of the premature infant. Insofar as it was possible, the School safeguarded the care of patients and the education of students by the essential faculty.

Not the least of the administrative problems in a school of nursing in a time of emergency is that of promoting and providing for faculty growth. The organization of the nursing faculty at Johns Hopkins created a regularized channel for reviewing current issues in nursing service and nursing education. The courses given at the Johns Hopkins University provided another aid to faculty development. For some time the University had offered to nurses courses in general education. In 1942 Jessie B. Black was appointed to teach the principles of supervision; in 1943 the University expanded its offerings to include courses in ward management and teaching, in principles and methods of teaching in nursing schools, and in evaluation and reorganization of nursing procedures. Members of the School faculty participated in the teaching of these courses: K. Virginia Betzold, Eleanor A. Hall, Martha Johnson, and Helen M. Schnetzer. The following year Margaret

F. Grainger gave the course in ward management and teaching. The staff was informed that to qualify for the position of head nurse the individual must either have had a course in ward management and teaching, or register for the one given at the University, or for one comparable to it. Seventy-six graduate nurses and thirty-five seniors registered for the course at Johns Hopkins University in the fall of 1944.

As it was possible, senior members of the faculty were given leaves of absence to pursue advanced study at a university. Many of the faculty served in various capacities in the state and national organizations. Among the more important offices held were: president of the Maryland States Nurses' Association, by Mildred Struve; president of the Maryland League of Nursing Education, by Miriam Ames; chairman of the Curriculum Committee of the National League of Nursing Education, by K. Virginia Betzold who was also a member of the League Committee on the Administration of the Accrediting Program. Anna D. Wolf was elected secretary of the National League of Nursing Education during the Forties; she was appointed to a number of national and international groups. She was advisor to the first federal nurse aid program, a member of the Committee to Study Proposals for a Student Nurse Corps, of the Advisory Committee for guiding the programs of the Nurse Training Act of 1943, of the Joint Committee on the Structure of National Nursing Organizations, and of the National Nursing Planning Committee. Miss Wolf testified at Congressional hearings on the proposed "Nurse Draft" legislation and on other legislative proposals concerned with nursing. Her Red Cross activities included membership on the National Committee on Red Cross Nursing Service and also on the Nursing Advisory Committee to the director, appointment to the Nursing Division of the American Red Cross Advisory Board on Health Services, and representation of the League of Red Cross Societies to the Grand Council of the Florence Nightingale International Foundation.

Between 1940 and 1950 the School lost faculty members who had served it for many years. One of these was Loula E. Kennedy. Miss Kennedy retired in 1946.

Loula E. Kennedy, of the class of 1903, was a graduate of Goucher College, Baltimore. She had been on the faculty continuously for twenty-five years. During twenty of these years she was director of theoretical instruction. In that capacity she exercised considerable influence on the development of the School. Her interests extended beyond curriculum considerations; she saw the School as a whole. She was convinced that the success of the program depended on the quality of the students admitted; that the total environment—health, social, counseling as well as instructional—was the determining factor in effective school conduct. She worked persistently for better hour schedules, for better health practices. Not only after her official appointment as counselor, but throughout her tenure she gave, without stint, sympathetic guidance and help to staff as well as to students. One of her major contributions was her work for the better organization of the library.

It is not easy to delineate the personality and character of Miss Kennedy. She fully enjoyed life and had a quiet sense of humor; she was modest, unassuming, and selfless, yet withal tenacious in matters affecting the welfare of students and the advancement of the School. Although never robust in appearance, she possessed great wells of vigor. Her resources lay in both her physical and her moral strengths. Miss Kennedy must have left on many of the more than two thousand students she taught an abiding influence of the spirit.

The School lost another long-time faculty member in the middle Forties. Early in 1945 Christina M. Dick, of the class of 1899, died after a brief illness. Most of Miss Dick's adult life had been spent at Hopkins. As residence director, a position she held for twenty-seven years, she will long be remembered.

Miss Dick was a handsome woman. She was tall, straight, well-proportioned. Her appearance might have created awe, had it not been for a ready smile and ofttime hearty laugh. She had an unusual personality and a great zest for life, was somewhat unpredictable and could, on occasions, be angry and severe. She was thoroughly interested in people. This interest manifested itself in a warmth of manner which, together with her natural sparkle and humor, created confidence in students. Her student reprimands usually took the form of jingles, which might be posted in the elevator of Hampton House or left in the bedroom of the student.

Above all Miss Dick wanted the residence to be truly a home, in spirit as well as mere physical accommodations. Her efforts to accomplish this end were unceasing. In 1931 the student publication, *Routine,* was dedicated to Miss Dick. The dedication reads:

"In acknowledgment of her wise counsel, in recognition of the continuance of her loyalty, in admiration of the charm and delightfulness of her individuality, the Senior Class gladly dedicates the Routine of 1931 to Miss Christina M. Dick."

Not only did the School lose faculty during the Forties, it also lost in Dr. Smith's retirement a staunch supporter and a friend.

Dr. Winford H. Smith retired on April 1, 1946 as director of the Johns Hopkins Hospital after thirty-five years of conspicuous service. He had been closely associated with eminent nurse educators before coming to Hopkins; he was general medical superintendent of Bellevue and Allied Hospitals while Annie W. Goodrich was director of nursing and also Clara D. Noyes. He was a member of the Committee for the Study of Nursing Education sponsored by the Rockefeller Foundation and of the Committee for the Grading of Nursing Schools. A number of renowned nursing leaders served on both of those committees.

To what extent, if any, these associations affected Dr. Smith's thinking with respect to nursing education cannot be known. This much is certain—Dr. Smith had his own convictions on the relationship that should exist between schools of nursing and their sponsoring hospitals. Speaking before the National League of Nursing Education in 1915 he said, "The point has been made by Mr. Flexner that hospitals owe a duty to medical education. . . . I would also make the point that hospitals owe a duty to nursing education. . . ." [14] Dr. Smith knew well and so stated in an editorial in the *Modern Hospital* [15] that the root of the opposition to better programs in nursing schools was financial; that nursing costs the hospital more as the educational standards of the nursing school are raised. By his own word he believed that "schools for

[14] *National League of Nursing Education Annual Report, 1915,* p. 165

[15] *Modern Hospital,* 1:34, Sept. 1913

nurses should be recognized as educational institutions, the graduates of which are professional women, who have important functions to perform in the interest of public welfare.[16]

Dr. Smith supported wholeheartedly the efforts of the Alumnae Association to provide an endowment for the School. He was proud of the School and earnestly desired the means to strengthen it and to give it financial stability. When Dr. Smith left Hopkins he took with him the deep respect and warm esteem of the many Hopkins nurses who had been associated with him for more than three decades.

Dr. Edwin L. Crosby succeeded Dr. Smith. Dr. Crosby had been officially connected with the Hospital as assistant director before his appointment as director. He began his tenure during the difficult period of transition from war to peace. Dr. Crosby's interest in the development of the School and his support made possible many important measures in both the program of the School and of the nursing service.

When Hester K. Frederick retired in 1941, Jessie B. Black was appointed as associate director of the School and the nursing service. Most of Miss Black's tenure was during the time when this country was at war. Not only did she make a contribution to the program of the School, but she also gave valuable war service as dean of the preclinical programs offered by Goucher College and as a temporary appointee on the recruitment staff for college students of the National Nursing Council for War Service.

When Miss Black resigned to be married in 1945, the dual position of associate director of the School and of the nursing service was abolished. This was significant action. Thereafter one associate to the director had the responsibility for the immediate administration of the total educational program, and another the responsibility for the immediate administration of the nursing service. Faye Whiteside, 1919, was appointed associate director of the nursing service early in 1945. Miss Whiteside had been associated with the Peiping Union Medical College, Peiping, China, for a number of years and, as superintendent of nurses, had given outstanding service. She was there on Pearl Harbor

[16] *Johns Hopkins Nurses Alumnae Magazine*, 18:113. Aug. 1919

day when the institution was taken over by the Japanese. In 1944 Miss Whiteside returned to this country. After devoting a year to study at Teachers College, Columbia University, she accepted the appointment at Hopkins.

K. Virginia Betzold returned as associate director of the School in 1943. Miss Betzold had been connected with the School continuously since 1934 except for several leaves of absence: one year as an international student to attend the Florence Nightingale International Foundation in London, England; eighteen months for study at Teachers College, Columbia University; and two summer terms to teach at the Bryn Mawr Summer School of Nursing.

As this history came to a close at the end of 1949 Miss Whiteside continued to hold the position of associate director of the nursing service and Miss Betzold, associate director of the School. Both Miss Whiteside and Miss Betzold rendered notable service during the difficult Forties: Miss Whiteside as a nursing service administrator thoroughly acquainted with the principles and problems of nursing service administration and, most important, experienced in meeting them; Miss Betzold as a nursing educator, possessed of keen insight and grasp of curriculum fundamentals, and well able to guide the new experimental program of the School.

The decade between 1940 and 1950 came to an end. The history of these ten years was a chronicle of global struggle. Events of great moment succeeded each other, world startling and cataclysmic. As always in war and in great social crisis, hospitals and nursing felt the thrust of events.

To head the program of the School and Hospital nursing service during the critical war and the postwar period required leadership of a high order. Anna D. Wolf was such a leader. Miss Wolf saw with clarity, undimmed by present urgencies, that the first purpose of any school, nursing or other, is to prepare its students for the profession of their choice; she just as clearly perceived that the first purpose of a hospital nursing service is to give its patients adequate care. She recognized that in time of war or other emergency the first purpose of a nursing school might temporarily

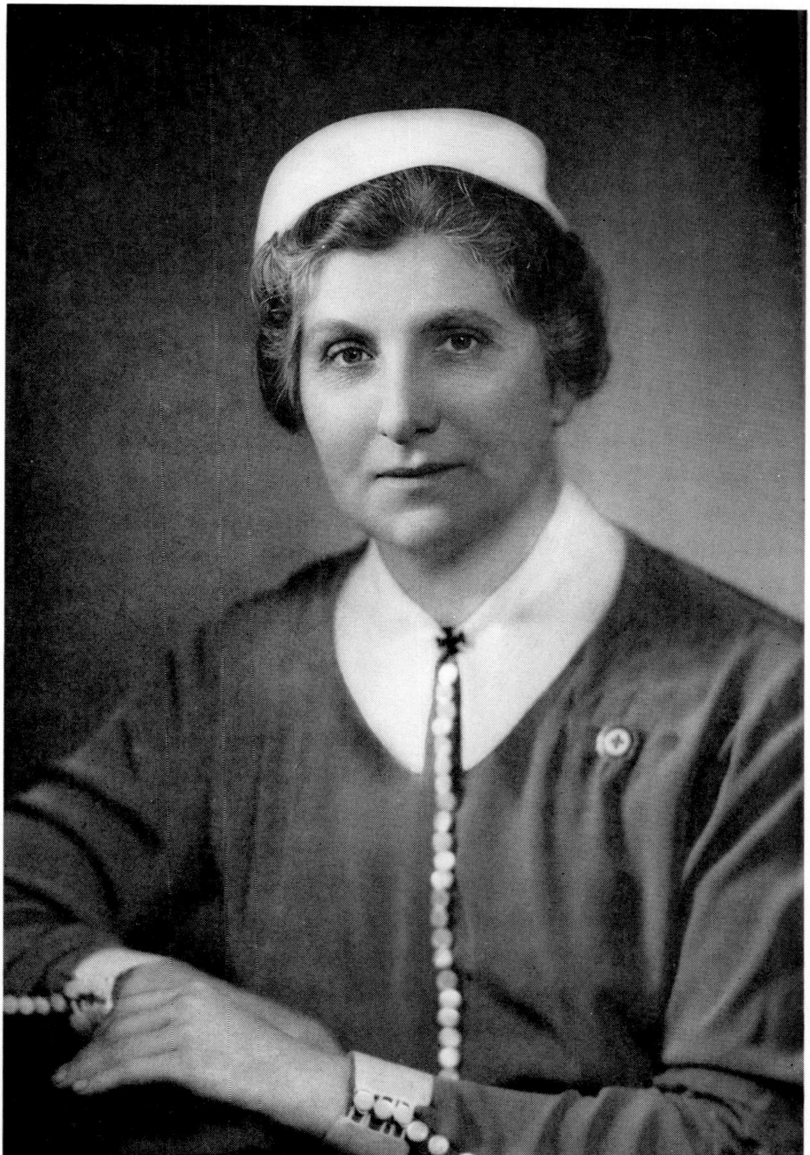

ANNA DRYDEN WOLF

Director, School of Nursing and Nursing Service, 1940–

BACHRACH

give way to the pressing urgencies of nursing service; she was convinced that when peace and normal conditions returned the School should regain its rightful educational status. In a dual position such as director of the School and of the nursing service, which Miss Wolf held at the Johns Hopkins Hospital, she knew that two designs were necessary—one for the School and one for the nursing service—and that each should maintain its essential identity and integrity and each contribute to the other. Her work testified to this knowledge, in practice as well as principle. Mary M. Roberts, editor of the *American Journal of Nursing*, described Miss Wolf as "one of the directors of schools of nursing who makes a real correlation between nursing education and nursing service."

Miss Wolf had a profound sense of nursing as a great human service. She believed that the Johns Hopkins Hospital School of Nursing had an historical obligation to send forth leaders aware of their social privileges, opportunities, and responsibilities. She always had visions for tomorrow. She was an individual "in whom the power of thought and the power of action are . . . balanced, conscious of the past, equal to the present, and reaching forward into the future."

The First Sixty Years

In the autumn of 1949, the Johns Hopkins Hospital School of Nursing was sixty years old. It was officially opened on October 9, 1889, five months after the formal inauguration of the Hospital, thirteen years after the University, and four years before the School of Medicine. Professional schools of nursing were still in their infancy; in the city of Baltimore "there had not as yet appeared a training school for nurses." As a pioneer in a new professional field in a locale where the field was little known, the School was peculiarly favored in the soil in which it took root. It was established in connection with a great new hospital, which was closely associated with a great new university. The Hospital and the University soon became famous throughout the world. The School of Nursing could do no less.

If it is true that history is largely affected by the work of individuals, then the Johns Hopkins Hospital School of Nursing was singularly fortunate in its first two principals, Isabel A. Hampton and M. Adelaide Nutting. Both were standard bearers of a young profession; both had high ideals of nursing, far-seeing vision, and a dream for the future. Their dream was a simple dream—a school built upon a bedrock of sound professional and cultural education. They sought to make the Johns Hopkins School of Nursing "looked to for what is best in nursing," as the University and the Hospital were looked to "for what is best in science." They set forth principles and introduced innovations; out of these principles and innovations came the character and traditions of the School.

Among the early innovations, that must have seemed radical at the time, were the reduction of the ward schedule from nine to eight hours, the extension of the course from two to three years, the abolition of cash allowances to students, and the establishment of a six-month preparatory course and a tuition fee to pay at least for part of the first-year instruction. But in withdrawing allowances and charging tuition, the School was not unmindful of "those poor but desirable women" who would not be able to receive the training without financial help. A certain number of scholarships was recommended and granted by the Hospital Trustees to students who demonstrated their worthiness. The principle of good bedside nursing was established by Miss Hampton in her address at the inauguration of the School. Said Miss Hampton, "It is not so much the great amount of work that she can accomplish . . . but the kind of work, and to render unto each patient under her care nursing in its best methods, and truest sense. . . ." Throughout the sixty years, bedside nursing in its "truest sense" has been emphasized as the foundation of all nursing and long ago became a tradition in the Johns Hopkins Hospital.

When Miss Nutting left Johns Hopkins in the spring of 1907, the School held a commanding position in the nursing schools of this country and in other countries—wherever schools were groping for new ways to better the existing nurse training systems. From home and abroad came a stream of visitors, continued to this day, to observe and to study the educational program. Out of the ideals, ideas, and determined efforts of Isabel Hampton and Adelaide Nutting a lusty young School had been born. The Johns Hopkins School of Nursing had become a symbol for progress.

Georgina C. Ross followed Miss Nutting but her tenure was too brief to leave a stamp upon the School. Elsie M. Lawler became principal in 1910 and continued in the office until she retired in 1940.

Looking over the years between 1910 and 1940 a new pattern is discerned. A study of events which followed one another in quick succession gives meaning to the pattern. The period between 1910 and 1920 was the great expansion period of the Hospital; it was also the period of war and epidemic. While the new departments in the Hospital brought new opportunities for training, the greater numbers of patients and the increased demands for student service militated against a satisfactory educational experience. Then came the war and the epidemic. Johns Hopkins rallied its nursing resources, largely student, to meet these two disasters. The School might preserve its present program, but it could not initiate new educational plans until the emergencies had subsided and the times were more nearly normal again.

With the end of World War I and the dawn of peace, a new spirit and new hope pervaded America. New trails were to be explored, new paths broken leading to a more humanitarian and more enlightened way of living. At the Johns Hopkins Hospital, the School of Nursing reacted to the rising tide of optimism by initiating the first of a series of studies. Other studies followed, culminating in an exhaustive survey of the School by a Special Committee of the Alumnae Association composed of distinguished Alumnae members. When the Special Committee submitted its report to the Hospital Trustees in 1928 it recommended affiliation with the Johns Hopkins University. A relationship was established in 1935, and in 1947 the relationship was amplified. As this history comes to a close the School of Nursing has not been reorganized into a collegiate school; it is still a hospital school. Many years ago President Gilman wrote, "All that belongs to medical instruction should be under the control of the University; all that belongs to the care of the sick and suffering and all that concerns admission to clinical opportunities . . . belongs to the Hospital. . . ." The philosophy inherent in this statement is yet to be applied to the School of Nursing.

While the Special Committee of the Alumnae Association focussed its recommendations upon affiliation with the University, it also dealt with current administrative and educational policies. A significant event that emerged from the report was the creation of the Advisory Board of the School of Nursing with the president of the Johns Hopkins University elected chairman. Now the School had an official group whose sole function was to advise upon all matters concerned with the School as an educational entity.

The establishment of the Advisory Board infused new interests and stimulated new deliberations of the School program. During the Thirties a good beginning was made on some vital aspects of the curriculum. These included concentration on clinical instruction and the appointment of the first full-time ward instructors, and, most important, the introduction into the curriculum of public health nursing, both class and practice. By the end of 1939 the library had been remodeled and reorganized, and a few years later the School boasted of a full-time librarian. With Miss Lawler's retirement in 1940 the second period of the first sixty years came to an end.

Anna D. Wolf succeeded Miss Lawler. When Miss Wolf took office the country was engaged in developing a national defense program; it would soon be engaged in the second World War. The problem of the Forties was two-fold: to admit large numbers of students to fill the gap left by the departure of graduate nurses for military service, and at the same time to maintain a sound educational program. Nevertheless during this decade occurred some of the most significant developments in the history of the School. The administrative and teaching staffs were organized as a faculty with clearly defined functions and responsibilities. Thereafter plans were evolved and recommendations made in faculty deliberations. About the same time the faculty was organized, the students formed the Student Association of the Johns Hopkins Hospital School of Nursing. The Association created an official channel for a cooperative working relationship between the students and the faculty. An educational experiment in clinical nursing was tried out in the postwar curriculum. The soundness of the experiment was demonstrated by the achievement of students who were graduated under the plan.

The Forties saw the passing of military discipline and the introduction of a counseling program planned to help students acquire self-direction and a sense of responsibility for themselves and others. In philosophy of discipline the School had travelled a long road in the sixty years of its existence. It had abandoned the discipline of unquestioning obedience and adopted a counseling design whereby *all* students shared in their manner of learning, growing, maturing, and living together.

Among the ideals held by the School from the day of its establishment was the admission of "women of superior education and cultivation." In 1905, the *Circular* of the School announced that applicants must show evidence of having been graduated from high school or of having received the educational equivalent, a requirement boldly in advance of the time. Such was the reputation of the School that it had always had more applicants than it could accept, with an increasing number whose educational background included one or more years of college. For four years during the Forties, a baccalaureate degree was required for admission; later the educational requirement reverted to high school graduation. But the large number of applications from candidates with college preparation continued. Of sixty-six students admitted in September 1949, seventeen had baccalaureate degrees; thirty-nine, two or three years of college work; two, one year of college; and eight only were high school graduates.

Another ideal, tenaciously held to through the years, was a shorter hour schedule for students. In 1896 reform in hours began. Some further gains were made in the Twenties, and in 1948 the 44-hour week, including both class and practice, became an accomplished fact for all students.

Not all of the names of the nurses who had faith in the School and who loyally supported it appear in the foregoing pages. Of those who are not mentioned there were many. Heads of departments, supervisors, instructors, head nurses, and general staff nurses rendered valiant service; their devotion to the care of patients and the fine character of their day by day work contributed in no small measure to maintaining the morale of the institution during difficult periods and in facilitating the transition from one administration to the other. At the time of the 1918 influenza epidemic and the two world wars, Alumnae members who were engaged in private nursing or were retired or married came back into the Hospital to give service where needed. Nor must one forget the nursing students who stoutheartedly shouldered their share of responsibility in times of stress.

So far this résumé has largely recorded evidence of progress during the first sixty years. But—what is progress? A series of achievements, specific and distinguishable? Or does progress also embrace durable faith, courage, resolution, ideals, from which is distilled a heritage of the spirit? The Johns Hopkins Hospital and the Johns Hopkins Hospital School of Nursing have such a heritage, inspired by the great men and women who founded them and were there when the doors were opened sixty years ago. A long procession of nurses have been graduated from the School since that day. They have benefited richly, not only by the skills and arts passed on to them, but by the inheritance of the spirit of the place. Many have won name and fame at home and abroad. Many more have contributed to nursing in the quiet, shadowed byways of the profession. The School is justly proud of its graduates. It is justly proud of its heritage, but it has not let pride in the past obscure the necessity of seeking new ideas, new truths, and new ways. It has labored to keep bright the promise of its birth and to strive constantly for new reaches. On the sixtieth anniversary of the School, it can be truly said that the Johns Hopkins Hospital School of Nursing is a school of high merit, built upon a solid foundation of education for service.

Studies of Special Aspects of the School

The Library

THE LIBRARY spark in the School of Nursing of the Johns Hopkins Hospital was kindled before the School actually came into existence. Dr. John S. Billings, speaking before a distinguished company assembled for the formal opening of the Hospital in May 1889, noted a library among the accommodations provided in the "large and handsome building," the Nurses' Home.[1] On the same occasion President Daniel C. Gilman referring to the library in the Hospital said: "One purpose of this central building is to afford opportunities for professional intercourse. Here are rooms set apart for the library that will presently be collected; here the medical journals will be taken in. . . ." [2] To the planners of the University and the Hospital, it was inconceivable that an institution dedicated to the spread of knowledge and human service should be without a library.

Uncertainty surrounds the exact location of the library in the Nurses' Home noted by Dr. Billings. But no uncertainty veils the idea of a library; the idea may also be found in the address of Isabel

[1] *Addresses at the Opening of the Hospital.* Baltimore, John Murphy & Co., Printers, 1889, p. 30

[2] *Ibid.*, p. 54

A. Hampton at the opening of the Nurses' Home and the inauguration of the Training School. Said Miss Hampton, ". . . we trust that in these rooms some bright, pleasant, social hours may be passed, and among the books, magazines and papers that are sure to find their way here, when the need for them is realized. . . ." [3]

Nor could "books, magazines and papers" have been long in finding "their way." Miss Hampton soon organized the Journal Club. It is recorded that the first meeting on January 28, 1891, was held in the "library." One of the declared purposes of the Club was "to keep in touch with what is being done in other schools and hospitals by means of reports and discussions drawn chiefly from English and American weekly and monthly nursing magazines, and to ensure a reading of such papers by all." Two programs of the Club are extant: one for the 1894–1895 and one for the 1895–1896 period. The subjects indicate that a wide array of medical and nursing magazines must have been available to the discussants.

From the historical fragments of the Training School library during the early Nineties, it appears that the first library materials largely grew out of the Journal Club needs and consisted mostly of magazines. There were then few text or reference books for pupil nurses, but the following volumes, now in the historical collection, were undoubtedly on the shelves of the School in the early days: *Textbook of Nursing* by Clara S. Weeks, published in 1885; *Materia Medica for Nurses* by Lavinia L. Dock, written before she came to Hopkins; *Nursing: Its Principles and Practice* by Isabel A. Hampton, published in 1893; *A Handbook of Invalid Cooking* by Mary A. Boland, instructor in cooking at the Johns Hopkins Hospital Training School, also published in 1893; *Textbook of Anatomy and Physiology* by Diana C. Kimber, first published in 1894. Ruth Brewster Sherman, 1901, remembers that during the time she was in the School shelves with text and reference books were along the wall of the classroom on the ground floor of the Nurses' Home.

[3] Isabel A. Hampton, "The Aims of the Johns Hopkins Hospital Training School for Nurses," *The Johns Hopkins Hospital Bulletin*, 1:7, Dec. 1889

Fifteen months after the inauguration of the School, Dr. Hurd wrote his annual report of the Hospital for the year ending January 31, 1891. In the section on "Acknowledgments" Dr. Hurd recorded with thanks gifts received during the past year. Thanks were given "to Miss Garrett for a supply of books to the library at the Nurses' Home. . . ." The next year Dr. Osler presented to the Nurses' Library a copy of his "Practice of Medicine," and the 1895 report of the Hospital stated that twenty-five volumes for the Nurses' Library were received from Mrs. William Osler. Other gifts of books were listed from time to time in the superintendent's annual reports with the names of the donors.

The first money contribution appeared in the 1904 report: "From Mrs. Dimmock and Mrs. Terson, to be used in the purchase of books for the Training School Library, $17.00." The next gifts of money were reported in 1907: $100 from Florence M. Patterson and $50 from Mrs. Marion Yates. Contributions came, too, from the School itself: from pupils for magazines and books, $64.50 were recorded in the 1907 report; the following year $122 from the officers and pupils of the Training School, also for magazines and books. It seems likely that during these early years many gifts in the form of books, magazines, and money were given by friends directly to the School through Miss Nutting.

Fortunately, several important sources exist which identify early library content and contributors: inscriptions in the volumes themselves and three accession books. One accession book begun in 1900 gives the general literature content during the Nineties and first decade of the present century; two, begun in 1905, the historical volumes for the same period. The two books dated 1905 have the same designation in gold lettering on their black cloth binding:

JOHNS HOPKINS HOSPITAL
SCHOOL FOR NURSES

THE HISTORY & LITERATURE
OF
NURSING

1905

The first 408 volumes recorded in "The History and Literature of Nursing" books are identical; after the 408th accession, differences occur, although many of the same volumes continue to appear in both records. The condition of the two books indicates that one was handled much more than the other. The more worn book contains 839 accessions, the less worn, 699. More than half of the entries in the worn book are in Georgina C. Ross' careful, beautiful handwriting,[4] as are all in the better preserved book. One wonders why two records were kept for the same volumes; perhaps that one might last for the future, if the other, used continuously as a reference source, should not survive the wear and tear of time.

The first two volumes accessioned in "The History and Literature of Nursing" book are "Notes on hospitals" and "Notes on nursing (etc.)," both by Florence Nightingale. Opposite "Notes on hospitals" and under the Source column is written "Council of Nightingale Fund" and under the Remarks column, the unembellished note—"Presented March 1875."

Two copies of *Notes on Hospitals,* both third editions published in 1863, are in the archives of the School. In one copy on the flyleaf facing the title page is inscribed in clear, bold handwriting:

PRESENTED TO THE COMMITTEE OF
THE "JOHNS HOPKINS HOSPITAL"
BALTIMORE
BY THE COUNCIL OF THE
"NIGHTINGALE FUND"
MARCH 1875

This volume undoubtedly is the copy of *Notes on Hospitals* sent by Mr. Bonham Carter, secretary of the Nightingale Fund, at the request of Florence S. Lees, to "Judge Brown, Trustee of the Johns Hopkins Hospital . . . for the use of the Trustees." [5]

[4] Loula E. Kennedy who knew Miss Ross well identified the writing as that of Miss Ross. The author compared entries in the accession books with Miss Ross' signatures in books she gave to the library. The entries and signatures appear to have been written by the same individual.

[5] See p. 23.

The second entry, "Notes on nursing (etc.)," was given by Miss Nutting. Lavinia L. Dock gave books and magazines to the historical library; President Gilman, Dr. Hurd, Dr. Smith, Helen S. Wilmer (Mrs. C. N. Athey), 1905, Miss Ross, Ada M. Carr, and Miss Lawler contributed. Some of the early historical volumes were purchased from a "Special Fund," probably a fund accumulated from the money contributions to the library noted in the reports of the Hospital superintendent.

The year 1905 saw the inauguration of "The Teresians." [6] With the historical library already begun how better could the School profit by the collection and at the same time share in its further development than through a society organized for "first, the study of the history of nursing; second, to aid in the building up of the historical library of the Johns Hopkins Hospital Training School for Nurses. . . ." At the first meeting of the society Miss Nutting referred to the historical volumes on nursing and hospitals "now being gathered together . . . which should ultimately prove of great interest and value, not only to our own school, but perhaps be given a much wider usefulness." While the new society doubtless stimulated new interest and acquisition of new materials, by 1905 the seed of the historical library of the Johns Hopkins Training School had been well planted. Miss Nutting's interest in the collection continued all her life and all her life she gave generously to it. When she left the School in 1907, a historical library was an accepted and esteemed responsibility of the School of Nursing. Its growth appears to have been steady over the years. During the Forties it was augmented by two important collections.

Dr. Howard A. Kelly, gynecologist-in-chief for many years at the Johns Hopkins Hospital and one of "The Four Doctors" in Sargent's famous painting, had long been a collector of books and other valuable memorabilia. Among Dr. Kelly's book collections was one that he called the "Florence Nightingale Collection." In a letter to Miss Lawler in 1920, Dr. Kelly described this collection and stated his intentions concerning it. That letter is here reproduced.

[6] The date of the last meeting of "The Teresians" is recorded as March 1925.

Library
Howard A. Kelly, M.D.
1406 Eutaw Place
Baltimore, Maryland

18 September
1920

Dear Miss Lawler,

I am accumulating a great deal of material—valuable books, letters and pictures—directly and indirectly relating to Florence Nightingale and her surroundings.

This collection is too large and important, and, if I may say so without being indelicate, too expensive, to be merged in any general library or put away where it is not likely to be seen and used frequently.

I write to enquire whether The Johns Hopkins Training School for Nurses would be ready to take charge of this collection, giving it distinction, and at the same time conferring distinction and honor on the School itself, by providing a special room for these memorials of the great founder of the nursing profession and the greatest woman of the last century.

If such assurance be forthcoming, I will collect henceforth with the specific intention of turning over all material accumulated to The Johns Hopkins Training School for Nurses.

Faithfully Yours
(s) Howard A. Kelly

Miss E. M. Lawler
Superintendent
The Johns Hopkins
Training School for Nurses

In 1920 the library of the School was neither organized nor administered to receive so large and valuable a collection. The William H. Welch Medical Library was ready for the installation of books in December 1928, and it must have been about this time that Dr. Kelly offered his Nightingale Collection to the Welch Library with the expressed wish it be kept intact. The Library Committee of Welch was sympathetic with Dr. Kelly's wish and provided a room to serve as a depository for the Nightingale books. Early in 1930 the Collection was received by the Welch Library.

In September 1941 a full-time professional librarian, Lillian Celmer, was appointed for the School of Nursing. By that time the School library had been remodeled and its physical facilities enlarged. Jessie B. Black was chairman of the Library Committee. Miss Black discussed with Dr. Kelly the transfer of the Florence Nightingale Collection from the Welch Library to the School of Nursing. From these discussions and from other unpublished documents, it is clear that Dr. Kelly wanted the Collection transferred to the School of Nursing library where it would be readily accessible to student nurses and members of the School faculty. By November 1942 the Nightingale Collection of 416 books was moved to the Nurses' Home. One year later at the age of eighty-five Dr. Kelly died. It must have given him satisfaction and pleasure to know that these volumes which he had gathered over many years and intended for the use of the nurses now reposed in the library of the School.

About the same time the Nightingale Collection was transferred from the Welch Library to the School of Nursing, another collection was moved to the Nurses' Home, first as a loan, later as an outright gift. This collection had been gathered by the Johns Hopkins Hospital Nurses' Alumnae Association. It included some 550 professional books, a bound set of the *Johns Hopkins Nurses Alumnae Magazine*, a set of the annual proceedings of the National League of Nursing Education (which is almost complete and very valuable because of the early numbers), a set of the annual reports of the director of the Johns Hopkins Hospital through June 30, 1932, and innumerable pamphlets, programs, announcements, and other items of historical interest. The School of Nursing is deeply indebted to the Alumnae Association for this collection and also to Ruth Brewster Sherman who so diligently watched over the Association library for many years.

The historical collection of the School of Nursing is thus comprised of books and other items from three main sources: the collection begun by the School in the early Nineties and largely assembled through the ceaseless efforts of Miss Nutting; the Florence Nightingale Collection, the gift of Dr. Kelly; and books, periodicals, and materials given by the Johns Hopkins Hospital Nurses' Alumnae Association. It also includes first editions of books written by Alumnae of the School. In 1949 the School collection consisted of twelve hundred books and was described as "probably the finest of its kind in the country, with the exception of the Nutting Collection at Teachers College, Columbia University." The pleasant room at the end of the east wing in the old Nurses' Home was given over to library use in 1946 and thereafter known as the "Historical Library." A large number of the historical volumes were moved to this room as were other historical items.

It is a great temptation to linger among the old books in the Historical Library, to examine their bindings, their type face, even their period-revealing advertisements, but most of all their handwritten inscriptions which give the names of long-gone and well-loved teachers, mentors, and friends. Time and space forbid but the briefest mention.

Miss Nutting's signature is written on the flyleaf of many of the books; her private library must have been the source of these particular volumes. Many of the books were published in London, which one might expect, since professional nursing as we know it today, was cradled in England. A gift of valuable Nightingaliana from Dr. Lida O. Meredith included *Notes on Nursing* by Florence Nightingale. On the title page of this volume is the handwritten inscription, "To my dear friend and 'Patroness' E. Herbert from F.N. July 1860." Below the inscription is the typewritten note, "The recipient was the wife of Sidney Herbert who, as Secretary for War, wrote and asked Florence Nightingale to take charge of nursing operations in the Crimea with the sequel that has made her world-famous."

If there could be any doubt that a library existed in the School of Nursing from its earliest beginnings, it should be dispelled by the inscription in a little volume called *Ministering Women*. At the top of the first page, otherwise covered by an advertisement listing the healing virtues of massage, is written in longhand, "Nurses' Library November 1891."

Two names that will always shine in the history of Hopkins are those of Dr. William Osler and M. Adelaide Nutting. The following inscription in a first edition of Florence Nightingale's *Notes on Nursing* is reproduced because both their names appear in it and because it shows the decisive handwriting of Miss Nutting.

In addition to books the School possesses other unique historical items. Especially should be mentioned the "Armchair," so noted on the plate, of Florence Nightingale. This roomy chair, a late Sheraton, early nineteenth century, was probably in the Nightingale home. Two large and strong side wheels, one small

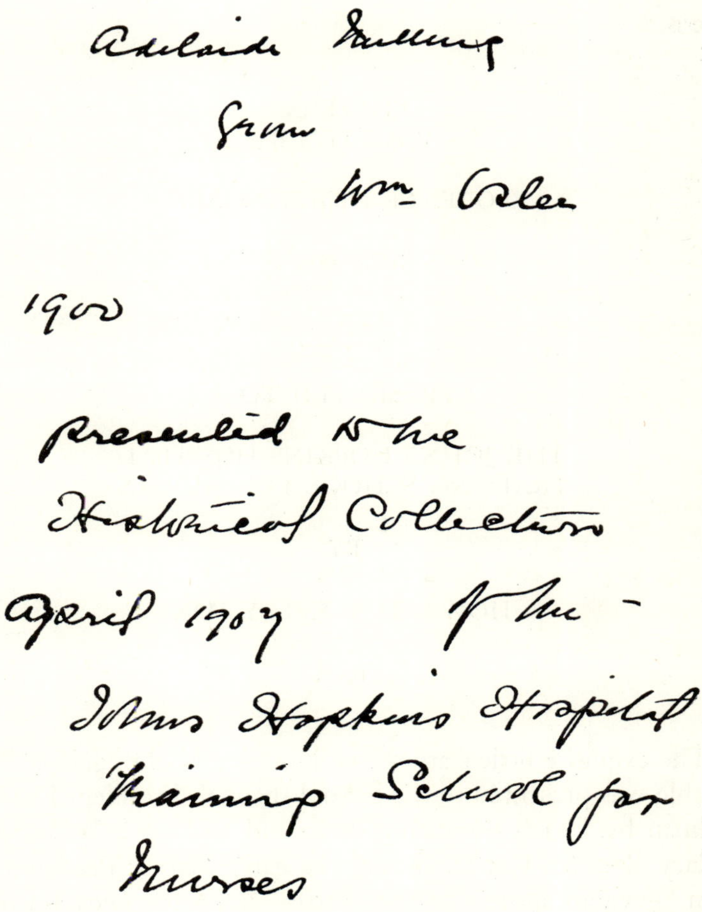
Adelaide Nutting
from
Wm Osler
1900
Presented to the
Historical Collection
April 1907 of the
Johns Hopkins Hospital
Training School for
Nurses

back wheel, and a small wooden footrest were attached, thus converting it into a wheel chair. Practically all of Miss Nightingale's later life was spent in that chair. Dr. Howard A. Kelly procured this memento with much trouble and expense and presented it to the School in 1921. In his letter accompanying the gift Dr. Kelly wrote, "If an inanimate object can convey a lesson and transmit an inspiration, may this chair suggest the spiritual presence of your great apostle of nursing and prove a blessing to the nursing school."

Another rare gift from Dr. Kelly is a collection of original Nightingale letters, which he had mounted in a beautiful, handmade book bound in Levant morocco. The inscription on the title page is:

LETTERS
WRITTEN BY

FLORENCE NIGHTINGALE

1865–1885

PRESENTED TO

THE JOHNS HOPKINS HOSPITAL
TRAINING SCHOOL FOR NURSES

BY

HOWARD A. KELLY M.D.

1917.

The exquisite little statuette of Florence Nightingale in Parian marble was presented to the School through President Daniel C. Gilman by Henry Bonham Carter and was made by his sister, Hilary Bonham Carter, during the early Sixties. President Gilman "gave an address to the Nurses" upon the occasion of the presentation.

Two fanback Windsor chairs, one a side chair and one a rocker, that were in the office of Isabel Hampton are in the Historical Library. A treasured piece is a small oak desk with a black leather top that "was owned and used by Mary Adelaide Nutting at The Johns Hopkins Hospital and at Teachers College Columbia University." On this desk Miss Nutting wrote *A History of Nursing*. It was given to the School by a friend, Isabel M. Stewart.

In the Historical Library, as the year 1949 ends, hang the photographs of the five directors of the School: Isabel A. Hampton, M. Adelaide Nutting, Georgina C. Ross, Elsie M. Lawler, and Anna D. Wolf. The Historical Library is indeed a fitting place for the photographs of these women. Each one of them has made history.

A major event in the development of the library was a gift of $3,850 secured through Christina M. Dick from Mrs. Annie M. Gill, a patient Miss Dick nursed. The gift is noted in the 1906 annual report of the superintendent of the Hospital as follows: "From the executors of the estate of Mrs. Annie M. Gill, to be used for the benefit of the Training School for Nurses. . . ." Miss Nutting had repeatedly called attention to a library as one of the necessary features of a good school. Doubtless, it was her decision that the "benefit" desired by Mrs. Gill should take the form of books. At first the income from the Gill Fund was used to augment the general literature library, which in 1905 consisted of a few hundred volumes; later it was diverted to the purchase of professional books.

The General Literature accession book, as previously noted, was begun in 1900. The last date of entries is March 1912. To glance over this record is like lifting a curtain on the reader's scene at the turn of the century. One sees the names of Shelley, Keats, Emerson, Dickens, Thackeray, Shakespeare, and others whose essays, poems, plays, and fiction are timeless. Edith Wharton is there too, Conrad, Galsworthy, Glasgow, and Mark Twain. The source of most of this collection is given as either the Library Fund or Gill Fund. Since books were bought with the Library Fund as far back as 1900, this fund must have preceded the Gill Fund, established in 1905. Of the many contributors who gave to the general literature library a few only can be mentioned, although one would like to name all. Dr. Osler, Dr. Hurd, Mrs. W. M. Ellicott, and the Hospital were among the early donors. The names of E. H. Sothern and Susan B. Anthony are listed as contributors. A gift of some two hundred books "to be known as the

Flack Collection" came from Anna Hoffman. Early graduates of the School who gave books of general interest were Miss Nutting, Miss Ross, Nancy P. Ellicott, 1903, and Florence M. Patterson; many of the later graduates also contributed. The class of 1899 presented a number of poetical works and the class of 1903 made a contribution of fiction. The best testimony that these books were read and enjoyed is found in notations such as those opposite the novels of George Eliot and Dickens—"Worn out and replaced by new."

The General Literature accession book includes some volumes having historical significance. Opposite such volumes is the notation, "Transferred to Historical Collection." In 1945 the general library was discontinued and all nonprofessional books, numbering more than twelve hundred, were sent to the Enoch Pratt Free Library of Baltimore City. The photograph of Mrs. Annie M. Gill, whose gift made possible so many delightful hours of reading for students and graduates, hangs in the reference library.

Loula E. Kennedy returned to the School in 1921, as director of theoretical instruction. Miss Kennedy, who believed that a well-selected, up-to-date, professional library was essential to a liberal professional education, at once set about putting the professional library in order. At that time the reference books were in two bookcases under the steps in the east wing of the Nurses' Home and the historical and general literature collection in the front room, then known as the "Nightingale Library," of the present (1949) library suite. Soon after Miss Kennedy arrived the reference books were moved to the back room of the present library, thus placing them in a better position to invite the attention of students.

One of Miss Kennedy's first acts was to check the reference volumes with the bibliographies given in the *Standard Curriculum for Schools of Nursing*, published in 1917 by the National League of Nursing Education. In an early report of the Department of Instruction is a record of the number of books comprising the reference library and the new references acquired during the year. According to that report there were then approximately five hundred reference volumes.

Evidently after the mid-Twenties the reference library steadily expanded. In November 1927 the teaching department occupied its new quarters in the old Surgical Building, a distance of several blocks from the Nurses' Home. To facilitate the use of reference books both for instructors and students, 490 references were moved to the classroom library in the new teaching department; seven hundred were left in the reference library in the Nurses' Home. Miss Kennedy wrote in her report for 1929–1930, "With about 1200 books beside the fiction and non-professional books, we think we have need of a librarian. . . ." That same report states that ninety-six new volumes were added to the reference library during the year and that many of these books were made possible by the Filler Fund. This fund was a bequest of $250 from William E. Filler to the Johns Hopkins Hospital to be designated for such purpose as his daughter, Mrs. Dorothy Filler McBride, named. Mrs. McBride "designated" the library of the School of Nursing.

In 1930 a library committee was appointed by Miss Lawler with the following members: Anna Beckwith, Christina M. Dick, Mabel N. Hay, 1925, and Loula E. Kennedy. Advice was sought from officials of the Enoch Pratt Free Library and the Welch Medical Library. Some months later the committee submitted a comprehensive report of the School's library facilities—book content, administration, funds available—and recommended that immediate steps be taken to procure a librarian, "a trained one, if possible," and that reference books be moved from the teaching department to the library in the old Nurses' Home. The following year the Department of Instruction recorded in its annual report, "The study of the nurses' library submitted last year has yielded no fruits due to the lack of funds."

Each year the Department of Instruction reported on the growth and needs of the library. The urgent need expressed in all these reports was the need of a full-time librarian. How could an expanding library of several thousand volumes be safeguarded and made accessible without the service of a trained librarian who would give her full time to the work? Then in March 1937 the library committee again sought advice and considered plans for the reorganization of the library. The recommendations made by the committee were essentially those made in 1931: that a full-time librarian be employed and that all reference books be moved to the library in the Nurses' Home where they would be available to a larger number.

The following autumn, Miss Lawler submitted the need of a full-time librarian to the Advisory Board of the School of Nursing. The Board appointed a special committee consisting of Miss Lawler, Miss Frederick, and Elma J. Hussey, 1923, to look further into the matter. In January 1938, the special committee rendered a report. Its recommendations included those made in 1931 and 1937: the appointment of a full-time librarian and the housing of all reference books in the Nurses' Home library. In addition the committee recommended that plans be developed for enlargement of the library.

Although a full-time librarian was not appointed for several years, plans for the enlargement of the library went forward rapidly. Dr. Joseph L. Wheeler, chief librarian of the Enoch Pratt Free Library, was consulted. Dr. Wheeler and members of his staff visited the School several times and advised concerning the rearrangement of rooms and the necessary new equipment and furnishings. The present reconstructed library suite consists of three rooms. One was formerly an open porch between the Nurses' Home and the Wilmer Clinic. The porch was enclosed on three sides with panels of glass about ten feet high and connected with the old library by a wide entrance cut through the north wall of the front room. This glass enclosed lounge became a general reading room. The two old library rooms were completely revamped; the back room was remodeled and provided with stacks, study desks and tables, catalogue and other files; the front room equipped with a magazine rack and a desk for the librarian. Later additional study tables and another magazine rack were placed in the front room. The remodeled library, completed by June 1939, was made possible by money accumulated from the Dickson Fund given with the proviso that it would be used "in promoting the comfort and welfare of the nurses. . . ." The new library did indeed promote the physical "comfort" of the nurses as well as their intellectual "welfare." Now there was a bright, cheerful reading lounge with comfortable chairs where one might spend a quiet hour perusing the day's news or a favorite magazine and also rooms with tables and desks for more serious reading and study. Soon after the new library was completed, all reference books were moved to it from the teaching department.

At this point it is in order to retrace the administration of the library over the sixty years of its existence. In the early days there can be little doubt that Miss Nutting guarded vigilantly the infant library, delegating to an assistant its immediate care. The first accession books bear witness to the considerable part Miss Ross played around 1900 in the library management. Later the official in charge of the Nurses' Home was responsible for all library books.

After the opening of the two new wings to the Nurses' Home in the autumn of 1907, the apartment of the superintendent of nurses, located at the right of the Home entrance, was moved to the end of the east wing, and the sitting room of the apartment made into "the much needed library." This room later became part of the library quarters as remodeled in 1939. An interesting, unsigned article, "Progress in the Hospital," published in the March 1908 issue of the *Johns Hopkins Nurses Alumnae Magazine* gives enlightening information on the School library at that time. The article states that three hundred books "comprise the Reference Library"; it describes the physical arrangements of the newly acquired library space and then goes on to say:

"The sitting room has made an exceeding comfortable and attractive library with its pictures and easy chairs. . . . The books have been catalogued according to the card system, and the cases are opened three evenings each week after five o'clock. The nurses are at liberty to take out any two books they wish, but must leave the cards with their name and date on it in the drawer. When the books are returned the name is crossed off and the card is placed in the book before being put on the shelf. This method has proved most satisfactory, as there has been a loss of only four books in six years. Each member in the school contributes one dollar a year to this library fund, part of which is spent in subscribing to about fifteen monthly and weekly magazines, the remaining is then spent by the Library Committee in the purchasing of books.

. . . The only restriction placed on any one in the library is that silence must be observed."

It is worthy of note that by 1908 a card system had been established for recording borrowed books, that *four books* only were lost in *six years*, and that a *library committee existed.* A few copies of "Library Rules" survive, which although undated must have been of the 1907–1908 period since they agree in substance with the above quotation. From these rules one learns that the library was open Tuesday, Thursday, and Saturday evenings from 6:30 to 8:00 o'clock; that a probationer was on duty in the library on those evenings; and that library books were not to be taken out of the Nurses' Home or the Nurses' Annex and "*never to the wards.*"

In 1921 Miss Kennedy assumed the responsibility for the reference library, and a probationer assisted her in keeping the books in order and in checking them daily. Sometime in the late Twenties the instructors took turns in keeping the library open in the evening. At that time there were no scheduled library hours; the hours the library was open depended largely on when the students wanted to use it.

During the Twenties, Harriet A. Blogg, who had been librarian at Goucher College, catalogued and accessioned books. Minnie W. Blogg, sister of Harriet Blogg, had been librarian in the Hospital for many years; when the content of the Hospital library was transferred to the Welch Medical Library she became reference librarian in Welch. After her retirement in 1936, Minnie Blogg gave one or two days of service to the School of Nursing library. Her activities were confined largely to accessioning books.

Finally in September 1941 the School had a full-time librarian, Lillian Celmer, and four years later, with the assistance of student nurses who were paid for their services, the library was kept open from 7:00 a.m. to 10:00 p.m. daily. Miss Celmer was graduated from the School of Library Science, Simmons College, Boston. Her tenure was short. Eager to take an active part in the war effort she left in March 1943 to join the Navy.

Trained librarians, like other professional personnel, were difficult to secure during the war. The School was fortunate in obtaining the services of Gertrude I. Bunting, 1911, in April 1943.

Miss Bunting had had no library training but was interested in library work. She gave valuable service during the war period and for several years thereafter.

The function of the library committee, appointed in 1930, seems to have been largely that of study: gathering information on other nursing school libraries, analyzing the needs of the School library, and making appropriate recommendations. When the faculty was organized in 1941, bylaws were drafted which provided for nine standing committees, one of which was the Committee on Library, Publications, and Illustrative Material. The functions of this committee as defined in the bylaws are here given: ". . . to regulate activities of the library; to determine all accessions and subscriptions to current literature; and to arrange for the use of teaching aids." The first chairman of this new faculty committee was Jessie B. Black. Its creation relieved Miss Kennedy of the general supervision of the library, a responsibility she had carried for twenty years. She was appointed a member of the new library committee.

The extent to which the library had expanded by the end of 1949 is indicated by the following record. The total book holdings then numbered five thousand of which approximately three-quarters were professional, and the other quarter, historical. During the year 1949, 265 reference books (218 different titles) were purchased; the School subscribed to fifty-three magazines, which included thirty-five nursing and related professional magazines and eighteen on recreational reading.

Of those who labored in the building of the library, the name of Loula E. Kennedy will always stand out. She toiled ceaselessly for the development of the professional library, and she gave of her time and her energies, not only to the gathering of reference books, but also in seeing to it that the library resources were made available to students and instructors alike. At the Homecoming of the Alumnae in May 1949, the School and the Alumnae Association joined hands in honoring Miss Kennedy by dedicating to her the library, henceforth to be known as the "Loula E. Kennedy Library." Prior to the dedication and without Miss

Kennedy's knowledge, Mrs. John W. Parsons, daughter of Isabella Stevens (Mrs. G. L. Hunner), 1900, painted Miss Kennedy's portrait from a recent photograph; a contest was held offering a prize for a bookplate, and a bronze plate placed at the entrance to the library. The inscription on the plate reads:

LOULA E. KENNEDY
LIBRARY

DEDICATED MAY 30, 1949 TO A
BELOVED ALUMNA, TEACHER AND COUNSELOR
OF THE
JOHNS HOPKINS HOSPITAL
SCHOOL OF NURSING

The specifications for the bookplate stated that it "should symbolize nursing, Hopkins, and teaching. . . ." The sketch selected was designed by Paul Bell, an art student at the Maryland Institute of Baltimore.

Miss Kennedy's portrait was hung in the professional library facing the entrance. Her name and her likeness, and perhaps through them her spirit, will thus endure, not only for those generations who knew Miss Kennedy but also for those who are to come and enjoy the "Loula E. Kennedy Library."

Nursing the Community

THE IDEA of providing trained nurses to care for people in their homes was echoed first by one, then by another of the founders of the Johns Hopkins Hospital and its Training School for Nurses. As far back as 1873, before a single visiting nursing agency existed in the United States, Johns Hopkins explicitly stated in a letter to his Trustees that he desired them "to establish . . . a training school for female nurses . . . to benefit the whole community. . . ." Francis T. King, first president of the Hospital Trustees, sailed for England in 1875 to discuss with Florence Nightingale the "new idea" of training nurses. Since Mr. King visited Miss Nightingale not once but a number of times, it is fairly certain that she did not miss the opportunity to expound to him an aspect of nursing in which she was deeply concerned—trained nursing for the sick poor in their homes. One can well believe that Mr. King brought back to his colleagues, engaged in establishing the Johns Hopkins Hospital, not only his discussions on the new nurse-training method but also a report of the district nursing movement in England.

At the formal opening of the Hospital, May 1889, both Dr. Billings and President Gilman asserted their conviction that the function of the nurse was outside as well as inside the hospital. Said Dr. Billings, "In a properly conducted hospital ward she is a necessity, but her field of usefulness and helpfulness is by no means limited to that. She is needed outside the hospital . . . in the home of the poor, to teach prevention as well as nursing." In his address President Gilman stated, "Our Hospital has such a department soon to be opened, where nurses will be trained, not only for their merciful offices within these walls but for household engagements and for visiting among the poor."

Five months later at the inauguration of the Training School for Nurses, Isabel Hampton, the newly appointed principal, proposed a plan of study providing that "a certain portion of each pupil's second year will be devoted to district nursing, among the poor, in their homes, under a competent head-nurse. . . ." Dr. Hurd's speech concluded the inauguration ceremony. In his closing paragraph he said, "Many hopes cluster about this Training School. . . . The poor of Baltimore in their homes, suffering for lack of proper nursing and adequate attention, look to this School for a solution of the problem of district nursing among the poor. . . ." Nor did Dr. Hurd cease to preach the gospel of district nursing with his address at the inauguration of the School. In his annual report to the Hospital Trustees in 1891 he wrote, "The need of district nursing among the poor as an adjunct to the work of the Dispensary is daily apparent. . . ." Dr. Howard A. Kelly took up the plea when he spoke before the second graduating class. Addressing part of his remarks directly to the Trustees and the public, Dr. Kelly said, "In the true spirit of their calling these graduates appeal to you as patrons for means to establish their work on such a wide basis that even the courts and the alley-ways shall be the daily beneficiaries of their skill." Miss Nutting, speaking at the commencement exercises in 1906, declared, "To many of us the best and most fruitful field for work is that occupied by the District and Visiting Nurse, and its finest development that which is making it a powerful instrument of social progress." Finally there was Dr. William H. Welch, appointed professor of pathology in the Johns Hopkins University in 1884 and later first director of the School of Hygiene and Public Health, whose work for sanitation and health reforms set the stage for community nursing in Baltimore and throughout the state. It seems conclusive that the founders and pioneer leaders in the School considered an experience of health teaching and nursing in the home an essential part of nurse training. One can only conjecture why this experience was deferred for almost forty-five years. The demands of an expanding hospital for student service, of a world war, and of a pandemic of influenza might postpone the inclusion of "district nursing" in the curriculum, but inevitably the day would arrive when the visions and the hopes of that early, far-seeing group would become a reality. In the meantime there were steps that could be taken.

A first step was the inclusion of health teaching in the curriculum. The first series of lectures, given in 1889–1890, provided instruction in "Ventilation." The junior lectures during 1890–1891 listed a course on "The Hygiene of Apartments" and among the subjects discussed were disinfection and preservation of food, milk, etc. Another course, "Children," included instruction in the care of healthy infants and infant feeding in health and in sickness. Miss Hampton stated in her yearly report, February 1891, that the "cooking school" had been opened the previous April. The following year she reported, "The Cooking School continues to prove valuable; the course has been increased to six weeks since last October, the last two weeks having special reference to instruction for District Nursing purposes." During 1899, the curriculum included eight lectures dealing with social conditions. Two years later the following announcement appeared in the *Alumnae Magazine:* "The nurses of the Visiting Nurse Association, as well as those of the Senior Class of the Johns Hopkins Hospital Training School, have been very kindly invited to attend the Course of Lectures on 'Home Life in Poor Neighborhoods,' given under the auspices of the Home Economics Section of the Arundell Club." In an article by Miss Nutting in 1902 on "The Hospital and Training School," she wrote:

"In our series of talks this year to the graduating class upon public and private charities and other similar matters, we have . . . had with us: Mrs. Florence Kelley, Secretary of the National Consumers' League, who took up the subject of Wage-Earning Children; Mr. Walter S. Ufford, General Secretary of the Charity

Organization Society, who outlined the purpose and scope of organized charities; and Mrs. John M. Glenn, who gave us a most interesting hour about Personal Work in Needy Homes. . . ." Miss Nutting went on to name other eminent lecturers who contributed to the series; one of these was Dr. Wilfred T. Grenfell, English medical missionary to Labrador.

The participation of the School in the young health movement was not limited to lectures. Evidently Miss Hampton and Miss Nutting stirred the imagination of their staffs and instilled in them a sense of obligation and desire to "carry a message to Garcia": a message of hygiene and healthful living into the homes of Baltimore. Between February 1895 and February 1896 reference is made in three reports of the Training School to the work of "our graduates" and "head nurses" in the community. The February 1895 report includes the statement, "The informal talks and demonstrations to the Women in Highlandtown have been given regularly each week by our Grad. Nurses." The following month the record states, "A little visiting among poor families has been done by 4 of the Head Nurses, in connection with the work of the Charity Organization. . . ." Then in February 1896 one finds the notation:

"At the request of different clergymen of the city, and for the help and teaching of the poor people of their parishes, several of the Head Nurses have undertaken to do similar work to that carried out last year in Highlandtown, and series of talks on the care of the sick in their own homes are now being given by these nurses in connection with four of the churches of the city."

With lectures being given to the pupils, with the head nurses visiting in the home, Miss Nutting saw to it that appropriate reading materials were available. In the archives of the Johns Hopkins Hospital School of Nursing are a number of pamphlets and bulletins of the period around 1900, dealing with the developments in the field of health nursing—nursing in the public school, in the home, tuberculosis nursing. Many of the publications have Miss Nutting's name on the outside cover with the terse request, "Please return." These materials, preserved more than fifty years, were evidently used as references for staff and pupils on the new and widening field of health at the turn of the century.

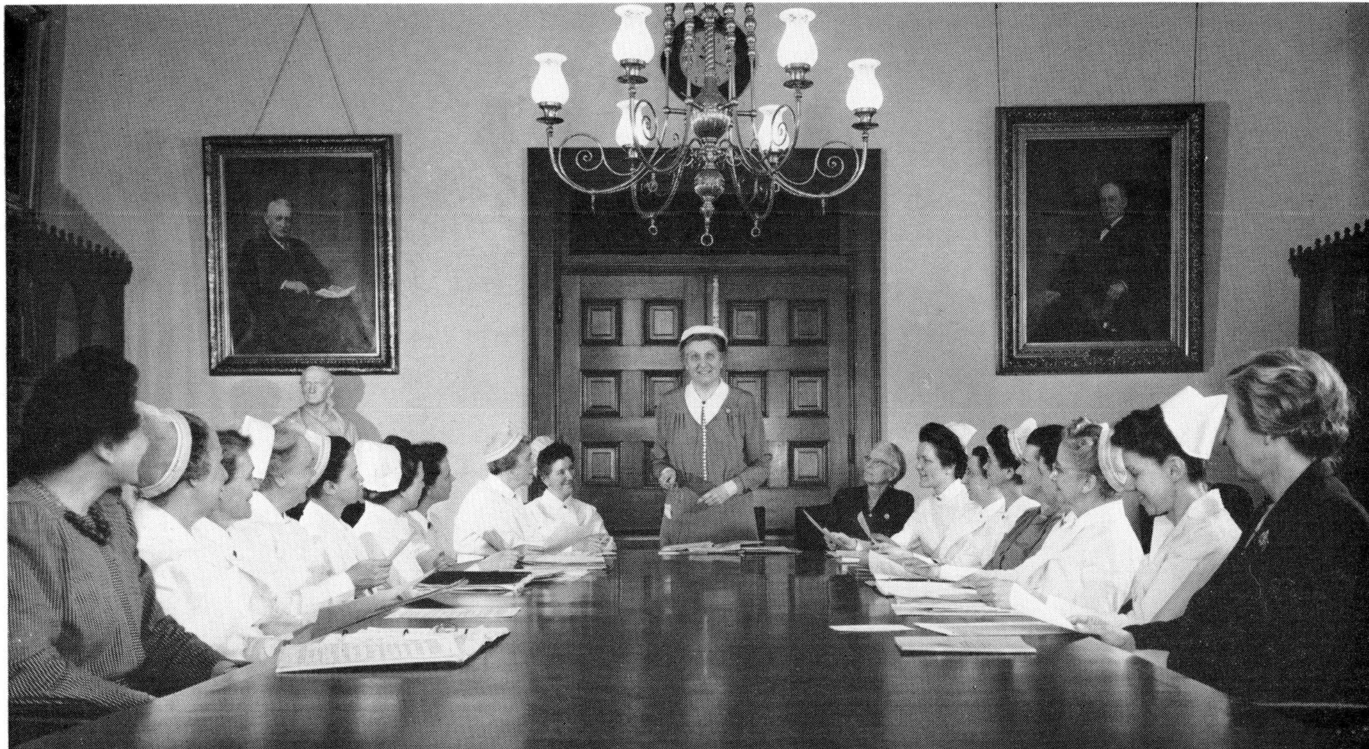

The Executive Committee of the Faculty of the School of Nursing, 1946

AUBREY BODINE

The public health education movement, begun in 1900, to spread the lesson of prevention and health, retreated into the background in the face of World War I. As the war ended there was evidence of renewed concern, especially in those instruments which would strengthen and vitalize public health activities.

One such instrument was the well-trained public health nurse. Soon after the close of the war, in December 1918, at the invitation of the Rockefeller Foundation, a conference was held in New York of individuals interested in the development of public health nursing. Out of this conference came the classic report, *Nursing and Nursing Education in the United States.*[1] The report dealt with all nursing fields and all patterns of nursing education: one highly important field, and the preparation therefor, was the field of public health nursing.

The Rockefeller study, which had nation-wide publicity, doubtless had its impact on curricula of nursing schools. Early in 1920 and again later during that year, Miss Lawler wrote to Dr. Smith urging the necessity of "providing some training as a preparation for public health work." About the same time Dr. Welch expressed himself in favor of endowments for schools of nursing, "not only for the better education of nurses for the sick but also to meet the crying need for the training of public health nurses. . . ."

The moment seemed favorable. Carolyn E. Gray was invited to survey the School. Miss Gray recommended two programs: a five-year program given in affiliation with the Johns Hopkins University, and a three-year program given entirely in the School of Nursing. Both programs provided for a four-month field experience in public health nursing, coordinated with systematic instruction in the subject. This was in 1924. Other events in the life of the School engaged the attention of the authorities and the Alumnae Association during the remaining years of the Twenties, and it was not until 1933 that a plan was outlined for incorporating in the curriculum public health nursing.

At the first meeting of the Advisory Board of the School of Nursing in December 1930, the Board appointed a committee,

[1] Committee for the Study of Nursing Education, *Nursing and Nursing Education in the United States.* New York, Macmillan Co., 1923

with Effie J. Taylor as chairman, to consider the purpose, scope, and function of the School of Nursing. Miss Taylor's report, submitted to the Board early in 1931, was based on the opinions of more than two dozen individuals, including outstanding nursing, medical, and public health educators, on the "function and scope of a high-class school of nursing." The group almost unanimously expressed the belief that "such a school should prepare students for all branches of sickness and health work . . . should concern itself with social and health movements . . . should plan its curriculum on changing community needs." Following Miss Taylor's report, Dr. Winford H. Smith, director of the Hospital, was instructed to present a request from the Advisory Board to the Trustees for authorization to invite Florence M. Patterson, then general director, Community Health Association in Boston, to survey the facilities available in Baltimore for the development of a public health nursing course in the basic curriculum.

Miss Patterson accepted the invitation. After an observation period of four days in Baltimore she submitted a report. Preliminary to more general discussion Miss Patterson said:

". . . it is assumed that the aim is to put public health into the general curriculum rather than to attempt to prepare nurses for the public health field. . . . Therefore the plan ought not to be thought of as a special emphasis in public health concentrated in a period of three or four months at the end of the senior year."

Miss Patterson then went on to say that further study was indicated to find out the possibilities of developing a satisfactory student field in the public health agencies of Baltimore. Heading all other recommendations was the recommendation: "That a new position be created in the teaching staff of the school as director of public health nursing education and as assistant to the Principal of the School."

Miss Patterson submitted her report in June 1931. The following October the Advisory Board considered financial sources in order to put Miss Patterson's recommendations into effect. Out of this consideration came the agreement that the Board approach the Endowment Fund Committee of the Alumnae Association for funds. Early in January 1932 a request was addressed to that committee for an appropriation of $4,000 "or such part of this sum as may be required," in order to secure the services of a highly qualified public health nurse for several months to work out in collaboration with the School of Nursing, the School of Medicine, and the School of Hygiene and Public Health, a definite plan. The plan would include the approximate cost of instruction in the Hospital and in the various clinics, and of supervised field experience in public health nursing.

The Endowment Fund Committee by a large majority recommended that the request of the Advisory Board be granted. An editorial in the *Alumnae Magazine* expressed satisfaction in the proposed plan. "We are sure," said the editorial, "our readers will be eager to learn the outcome of a study that anticipates the fulfillment of the desires of those responsible for the educational program of the student, as well as those graduates who have felt for years that the students should have some experience in the field of public health nursing."

The School authorities acted promptly and were fortunate in securing the interest of Marion G. Howell, director, Course in Public Health Nursing, Western Reserve University. In May 1932 Miss Howell came to Baltimore for a week to begin consideration of a plan "for a proposed public health program in the School of Nursing." In November she and her assistant, Irene Bower, returned to continue the study.

Early in 1933, and before submitting her final report, Miss Howell stated in a letter to Miss Lawler that the first step in the development of public health nursing in the undergraduate curriculum was the appointment of a well-prepared public health nurse on the staff of the School of Nursing. She defined the immediate task of this nurse as giving instruction in public health nursing, with such application of the subject as the facilities of the School and Hospital afforded.

The Johns Hopkins University School of Hygiene and Public Health had been established under an endowment from the Rockefeller Foundation. During 1932, the period of Miss Howell's study, the Foundation made an additional grant for the establishment of the Eastern Health District, "organized as a field study and training area in cooperation with the City Health Department, and other agencies actively engaged in public health work."

The District immediately surrounded the School of Hygiene and Public Health and the Hospital and served a population of fifty-six thousand; it provided facilities for students in the School of Hygiene for field experience in the administration of public health work. For the School of Nursing the establishment of the District was timely; the School could now inaugurate a program of public health nursing which would include experience in a properly controlled field.

In March 1933 the "long looked for report" arrived. Miss Howell gave much space in the body of the report in illustrating the rich opportunities for developing preventive and health teaching in the Hospital and the clinics of the Dispensary. She also pointed up the need of courses specifically designed to teach the public health aspects of nursing. Included in her recommendations were the following: (1) that the School of Nursing affiliate with the School of Hygiene and Public Health for special lectures in Public Health Science—a series of at least fifteen lectures to be carefully planned and executed with such field trips to local agencies and plants as seem advisable; (2) that an affiliation be established with the new teaching center, the Eastern Health District, permitting senior students to have a period of two or three months in a generalized community service, their time being divided between the clinics of the Johns Hopkins Hospital outpatient department and home visiting in the special area of the center; (3) that additional well-qualified personnel be secured in developing the teaching facilities in the outpatient department, working largely through the head nurse of each clinic and in very close relationship with the medical social service department and with the wards.

As already noted, before Miss Howell submitted her final report she suggested that a well-prepared public health nurse be appointed to the School staff. The Advisory Board again approached the Endowment Fund Committee for financial support. The committee again complied and agreed to pay the salary of an instructor in public health nursing for a two-year period; later the committee underwrote the salary for a third year. In a few months Miss Lawler could report at commencement "definite progress": arrangements for a course in public health and sanitation with the School of Hygiene and Public Health; affiliation for field experience with the Eastern Health District; appointment of Miriam Ames as instructor in public health nursing.

Miriam Ames was graduated from the Johns Hopkins Hospital School of Nursing in 1914. Following her graduation she had a broad and varied experience in the public health nursing field. Just before coming to Hopkins she pursued a program of study in public health nursing at Teachers College, Columbia University. In October 1933 Miss Ames began her work at Hopkins. She brought to the newly created office interest and enthusiasm, vision, and a well-seasoned experience.

Three months after her arrival Miss Ames presented a plan for the introduction of public health nursing in the undergraduate program. In the meantime she had become acquainted with the local situation—the people, the School, the Hospital, the School of Hygiene and Public Health, the Eastern Health District and other community agencies. After listing the objectives of public health nursing services and briefly discussing the foundation and techniques essential to making these objectives effective, Miss Ames pointed out how public health nursing could be developed in the various departments of the Hospital. She then submitted sixteen recommendations. These recommendations, Miss Ames said, were "evolutionary rather than revolutionary" and added that she believed the majority were immediately workable. The correctness of her views was substantiated by the promptness with which most of them were introduced into the program.

Among Miss Ames' recommendations were: (1) that preliminary students have at least one-half day of observation in the outpatient department and one-half day in home visiting, preceded by an orientation conference with the outpatient supervisor and followed by a second conference with the director of public health nursing; (2) that group conferences of the public health nursing director, instructors, and head nurses be held regularly to discuss public health aspects of the care of patients in the wards; (3) that in *all* clinics the preventive aspects of disease be taught by conferences of head nurses and students; (4) that supplementary instruction be given in the social and economic aspects of health and disease; (5) that a close working relationship be maintained between the Eastern Health District and the School and Hospital.

While Miss Ames was orienting herself to the opportunities for public health nursing in the School program, the first student nurses were sent to the Eastern Health District for a two-month assignment. The District advised the School that its facilities could not accommodate more than six students at one time. Under these circumstances only about half of the senior group could receive experience in the course of a year.

As a result of the limitations of the training facilities of the Eastern Health District, the Dispensary Visiting Nurse Service, in connection with the outpatient department of the Hospital, was inaugurated in September 1934. Its inauguration made possible field experience for all students. The following quotation is from an article by Miss Ames in the January 1935 issue of the *Alumnae Magazine:* ". . . its [the Dispensary Visiting Nurse Service] purpose is to offer a restricted and selective field wherein a clinic bedside nursing service may be developed, first for the need of the patient and second for teaching material. . . ."

At the time the Dispensary Visiting Nurse Service was proposed Miss Lawler presented the need for a second public health nurse whose particular function would be the supervision of students in the D.V.N.S. area. Four years later an assistant to the director of public health nursing was appointed, "an outstanding event of this year."

Reference has been made to the establishment of the outside obstetric service.[2] This service was used almost continuously for student nurse experience in obstetric nursing since 1895; in the beginning for experience of Hopkins students, then for some years for students from affiliating schools. In 1929 Hopkins again assigned students to the outside obstetric service, and in 1931 Louise M. Sheddan (Mrs. W. H. Ewert), 1926, who had had several years of public health nursing experience, was appointed supervisor of the service. Miss Ames referred to this outside service in her plan for introducing public health nursing in the program as a highly important phase of family health work. Ten

[2] See page 117.

months later she stated, "It is . . . good news to report that each student will have a month in the Outside Obstetrical Service. . . . This experience is invaluable since every nurse should have an opportunity to care for mothers and babies in their homes." The obstetric home experience was given during the intermediate year and in addition to the two-month field assignment in public health nursing during the senior year. In September 1940 when the service was closed after forty-five years of continuous performance Miss Ames wrote: "It is impossible to estimate the worth of the experience to the student . . . without it we feel we have lost one of our most valuable teaching aids. There is, of course, lamentation on the part of many of the patients." Thus passed into the pages of history another of the pioneer community activities of the Johns Hopkins Hospital.

With the great increase in admissions during the early period of World War II, the Eastern Health District and the Dispensary Visiting Nurse Service could no longer accommodate the larger classes for field experience. The executive committee of the School faculty recommended an eight-week affiliation with the Instructive Visiting Nurse Association of Baltimore. The Hospital Trustees approved the recommendation, and the new arrangement enabled all senior students to have the benefits of public health nursing field work. A tuition fee of $25 was required. Members of the U.S. Cadet Nurse Corps were assigned to the I.V.N.A.; the fee was thus paid through federal funds. Students assigned to this agency were under the immediate supervision of its educational director; they continued to have their classes with the director of public health nursing of the School and members of the Eastern Health District. It is of interest to note that many of the Alumnae of the School rendered notable service to the Instructive Visiting Nurse Association; also that it was the first time during the almost half-century of its existence the Association received for affiliation Hopkins students or students from any nursing school. The affiliation began in October 1943; it terminated in June 1945.

Much space is given in this study to the efforts of the School for securing and developing field facilities for student experience.

While such facilities are highly important in a well-rounded public health program, in a school such as Hopkins the hospital resources, inpatient and outpatient, offer a wealth of opportunity for implementing health teaching in the curriculum. Miss Patterson had emphasized this fact, as had also Miss Howell. Miss Ames dwelt lengthily upon it; most of her "Plan" dealt with techniques for developing the preventive and health aspects of nursing in the Hospital.

One channel, of which Miss Ames took full advantage, was the existing system of conferences of the various staff groups. Within a year of her arrival she wrote, "The mechanics of keeping the graduate nurses informed in regard to public health activities has been relatively easy owing to the regular group conferences for staff, head nurses, general duty nurses and instructors." The head nurses and instructors were in daily contact with students. It was important that they recognize the occasions in the wards and the clinics where simple rules of hygiene and health could be taught to patients. It was also important that they understand and appreciate the significance of their role in making effective the principles of public health in the School program.

While a major objective was to incorporate naturally the health aspects throughout the curriculum, from 1933 on instruction was added specifically directed toward a community health program. One such course was Social and Economic Aspects of Nursing. Another course of approximately twenty-six hours of classes, demonstrations, conferences, and clinics in public health nursing was begun at the Eastern Health District when the affiliation with that agency was initiated. The course, Public Health and Sanitation, included in the curriculum before 1933, was continued under the auspices of the School of Hygiene and Public Health. As the public health nursing program developed, changes were necessarily made in public health and related instruction.

The Dispensary was opened the same month as the wards of the Hospital, May 1889. Between that May and January 31, 1890, thirty-nine thousand patient visits are recorded in the clinics. In the clinics, as in the wards, the infant School found itself confronted with a considerable service to staff.

It appears from the School records that one graduate nurse was assigned to the Dispensary from the day it opened its doors to the sick and poor of East Baltimore. Miss Hampton noted in her first annual report, "Miss Greenwood, dispensary nurse resigned. . . ." The next year she recorded, "The School now numbers seven ward head-nurses, two operating room head-nurses, one dispensary. . . ." For many years this one nurse constituted the Dispensary graduate staff. By 1910 patient visits had more than doubled, the staff still consisted of one head nurse; by 1916 the visits had more than tripled, the staff then included the services of a head nurse and an assistant. By the middle Twenties the graduate group increased to a supervisor and six head nurses.

From the record it appears that the first pupil was assigned to the Dispensary in September 1889, four months after the opening of the Hospital; the record also indicates that one pupil was in the Dispensary most of the time for the next eight years. Then the number was increased to two. Wrote Miss Nutting in 1897, "The growing needs of the Dispensary have really demanded the services of a second pupil nurse. . . ."

For many years one finds practically no reference in the School reports to the duties of pupils in the Dispensary, to the supervision given them, to the learning expected from the experience. Until 1916 the graduate staff consisted of one head nurse; it is hardly likely that in her busy day she had time to give more than the barest directions in the daily routines of the department. The duties of pupils seem to have consisted largely of dusting, of seeing to it that the proper equipment and supplies were in the clinic rooms before the clinics began and putting rooms in order after the clinics were over, of giving assistance in preparing patients for examinations and attending women during examinations, and of helping with surgical dressings. Doubtless the alert and socially-minded pupils perceived that patients in the Hospital, divested of their own clothes and separated from their families, were somehow *different persons* from the ones they met later in the Dispensary. Doubtless they recognized that all could not be well for these patients; the habits and appearance of the children and the parents, and their ignorance, too often, of the simpler rules of hygiene, gave stark testimony to the social and economic inadequacies of their daily life.

The first outpatient service connected with a hospital was established in this country in 1752.[3] More than another hundred years were to pass before the birth of a professional nursing school in America, and still another fifty before recognition of the outpatient department as a health service center for the community and a valuable practice field for students to learn prevention and health. It was not until the Nineteen Twenties that the educational opportunities of the outpatient department were emphasized in nursing literature. An early article, written by Mary B. Hulsizer, 1920, on "Developing the Teaching Material in the Out-Patient Department" was published in the 1923 annual report of the National League of Nursing Education. In the next six years more articles and several studies bearing on the subject appeared.

Miss Ames' "Plan" for introducing public health nursing into the curriculum included a number of recommendations intended to develop and utilize the outpatient field for student instruction and experience. Some of her recommendations were described as goals to be reached; others, she stated, could be implemented without delay by taking advantage of already existing learning situations. As already noted, one recommendation was that preliminary students have at least one-half day of observation in the outpatient department and one-half day in home visiting, with conferences preceding and following the observations. This recommendation was promptly put into effect. Otherwise the lag in introducing an educational program in the Dispensary continued until 1939. At that time the outpatient supervisor, Mrs. Sophie Booker Packer, 1918, presented a plan which included rearrangement of experience, formal instruction, and conferences. The plan was generally adopted.

Martha Johnson, a nurse with considerable experience in outpatient nursing, was appointed head of the department in 1942. Miss Johnson had a well-defined philosophy of nursing in the outpatient service; she regarded it as unique and different from nurs-

[3] Henry M. Hurd, "Hospitals, Dispensaries, and Nursing," *Charities Review*, 10:408, Nov. 1900

ing either in the home or hospital, and she sought to develop in students an awareness of this uniqueness and difference. In a dispensary the patient is ambulatory, a very different person from the bed-confined patient. In a dispensary, such as at Hopkins where more than a thousand patients were cared for daily, the students saw ailing human beings en masse. The great numbers of patients, it was hoped, would arouse a realization of the magnitude of the problem of disease control and community health. The social urgency to reach and to help the patients was impressed upon the students; also the importance of an unhurried, sympathetic manner to gain their attention and confidence. In order to make a considered approach, it was essential that students be free from the pressures of nursing service to spend whatever time with the patient the occasion indicated. To accomplish this objective the department was sufficiently staffed with graduates to enable it to operate without students, although their contribution to an effective service was a real one, and it was so emphasized to them. Altogether students had ten weeks of guided outpatient experience correlated with individual and group conferences; four in the medical and surgical, and six in the obstetric, gynecological, and pediatric clinics.

When Miss Ames resigned in 1949 after sixteen years of unfaltering faith in the great possibilities at Hopkins for emphasizing the public health aspects of nursing, the extent to which public health had been infused throughout the curriculum must have been a great satisfaction to her. Head nurses, instructors, and heads of departments had all contributed to the rich development of the program. The hope of the founders was now fulfilled. Johns Hopkins nurses were prepared to nurse and to teach health in the homes and "to benefit the whole community."

Life in the School

Winding over the hills and through the valleys of the past brings to the mind and heart of every Hopkins nurse a host of memories. The days spent in the School and Hospital were all too short and filled to overflowing; life was teeming with experience. Some of that experience we acquired in the classroom, some in the wards, and some just by living and playing together as young, ardent pupils traveling along a common road.

In the wards we learned about people—all kinds of people—which was important for us in order *to become people.* Early in our training we learned that the patient was the core person surrounded by layers of other persons. There were the doctors, and since they were also people, they possessed in varying degrees the attributes of dignity, kindliness, humor, and courtesy. Then came the nurses, and they had the same personal attributes in the same varying degrees as the doctors. The doctors and the nurses each formed a hierarchy in which each individual, including medical and nursing students, had his ranking niche, and woe betide the student who, preoccupied with less important matters, strayed from his niche. Together they, the doctors and nurses, labored for the recovery in body and mind of the patient.

In the course of this labor there were occasions that caused in the nursing student apprehension tinctured with excitement. One such was the ceremony of rounds. When rounds were scheduled the patient ceased, for a brief time, to be the core of the Hospital universe, in that baths and other routines served merely as a prologue to the goal of "being ready for rounds." The big, heavy, three-winged screens, used in other days, were swung from bed to bed and the task of preparing patients, of hanging charts, of straightening the patient-unit went forward with unbelievable speed. Not to be ready for rounds was an unendurable disgrace. But always, that is *almost* always, everything was in readiness when the chief with his retinue of resident, assistant residents, internes, medical students, and perhaps a visitor or two, came over the bridge (when the bridge was still there) into the ward. The ceremony was begun.

And it was indeed a ceremony, formal and impressive, an intellectual feast presided over by great teachers. The head nurse, accompanied by a senior pupil, became part of the group once it entered the ward. As rounds proceeded from bed to bed, the patients who were well enough also became part of the group, and a most interested part. After all they were essential to the ceremony and it afforded them a glimpse into another world, if unknown still important to them, and it also tempered their long, monotonous day. As to the pupil nurse, who assisted with the patient and performed other necessary duties, her emotions were mixed. She was fearful that she might not measure up to her responsibilities and she knew, on occasion, that she was in the company of great physicians and that the event was one to be stored in her memory.

Stories are told of the chiefs. Dr. Lewellys F. Barker occasionally took a puckish delight in mispronouncing words and confounding his listeners. One day when the rounds procession was going from one patient in one corner of Ward C to another patient in another corner of that ward, Dr. Barker remarked, "We are going from Dan to Ber-sheb′-ba." Whereupon the resident asked the assistant resident, "What did he say?" The assistant resident passed the question to the interne who in turn passed it to the head nurse. The head nurse, who happened to be Elizabeth

Thomas, was aware of Dr. Barker's occasional excursion from the field of medicine to the field of phonetics, informed the interne that Dr. Barker had said "We are going from Dan to *Be'er she'ba!*" Stories are told, too, of other chiefs, especially of Dr. Osler, "The Gay of Heart." [1] But this chronicle must go on.

"There are two things," wrote Nell Pottenger (Mrs. L. C. Maxwell), of the class of 1912, "I would like to do again— One is to be back at J.H.H. on Christmas morning for the carols. The other is to attend morning prayers."

From the time of the opening of the Johns Hopkins University, morning prayers were held regularly. In the early days, President Gilman conducted the service in a classroom, the attendance of students and faculty being voluntary. The service as led by the President "usually consisted of scripture reading, a brief talk, and the reading of one of a collection of printed prayers which seemed to him appropriate."

In the School of Nursing the custom of having prayers after breakfast and before going "on duty" was begun by Miss Hampton. It is possible she knew that morning prayers were held in the University; it is probable that the impulse which led her to begin the day with prayer arose out of her own faith and desire to bring her group together for a few brief minutes in a communion of spiritual fellowship.

At the beginning, the School gathered in the parlor. Miss Hampton read a prayer and a hymn was sung. As the School grew morning prayers became more formalized. Since the entire School except the night nurses attended, it was an opportune time for making routine and special announcements. The pupils assembled promptly at 6:50 a.m. and stood on three sides of the square entrance hall of the Nurses' Home, now known as the Main Residence; the head nurses and other members of the graduate staff ranged themselves on the fourth side of the hall. After the gathering of these groups there was a silent moment of ex-

[1] Dr. Thomas S. Cullen wrote an article, "The Gay of Heart," in the Sir William Osler Memorial Number of *Archives of Internal Medicine*, published by the American Medical Association, July 1949. In this article he described the pranks of Dr. Osler.

pectation, then the assistant, stiffly starched and awesomely inscrutable, who was conducting prayers that day, appeared and took her place before the small table in front of the head nurses. The principal of the School was present only on special occasions.

The morning prayer service consisted of a reading from the Bible, singing of a hymn, and reciting the Lord's Prayer. Following these devotions came the announcements: changes in assignments and special notices were read. This was the order of the service and since it occurred day after day it might have become another routine. It never did. If we, the pupils, were laggards in rising and missed our breakfasts we still got to morning assembly, often in a breath-taking rush. For we liked the feeling of "oneness" and "belonging" that the morning gathering gave, we had an abiding, if unspoken, belief in the goodness of prayer, and—we had a consuming eagerness to hear the announcements of the day.

The assistant who led the service selected her own scripture reading. One assistant tells how she labored in selecting the scripture that seemed to her appropriate. The students chose the hymn. They, too, labored to find the hymn in keeping with the events of the day. The first line of one favorite, which appeared particularly fitting most times, was "Work, for the night is coming." Another favorite, which seemed to breathe a land of repose and less arduous labors, began "From Greenland's icy mountains, From India's coral strand."

The announcements! The memories of them are personal and exciting. Monday was the day for the announcement of new assignments of nursing practice. If it so happened that our present assignment was completed, on what new experience were we about to be launched? Were we to be initiated into the mysteries of "special assignments," such as operating room, or were we to be invested with the responsibility of our first night duty? Or, dreary thought, were we just to be transferred from one medical ward to another? Monday morning assembly was a time of adventure, and where that adventure would take us only the voice, final and inexorable, of the presiding assistant would tell.

Other and more earthy things took place at the end of the morning gathering. As we passed through the door of the Home, the assistant inspected our uniforms, our shoes, our hair, and our caps. Woe unto the pupil whose apron did not reach to the bottom of her skirt, whose heels were run down, whose hair was untidy, whose cap was tilted at the wrong angle. For her one of life's darkest moments was at hand.

Leaving the hall at the close of assembly the pupils made an unforgettable picture. They proceeded to their places of assignment in order of seniority: seniors first, then intermediates, juniors, and probationers. All except the probationers wore blue uniforms with white aprons, the probationers wore pink,[2] also with white aprons. It was an inspiring and moving sight to watch that long line of students, in blue tipped with pink, two abreast, marching down the long hospital corridor to their posts of duty. They were indeed recruits in the army that fought the cause for a happier, healthier world.

Morning prayers as a daily event gradually ceased during the early Forties. The School had grown, and by 1941 it numbered more than three hundred students. The entrance hall in the old Nurses' Home, where prayers had been held for so many years, could no longer accommodate the greatly increased student body. The place of assembly was moved to the pleasant and quiet reading room adjoining the hall. At the same time, following the changing discipline tide, innovations were made in the ceremony. The assistants to the principal ceased to be the sole presiders; nursing heads of departments and students also conducted the prayers.

But other times, other cultures had their impact on the daily assembling for prayer. The attendance dropped to a point where it was plain that the gathering had lost its significance except for a very few. Regular morning devotions were discontinued in 1942. Students were told they could resume the morning prayer service under their own leadership at any time and also hold services on particular occasions. As this chronicle ended morning prayers, although not held daily, still continued on days of special events. On Christmas morning the students and everyone in the Hospital were invited to meet in the lounge of Hampton House for coffee followed by prayers before the traditional singing of

[2] Probationers wore the pink uniforms until late in the Twenties.

carols; on the day of commencement, a day of solemnity and triumph for the outgoing class, also was held the old ceremony of morning prayers.

Christmas carols—treasured memories—the hour of carols before dawn on Christmas day! Unlike morning prayers Christmas carols did not begin with the beginning of the School. One Christmas, early in the Nineties, the nurses celebrated by performing Haydn's "Toy Symphony." Later was begun the singing of Christmas carols, to become a beloved tradition.

Through the years the caroling changed but little—the ringing of the rising bell, the quick response and upsurge of spirits, the gathering for brief prayers, for long in the entrance hall of the old Nurses' Home, later in Hampton House. From the Home the nurses moved to the rotunda in the Administration Building where they were joined during the early years by the doctors, and sometimes by Dr. and Mrs. Winford H. Smith. One Christmas, it is recorded, "Two-hundred and sixty-five nurses and doctors . . . met according to the old custom around the statue in the Administration Building. . . ." Some of the older graduates will remember that faraway time when a small organ mounted on a movable platform, large enough to accommodate the organist, accompanied the carolers.

Once the group was gathered in the Administration Building, the singing began with the national anthem and one or two carols. Then the procession proceeded to the wards, stopping at each in turn. To see again in the mind's eye the carolers moving over the bridge from one pavilion to the other in the early starlit morn of a clear, frosty Christmas, sometimes singing as they went, sometimes approaching silently with a rising of the old carols at the entrance to the ward, is to recapture an experience of great joy, shared with the patients, who somehow knew the carolers were coming and who sometimes joined in the singing. The caroling ended where it began, in the rotunda of the Administration Building. There around the compassionate figure of "Christus Consolator," [3] carols and the national anthem were again sung,

[3] In his address at the opening of the Hospital, President Daniel C. Gilman expressed the hope that "some friend of this hospital place beneath

and one more enduring moment was forged into the lives of all the nurses and into the history of the School.

Other Christmas singing lingers in our memories. It was through William Edward Thomas, doorman at the Hospital since the day it was opened, that the senior choir of the Memorial Baptist Church first sang at Hopkins in the late Twenties on Christmas Eve. Yearly thereafter this choir came and yearly they gathered in the early evening in front of the Christus to sing the Hallelujah Chorus from the Messiah; then they proceeded to the Hospital wards, trailed silently by doctors, nurses, other Hospital personnel, and visitors. The rich cadence of their voices echoed in the stillness as they sang the old Yuletide carols.

We who were in old Wards M and O will remember the spirituals sung there by the Negro patients. They raised their voices in the early golden summer dawn and again in the long purple summer twilight. In minor harmony they sang of their hopes on earth and of their faith in heaven after earth: "Swing low, sweet chariot, /Comin' for to carry me home."

Once upon a time, the young, the gay, the uninitiated, otherwise known as the probationer, wore a nondescript cotton dress, next she donned a pink uniform *but no cap*. For one, then two, then for six long months the probationer was on "trial." The bright probationer, the one who emerged triumphantly from the trial period received her due reward—the blue uniform and cap. And so the ceremony of "capping" began.

Capping was not always an official affair. At one time the silent and awed probationer stood before a member of the School staff, who tried caps of different sizes on her and instructed her in the proper angle at which the cap should be worn. Official or unofficial, the great day had arrived and henceforth the probationer dwelt in the company of "blue nurses," and wore the coveted cap.

Then in the early Thirties capping was given recognition and ceremonial pomp. According to a record left by Myrtle R. Grande (Mrs. Theo. Winship), 1930: "This momentous occasion

this dome a copy of Thorwaldsen's Christus Consolator." William Wallace Spence presented to the Hospital in 1896 a marble reproduction by Stein of Copenhagen of the Statue.

has, at last its ceremony. . . . Miss Kennedy led in the group of young nurses who sat primly in the front rows—new cuffs conspicuous—aprons white and stiff—faces glowing and solemn. A small chorus of Staff Members led the singing of a few hymns before the group filed down to have either Miss Frederick or Miss C. Dick place their first organdy caps on their heads. It was, as Miss Lawler said, one time when we might see caps placed as they should be instead of in the almost invisible posterior position they have assumed on the heads of the present generation."

Late in 1941, capping passed into the yesterdays of Hopkins. A new and common uniform was adopted for all students: those in the first six months of their course as well as those in the later period. The new uniform was trim and tailored, of the familiar blue, short-sleeved with white cuffs and collar and apronless; tan shoes took the place of black. And finally it provided for a "most becoming" white muslin cap, marked by a design having the outline and the letters, J.H.H., embroidered in blue. The design was drawn by Jessie B. Black. This uniform, complete in all details, including cap, was bestowed on a class a few months after it entered the School.

The old uniform was duly mourned. The new uniform, with its simplicity and "antiseptic" features, was soon in high favor. Upon the request of the Student Association the "Candlelight Service" was introduced at the time the new class was given the School uniform. Candlelight Service was held in Hurd Hall and participated in by both faculty and students. During the ceremony the newly-admitted students accepted the principles and honor code of the Student Association. Each new student carried a candle which was lit by an older student. Hall lights were extinguished during the lighting. In the darkened halls the bright glow of the flames from sixty-five or more candles held by sixty-five or more young and eager students spoke promise for the future. Nursing would carry on.

Remember Teenie? As the year 1949 came to an end, Teenie had been in service in various positions in the School for fifty-five years. Teenie's real name is Josephine Waldhauser, but everybody called her "Teenie." For twenty-seven years Teenie was head waitress in the dining room of the Nurses' Home and as such she served Miss Nutting, later Miss Ross, and later Miss Lawler.

In appearance Teenie belied the affectionate nickname she acquired soon after coming to Hopkins. She was short and plump and plump she was still in 1949. Then past seventy years of age, Teenie had the same expressive blue eyes, the same mental alertness. Possessed of a photographic memory, she could recall individuals, happenings, and customs in the School from the time she came to Johns Hopkins in 1895. Her motherliness and goodness to many young Hopkins pupils will not be forgotten by them.

Sherwood Forest! Happy, care-free memories evoked in many of us by that name—Dick Cottage, perched high on a hill dropping sharply to the river, the greenwood embracing it, shading it, and casting long shadows around it at day's end.

Sherwood Forest on the Severn River, less than an hour's drive from Baltimore, is in the Chesapeake Bay country and covers 850 acres of hilly, virgin woodland. In 1916, through the suggestion of Dr. Smith, the vacation cottage in Sherwood Forest came to the School as a gift from Dr. Hugh H. Young and three Trustees of the Hospital—George Cator, George K. McGaw, and Richard J. White, a great nephew of Johns Hopkins.

Never was a gift more welcome. Now we could escape from the humid heat of east-end Baltimore to the refreshing cool of Sherwood Forest. There we could swim in the Severn River, go boating, crabbing, or, if preferred, ride a bicycle, play tennis, or just loaf in the sun. In the long summer twilight, after a capacious meal, we sat on the porch overlooking the river, and we marveled at the changing color of the sky as the sun dropped in the west, and the fireflies lighting the night. Or in the cool fall evenings we gathered around the glowing fireplace in the living room and recounted our exploits of the day. Later—much later in the early hours of dawn we were awakened by the rustling of the wind through the trees. Half asleep, half awake, our imagination leaped the space of six centuries, and we fairly tingled with the thought that the rustling we heard was the rustling of Robin Hood, Little John, Friar Tuck, and all the men come home to their retreat in

Sherwood Forest. As daylight came Robin Hood was again a legend; we were brought back to reality and, perhaps, to the station wagon turned toward Baltimore.

The Ford station wagon was the gift of the Gate House Shop in 1946. No more would trains be caught (and missed) or busses chartered. A second event during the Forties was the naming of the cottage. "Dick Cottage" it was to be for all time as a memorial to Christina M. Dick, who, for so many years, was custodian of the key to the little green house; who saw to it that the cottage in Sherwood Forest on Nottingham Hill should be a place of fun and relaxation for all students and a place of inspiration for some.

No one ever doubted the "fun and relaxation," although a few might question the "inspiration." But inspirational it was and for the doubters are quoted lines from "Sherwood Forest," printed in *Routine*, 1923.

In the heart of Sherwood Forest
By the shining River Severn,
Stands the wigwam of Johns Hopkins,

. . . .

All around it grows the forest,
Grows the green and swaying spruce tree,
Grows the pine with needles on it,
Smooth below it lies the water,

. . . .

Lies the shining River Severn.
Here the nurses of Johns Hopkins
Spend their leisure time in summer;

. . . .

Wander far upon the hillside,
Spy the sail boat on the water,

. . . .

But when twilight dims the landscape
Come they back into the wigwam
To prepare the evening banquet;
To prepare the place for dancing,

. . . .

Then grown weary of this pastime,
Sit around the open doorway,
Telling weird and ghostly stories

. . . .

Thus for many days each summer,
Gay and clear these joyous voices
Echo through the boundless forest,

. . . .

Voices of the true light-hearted,
Young again with life in wildwood,

. . . .

Happy in the heart of Nature,
Happy in dear Sherwood Forest.
—*Anon.*

The Work of the Endowment Fund Committee

NURSING education, in the total scheme of education, has presented and still presents a financial anomaly and an outmoded system. Schools of nursing generally derive their support from services rendered by students in the process of learning nursing and from such funds as are allowed them by their sponsoring institution. As late as 1949, the closing year of this chronicle, most schools of nursing had no clear-cut income, did not know their expenditures, and did not have budgets.

At the beginning of the twentieth century, Miss Nutting and Dr. Hurd were keenly aware of the inequities of a system which (1) placed on students the burden of financing their schools and of contributing to the support of the hospital through long hours of service and (2) failed to give the principal a knowledge of the funds available for the school's development during the current year. They both affirmed the principle that educational growth requires educational freedom and educational freedom a modicum of financial independence. As early as 1906, the title of an address given by Dr. Hurd was, "Shall Training Schools Be Endowed?" [1] In this Dr. Hurd asserted that training schools for

[1] Henry M. Hurd, "Shall Training Schools Be Endowed?" *American Journal of Nursing*, 6:843–54, Sept. 1906

nurses, along with medical schools, must have ample endowment.

On the twenty-fifth anniversary of the Hospital and the School of Nursing, October 1914, Miss Nutting said:

"Some of the largest and most fundamental problems in nursing are as yet untouched. Take one of them: there is not one single endowed training school in the whole wide world.[2] All training schools are self-supporting institutions and most of them are ample contributors to hospital support. . . . Could the Twenty-Fifth Anniversary of the Johns Hopkins Hospital Training School be more appropriately or more justly celebrated than by beginning to provide her with a suitable endowment? . . . How fitting it would be to have this School lead the way in this essential advance. Our large and important alumnae could render no higher tribute to their school than to help it serve better the profession we all so love and cherish." [3]

One can be certain that long before 1914 Miss Nutting was convinced that an endowment was a necessity; that it was indispensable to the substance and vitality of nursing education. From 1894 to 1907 she had had daily association with Dr. Hurd who had recorded in both the spoken and the written word his conviction of the need of a nursing school fund. In Miss Nutting's report given at the commencement exercises of the School in 1903 is the statement:

"What a benefactor would he be who should for once so equip a training school for Nurses that its work might be carried on in the way in which the work of other schools, general and professional, of no greater importance to the community than ours, is always carried on." [4]

One can only conjecture why she had not earlier broached the

[2] An error must have occurred in printing the statement, "there is not one single endowed training school in the whole wide world." Amy P. Miller in her article, "Twenty Years Later," published in the *Johns Hopkins Nurses Alumnae Magazine*, April 1934, quotes Miss Nutting as saying on the twenty-fifth anniversary that there was not one endowed training school in the whole wide world with the exception of the first school for nursing at St. Thomas' Hospital in London.

[3] M. Adelaide Nutting, "The Work of the Johns Hopkins School for Nurses," *Johns Hopkins Nurses Alumnae Magazine*, 14:6–18, Jan. 1915

[4] "Commencement Exercises," *Johns Hopkins Nurses Alumnae Magazine*, 2:76–78, Aug. 1903

subject to the Alumnae Association. Miss Nutting was a statesman and it may be she was biding her time for the proper moment.

In any event in October 1914 Miss Nutting sounded the call. Promptly and with zeal the Alumnae Association responded. One month later one reads in the report of the quarterly meeting that Emma J. Beckwith (Mrs. Thomas S. Cullen), 1896, repeated her motion, made at the twenty-fifth anniversary, to mark the occasion "by collecting a fund for the Training School." At the following annual meeting of the Association, May 27, 1915, Mrs. Isabella Stevens Hunner, then president, announced she had received a special delivery on the previous day from Miss Nutting, accepting the chairmanship of the Endowment Fund Committee on one condition—that she be permitted to choose her own associates.

The first meeting of the committee was held on December 3, 1915 in the Nurses' Home. Those present were: M. Adelaide Nutting, 1891, professor of nursing and health, Teachers College, Columbia University, New York, N.Y.; Georgia M. Nevins, 1891, superintendent of nurses, Garfield Hospital, Washington, D.C.; Helen C. Bartlett, 1894, president, State Board Nurse Examiners, Maryland; Clara D. Noyes, 1896, general superintendent of training schools, Bellevue and Allied Hospitals, New York, N.Y.; Helen S. Hutchinson (Mrs. Martin Caples), 1896, former assistant superintendent, Johns Hopkins Hospital Training School; Yssabella G. Waters, 1897, member of Henry Street Nurses Settlement, New York, N.Y.; Elsie M. Lawler, 1899, superintendent of nurses and principal, Training School for Nurses, Johns Hopkins Hospital; Mrs. Agnes C. Hartridge, 1900, superintendent of nurses, Pine Heights Sanatorium, North Augusta, Georgia; Margaret B. Hoyt, 1902, president, Johns Hopkins Hospital Nurses' Alumnae Association; Mary Bartlett Dixon (later Mrs. Thomas S. Cullen), 1903, editor, *Johns Hopkins Nurses Alumnae Magazine;* Mrs. Helen Wilmer Athey, 1905, chairman, Ways and Means Committee, Johns Hopkins Hospital Nurses' Alumnae Association; Effie J. Taylor, 1907, supervisor, Henry Phipps Psychiatric Clinic, Johns Hopkins Hospital.

Two members, Florence M. Patterson, 1907, field secretary for the State Committee for the Blind, Boston, and Mrs. Isabella

Stevens Hunner, 1900, were unable to attend. Voted into membership at the meeting were: Helena Barnard, 1892, Anna C. Jammé, 1897, and Amy P. Miller, 1900.

Dr. Winford H. Smith, superintendent of the Johns Hopkins Hospital, was present at the historic session on December 3. He gave his cordial approval to the endowment proposal. In her remarks to the committee, Miss Nutting said, "I am happy to tell you that we can begin our work under favorable auspices. We have the sanction and good will of the Trustees and the superintendent of the Hospital. . . ."

The first act of the Endowment Fund Committee was to express its approval of the proposal to raise a suitable endowment for the Johns Hopkins Hospital Training School and to put itself on record "as unanimously and heartily in favor of the principle involved in the provision of adequate financial support as a necessary basis for all training school work." An endowment of not less than one million dollars, according to the committee, would ultimately be required to maintain a training school such as the Johns Hopkins School. The committee specified by formal action that the income from the endowment fund secured through the Alumnae Association "shall be applied solely to the educational work of the School, but that it be unrestricted in meeting educational needs." Then the committee proceeded to safeguard whatever moneys would be collected by creating an advisory committee for advice on the investing and handling of funds. The chairman of the Endowment Fund Committee and the principal of the Training School were authorized to confer with the president of the Board of Trustees and the superintendent of the Hospital regarding advisory committee personnel. Yssabella G. Waters was elected secretary of the Endowment Fund Committee, Mary B. Dixon, treasurer, and an executive committee was organized. Before adjourning it was formally voted that the committee should proceed with plans for building an endowment.

Thus was launched the endowment. Its story is one of heroic vision and magnificent effort. At the beginning the Alumnae Association confined its endeavors to establishing a school fund. But time and changes in the social and educational structure of nursing had their impact. The recorded facts disclose that certain fundamental movements—analysis of the organization and of the functioning of the School, effort to place the School under university direction—were, to a considerable degree, outgrowths of the Endowment Fund Committee's labors. The cornerstone of the committee's work was laid at its first meeting; on that occasion the seeds were cast which were to have a profound effect on the life of the School.

When does the history of a movement begin? When the germ of the idea behind the movement is born, even though not recognized or formulated? When the idea is first expressed in the spoken or written word? When the idea begins to take shape in an organized movement? Or when the idea is projected into planned action?

Catherine Drinker Bowen in her brilliant study of John Adams quotes Adams, ripe in age and wisdom, at eighty as saying:

"What do we mean by the revolution? The war with Britain? That was no part of the revolution; it was only the effect and consequence of it. The revolution was in the minds and hearts of the people, and this was effected from 1760 to 1775, in the course of fifteen years, before a drop of blood was shed at Lexington." [5]

When did the endowment for the School begin? Can one say categorically the exact day, month, and year? To so state would be contrary to the subtle, the fragmentary, and the formless beginning of the things that make history. Miss Hampton and Miss Nutting both knew of the expanding demands on the Hospital resources and the limit of those resources which might be expected for the School. One can easily believe that they, with their vision for nursing, discussed together the need of an independent fund to make that vision a reality. Sometime in the early Nineties when these two women were closely associated the germ of the idea of the endowment must have been born. As already cited, in 1903, Miss Nutting stated the need of a benefactor to equip a training school for the proper conduct of its work, although she did not then use the word, "endowment." But in October 1914, she unmistakably and explicitly asked that a fund be established,

[5] Catherine D. Bowen, *John Adams and the American Revolution.* Boston, Little, Brown & Co., 1950, p. xiv

and she placed before the Alumnae their responsibility and their privilege, as graduates of the School, to initiate an endowment. The Alumnae responded at the quarterly meeting the following month in an organized movement which culminated, May 1915, in the acceptance by Miss Nutting of the chairmanship of the Endowment Fund Committee of the Johns Hopkins Hospital Nurses' Alumnae Association. On December 3, 1915 the newly created committee met, and the idea born long ago was projected into a declaration of principle and a working organization. In expressed words and in expressed group action, the effort for securing a School endowment began in the fall of 1914; the Endowment Fund Committee actually began its work December 1915.

Since 1901 the Johns Hopkins Hospital Nurses' Alumnae Association had published a magazine four times yearly. It was indeed a fortunate circumstance to have a well-established quarterly when the endowment was begun. Owned and published by the Alumnae Association, edited by graduates of the School who were deeply interested in the project, sent automatically to every Alumnae member, the *Magazine* offered a perfect instrument for keeping before the Association the endowment program and its progress.

And the Endowment Fund Committee and the successive editors made effective use of this instrument. One cannot help speculating on the fate of the endowment without the *Magazine*. In its pages is the history of the endowment: the exhortations of the chairmen, the reports of the secretaries, the reports of the treasurers, and the many fine articles and stirring editorials through the years.

The Alumnae Association lost no time in spreading over the printed page the gospel of the endowment. In the January 1915 issue, the leading editorial written by Dr. Hurd set forth the reasons for endowments for training schools. The report of the November 1914 meeting of the Alumnae Association containing reference to the endowment, and the paper which Miss Nutting gave at the twenty-fifth anniversary proclaiming the necessity of endowment, were published in the same number. The first report of the treasurer of the Endowment Fund Committee was printed in the May 1916 issue and thereafter until 1929, with few exceptions, each quarterly contained a reference to the financial status of the fund and new subscriptions. A full financial statement was published annually by the committee until the fund was transferred from the Alumnae Association to the Board of Trustees of the Hospital in 1937. From 1916 to 1943, not one single year passed without one report from the committee; during years of activity the reports increased to three, four, or more. There were few years when the *Magazine* did not make its own pronouncements in one or several editorials from the year 1915 to the year 1940. During the committee's active life the reports, editorials, articles, and other items numbered some three hundred. Quantity, however, is only half of the story. The other half is the quality of the published material—its frankness, its vigor, its persistence, and its conviction of the educational need and the responsibility of both professional and lay groups to see to it that an endowment for the Training School should be established. The reports of the committee were full and informative; the Association took the entire membership into its confidence. But the voice of the Alumnae was not the only voice that spoke for the endowment. Other voices were raised and of these more will be told later.

Four months after its first meeting, the Endowment Fund Committee laid the groundwork for the first campaign. Under date of April 18, 1916, the Executive Committee of the Endowment Fund Committee sent a letter with a questionnaire to 716 graduates of the School, asking for expressions of faith in the undertaking and suggestions for carrying it out. The letter is a masterly summary not only of the educational program and economics of nursing education in the Johns Hopkins Hospital Training School, but also in other high-ranking schools of the time.

One by one the committee described the changes that were essential in training schools in order to graduate nurses qualified to keep pace with the growing demand in public health nursing, mental hygiene nursing, and other newly developed health fields. The financial dependence of the school upon the hospital was discussed. "Everywhere," said the committee, "there has been the necessity for weighing the needs of the hospitals against those of the schools of nursing, and usually the balance of the scale bears far down on the side of the hospitals." This was not questioned by the committee. Its members categorically believed that the primary purpose of hospitals is to give medical and nursing care, even though they assume partial or full responsibility for education. But the committee did ask, "What then should be done?" Why should not schools of nursing be considered in the same category as colleges and professional schools which fit women for special work? Those schools are meeting their problems by endowment and various forms of state and municipal aid. "This then," said the committee, "must be the solution of the problems of schools of nursing, for they stand today as educational institutions supported largely, and in most instances entirely, by the labor of the students." The committee charged the Alumnae Association to see to it that future graduates of the Johns Hopkins Hospital School of Nursing were properly equipped for whatever kind of work was demanded of them. An urgent appeal was made for the help of Alumnae members: help in the form of giving from their earnings, help by asking their classmates and friends for contributions, help by telling their patients of the proposed endowment and of the great need of the School. The letter ended by asking for "material evidence" of interest in the endowment plan.

One month after the circulation of the letter, the annual meeting of the Alumnae Association was held. The reports and discussion of the endowment occupy considerable space in the records of that session. Miss Nutting came to Baltimore for the occasion, even though it meant an "extraordinary effort." She reviewed briefly the achievements of the committee, then she read excerpts of letters received from Alumnae members in reply to the communication from the Executive Committee. These letters rang with pride in the fact that the Alumnae Association had initiated an endowment; the "material evidence" they contained gave proof of the writers' unqualified approval. Miss Nutting again expounded to her fellow Alumnae the limitations of the Training School, the urgency of educational reform, and the inability of the School to effect needed reform because of lack of funds.

"When I left you and went away . . . ," said Miss Nutting, "nothing amazed me more than to see the ease with which people get money for almost anything in the way of education." She then gave a list of recent gifts to colleges and universities, amounting to "six or seven millions." Miss Nutting stated it was the committee's opinion that a collection through each class was desirable; that this is a common practice in colleges. The Association thereupon voted that class collections should be one means of raising the endowment. Another method suggested was that of seeking contributions from physicians and persons likely to give to the fund. It was agreed that the names of such individuals should be sent to the secretary, as it was thought that the appeal would be more impressive if it came from the committee. Plainly, however, the first task the committee set for itself was to enlist the interest and convince the Alumnae of the urgency of an endowment for the School. "For the idea . . . that Training Schools cannot exist as schools without money is a new one in nursing affairs, and it takes time for most of us to grapple with and accept a new idea." But there were those who already were convinced. Wrote Marion L. Vannier, 1905, "The general educational standards of the school fluctuate with the rise and fall of the hospital income."

The first gift to the endowment fund of $50 by Annie C. Bonneville, 1910, must have been given sometime before May 1915, since it was announced at that time by the president of the Alumnae Association in her annual address. The first report of the treasurer of the Endowment Fund Committee was published about the time of the launching of the first campaign, April 1916. To that date there had been no solicitation of funds. Nevertheless, the moneys already received amounted to $2,950, pledges, $3,000.

It will be recalled that an Advisory Committee was created at the first meeting of the Endowment Fund Committee for advising on the investing and handling of funds. In January 1916 at the quarterly meeting of the Alumnae Association, Miss Nutting announced that Judge Henry D. Harlan, president of the Board of Trustees of the Hospital, and Dr. Winford H. Smith, superintendent of the Hospital, had accepted membership on the Advisory Committee; it was hoped, she added, that Dr. William H.

Welch would be the third member. Dr. Welch did accept the invitation to serve on that committee.

The Endowment Fund Committee lost no time in seeking the counsel of its Advisory Committee. The report of the treasurer, as of July 23, 1916, records the sum of $1,665 expended for United Railway and Electric Co., 1st Consolidated 4% Bonds. In this same report the total moneys received are given as $3,550. The practice of listing the names of those making cash contributions and those making pledges according to classes was begun with this report and continued for the next twelve years. The contributions of physicians and the "public" were also given in these lists.

Miss Waters, secretary of the Endowment Fund Committee, must have believed in the power of graphic reporting to spur into action. At the annual meeting of the Alumnae Association, May 1917, she presented two bar diagrams, one showing the total number of members in each class from 1891 to 1917 inclusive and the number that had contributed to the endowment; the other, the amount pledged by each class and the sum already paid on the pledge. That stalwart first class of 1891 had pledged the largest amount, and more than half of its members had already contributed to the fund. Every class had either contributed or pledged or done both. The record testified to the vigorous work of the committee. It was made clear that the purpose of the charts was not only to show what had been accomplished, but also *how much more was to be done*.

The secretary reported that all preparations had been made to mail the letter, proposed at the last annual meeting, to Johns Hopkins physicians. The mailing was delayed from week to week because of the unsettled conditions of the time. The committee thought it wise to wait for a more favorable moment; then the United States entered the European war. Nevertheless, it was urged that individual effort go on.

The secretary also reported she had recently returned from the 1917 national nursing convention in Philadelphia. One of the most heartening reports she brought back was that endowments for nursing schools were being begun by other schools in other states. Upon the solicitation of Mrs. A. C. Hartridge, a member

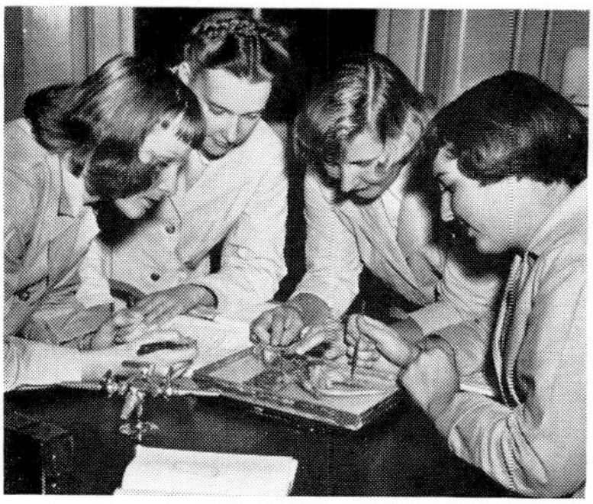

Class Room

JACK ENGEMAN

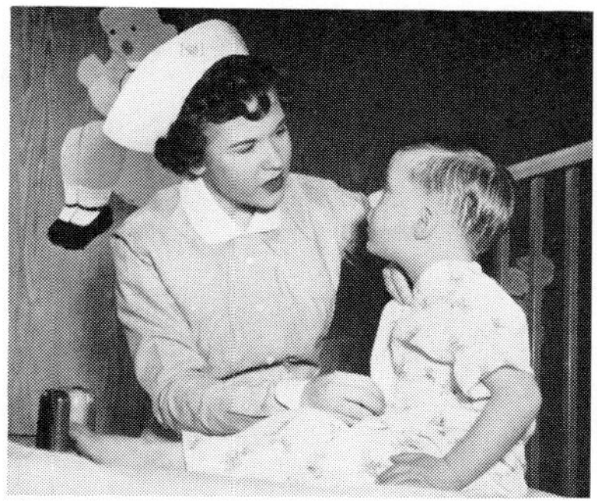

Ward
[U.S. Children's Bureau]

GEORGE JONES

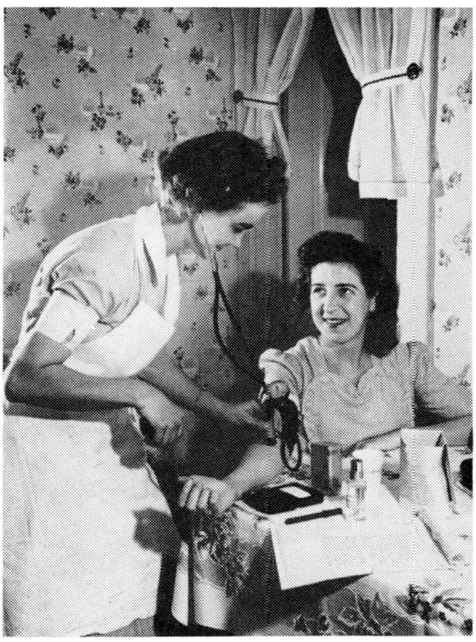

Community

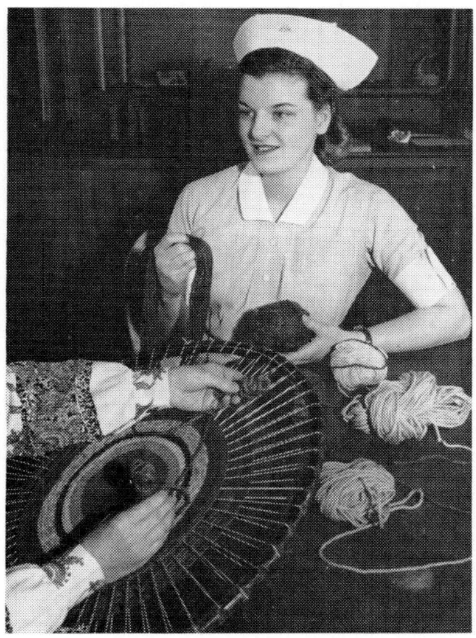

Occupational Therapy

CURRICULAR ACTIVITIES

of the Endowment Fund Committee and principal of the University Hospital School of Nursing in Georgia, a wealthy citizen had made a substantial contribution as a nucleus of an endowment for the Georgia school. The first gift to an endowment fund for the Massachusetts General Hospital School of Nursing was made by one of its graduates during the summer of 1915; in 1916 the Alumnae of that school took up the matter. A second school in Massachusetts had started its fund and a large school in New York was beginning an endowment campaign. On the memorable occasion of the twenty-fifth anniversary, Miss Nutting had said, "How fitting it would be to have this school lead the way in this essential advance." Well, the doctrine of endowment had spread since that October day in 1914, less than three years ago.

The Endowment Fund Committee promptly saw to it that its financial activities were operated according to correct business methods. The second of the yearly reports of the treasurer, submitted in May 1917, bore the notation, "Audited and found correct. Thomas M. Bartlett." Mr. Bartlett was cashier, Easton National Bank.

Early in 1918, an editorial in the *Alumnae Magazine* informed its readers that every cent contributed to the endowment until the end of the war would be invested in Liberty Bonds. Nurses who gave to the fund would have a double satisfaction; they would be helping to maintain professional standards and to win the war by lending their money to the government.

By May 1918 approximately $13,000 in cash and pledges had been subscribed to the fund. But that was not enough—far, far from enough. The secretary again used diagrams to drive home the fact that much more could be done by the Alumnae. Of the 858 graduates less than 25 per cent had contributed and pledged to the fund. Other sources of giving, said the secretary, which had barely been tapped were patients and friends. From this group, only fourteen different people had made contributions, amounting to $850.

In October 1918 Olive Schureman, class of 1916, died of pneumonia at Camp Meade in the service of her country. Realizing the possibility of death, she gave instructions for the disposal of her possessions and provided that $500 be given to the endowment fund of the School. In this final act, Miss Schureman poignantly symbolized the hope and the faith of her sister Alumnae.

World War I had begun in August 1914, the organized movement to raise a fund for the School, November 1914. The endowment campaign was actually launched in April 1916; one year later the United States entered the European war. The emotional strains which engulf a nation in the grip of a world-wide conflict and the financial drain upon its resources, inevitably react unfavorably upon any effort designed to raise money for purposes other than those directly related to the war. On November 11, 1918 the armistice took place. On November 28, 1919 the Executive Committee of the Endowment Fund Committee met. The endowment cash receipts were still less than $10,000. Now that hostilities had ceased, peaceful interests and peaceful pursuits were again in order, and the world would again lend its ear to an endowment movement so vital to the health of the nation. The time had come, the committee decided, to start afresh the work on the endowment fund.

Having agreed to renew the work on the endowment, the committee proceeded to act. In the early Twenties a new interest was being manifested in nursing, particularly in public health nursing. Large foundations were giving of their means to health programs and those related to health; the study, *Nursing and Nursing Education in the United States*, sponsored by a distinguished committee and financed by the Rockefeller Foundation was then in progress.[6] It seemed an auspicious moment to seek foundation aid. The Rockefeller Foundation was approached by the chairman of the Endowment Fund Committee; the Foundation officials were sympathetic, but they gave no promise of help.

Undaunted the committee turned its zeal in other directions. Colleges and universities either had raised or were raising large sums of money: Wellesley, two million dollars; Smith, four million; Bryn Mawr, two million; Harvard, fifteen million. Letters were sent to some seventeen well-known colleges and universities requesting information on their campaign methods. Sixteen re-

[6] Committee for the Study of Nursing Education, *Nursing and Nursing Education in the United States*. New York, Macmillan Co., 1923

plied; their answers were courteous and helpful. The more common features of their campaigns were alumnae sponsorship, class and regional organization, and an extensive publicity program. In some instances a professional firm was responsible for the drive. The John Price Jones Corporation of New York was conducting the Harvard campaign; it was also concerned with the campaigns of Smith, Bryn Mawr, and Mt. Holyoke. The logical next step was to inquire into the possibilities of utilizing the services of that corporation.

Promptly the secretary of the Endowment Fund Committee had an interview with Mr. Jones. Mr. Jones' best estimate was that it would cost $25,000 to raise one million. But where and how was the committee to find $25,000? Endowment receipts now amounted to $12,000. The Alumnae Association forthwith gave evidence of its faith in the committee and its unshakable conviction of the essential need of independent school funds. It voted to authorize the Executive Committee of the Endowment Fund Committee to take whatever steps necessary to implement the drive and to finance it with funds already collected.

Alert to its responsibility in preparing the soil, the *Alumnae Magazine* published in the November 1920 issue the full text of letters from Judge Henry D. Harlan, Dr. William H. Welch, Dr. Henry M. Hurd, and Dr. C.-E. A. Winslow. Each of these letters expressed sympathy, support, and confidence in the success of the campaign. Wrote Judge Harlan, "Our training school has stood in the front rank. . . . We wish . . . to keep it in the front rank. . . . I have an abiding confidence that you will not only embark upon this undertaking with enthusiasm, but that you will fully accomplish it." Dr. Welch said, "I consider the endowment of training schools for nurses one of the most urgent needs of the present day, not only for the better education of nurses for the sick but also to meet the crying need for the training of public health nurses. . . ." In his usual meticulous manner, Dr. Hurd outlined in detail the changes essential in the training program to meet new health needs and new opportunities and the necessity of an endowment to finance them. Dr. Winslow was plainly delighted and said so. "I think," said he, "there is nothing more important in the whole field of public health than the development of a few strong endowed schools of nursing, for it is only by obtaining adequate endowments that nursing schools will be able to realize their true educational possibilities."

Three meetings of the Endowment Committee and its executive body were held between the fourth and twenty-fourth of November 1920. Judge Harlan was present at the first meeting. The committee at once mapped out a tentative plan of procedure, began the reorganization of its forces, and empowered Miss Nutting to secure a trained publicity worker. At the quarterly meeting of the Alumnae Association in the same month. Miss Nutting announced that this second campaign would not be restricted to Alumnae members, physicians, and friends. "We are now strongly urged," said she, "not to limit ourselves to any such group, but to realize that the entire public is concerned with the education of nurses. . . ." Miss Nutting added that the committee had turned to Smith College for advice; that Mrs. Alice T. L. Parsons, chairman of the publicity committee of the Smith campaign, was present and would speak to the group.

Mrs. Parsons described how Smith had organized the campaign. A chairman was appointed with the privilege of choosing her committee personnel to conduct the campaign. The work was divided into several subdivisions: publicity, work with classes, work with potential donors—a potential donor being a person who could be asked to give more than five thousand dollars. Mrs. Parsons stressed the importance of publicity in newspapers and other publications. She declared, ". . . the thing which you are striving for is to make a whole world of givers know that good health means good nurses, good nurses mean Johns Hopkins Training School for Nurses, and Johns Hopkins Training School for Nurses means a million dollar endowment." The practical benefit of Mrs. Parsons' advice was reflected in the reorganization of the Endowment Fund Committee and the general conduct of the campaign.

By February 1921, the reorganization was complete. A finance committee with Mrs. Cullen as chairman was created and its function defined. Mrs. Cullen had been treasurer of the endowment fund since its beginning; she was well-qualified to take over the responsibilities of this new committee. At the same time, John C.

Thomas, treasurer of the Johns Hopkins Hospital, accepted the office of treasurer of the campaign. A men's advisory council was organized and also a women's committee. Mrs. Marie de Montalvo, a newspaper expert, was engaged. The membership of the campaign organization was an impressive one, as is shown in the list given in the Appendix, page 390.

Early in February 1921,[7] the *Sun* of Baltimore, which has ever espoused the causes for a better life, raised the campaign banner. Referring to the nurse, the *Sun* editorial said:

"She is a moral and physical necessity, and it is to the interest of the poor, even more than of the rich, that her tribe should increase, and that there should be enough of her to go around. . . . For this reason the nation-wide campaign to raise an endowment fund of $1,000,000 for the Johns Hopkins School of Nursing . . . is everybody's business. . . . Such an endowment is an endowment for ourselves."

The campaign was formally launched at a reception in the Nurses' Home on February 26, 1921. The Home with its spacious simplicity—high ceilings, long drawing room, wide entrance hall, and broad stairway—was attractively decorated with roses and pink snapdragons. Color was added by the white, blue, and pink uniforms of the graduates and students. The day began cloudy with melting snow and sleet in the streets. Around noon faint rays of sunshine broke through the clouds, as though trying to lend to the event brightness and cheer; by four o'clock the sun had again completely disappeared, and Baltimore settled into an early gray twilight. But if outside there were gloom and darkening skies, inside was the warm friendliness of people come together with a common purpose and a common belief. Enthusiasm and confidence were in the air. To the Johns Hopkins nurses it was a dedicated occasion.

The guests at the reception included representatives of the Men's Advisory Council, the Women's Committee, the Alumnae Association, and the School. Among those who voiced the need of an endowment on that occasion were Dr. Frank J. Goodnow, president of the Johns Hopkins University; Dr. William H. Welch, director of the School of Hygiene and Public Health,

[7] Feb. 8

Johns Hopkins University; Judge Henry D. Harlan, president, Board of Trustees, the Johns Hopkins Hospital; Dr. Winford H. Smith, director, the Johns Hopkins Hospital; Elsie M. Lawler, principal, the Johns Hopkins Hospital School of Nursing; and that long friend of nursing education, Dr. Henry M. Hurd.

"No educational institution can exist without adequate funds," said President Goodnow. Dr. Welch emphasized the necessity "to change the system completely to a new and better system. . . . If we are to make these changes an endowment is necessary, and our school should take the lead . . . as it has taken the lead in other things." Judge Harlan deplored the fact that the School lacked classrooms and essential equipment but stated that the Trustees had no more money to spend on it than they were now spending. "So money will have to come from somewhere else," said Judge Harlan, "if the nurses are to get what they must have." Miss Lawler declared, "One thing we do know, we are definitely faced with the fact that with the present organization of our school, we are neither utilizing the abundant facilities within our reach, nor yet are we fulfilling our obligation to the public."

The impetus given at the launching reception swept the various committees into vigorous action. The secretary, Yssabella Waters, always alert to the effect of facts and figures, published in the May 1921 *Alumnae Magazine* the number that had been graduated from each class (in the case of two classes still in the School, the number in each class), the number from each class that already had subscribed, and the amount subscribed. Since the inception of the fund, somewhat more than half of all the graduates had given to it $43,000. Somewhat less than half were still to make their offerings; with a well-aimed barrage of the spoken and written word, they, too, would pay tribute to their School.

And the barrage was promptly forthcoming. By May the campaign office staff which consisted of five paid workers—the publicity expert and four stenographers—and volunteers, mostly graduates of the School, had sent out thirty thousand pieces of literature and more than eleven thousand letters. From the public at large, which was looked to for the greater part of the million, so far there had been little response. But the Potential Donors Committee, whose particular function it was to canvass possible donors of one thousand dollars and over, was gearing its forces and making every effort to build up strong sectional committees in every part of the country. The Regional Committee and the Class Organization Committee were exerting their utmost to have nation-wide representation. During the two months between February 25 and April 24, cash contributions and pledges amounted to $22,000.

Of all the episodes in the history of the endowment, none is more gallant than that of the Gate House Shop. Somehow the Shop reached into the hearts and, most important, into the purses of Johns Hopkins graduates in America, Europe, and Asia. The little house, well-known to every Hopkins man and woman, stands at the gate of the Hospital. Included in the plans of the hospital architects, Cabot and Chandler of Boston, "to produce the effect of a lodge at the entrance to an estate," it had served various purposes. At one time it was used by orderlies. Then rumor had it that the house was haunted; so said old Ben, doorman at the Hospital since it was opened in 1889.[8] Not liking ghosts, the orderlies abandoned the little house; for a long time it was empty.

One of the proposals to raise money for the endowment was a bazaar. The location of the bazaar was important. Dr. Smith gave permission to install a counter behind the statue in the rotunda of the Hospital where the telephone booths now stand. Then Mary E. Lent, 1895, suggested the gate house. To this suggestion the Hospital authorities gave their consent. In May 1921 the Gate House Shop opened its doors.

How the Shop grew, the interest and generosity of the nurses in supplying it with attractive, saleable articles, is a story in itself. Here let it suffice to say that the Shop worked for the endowment almost eight years and at the end of that time turned over to the fund $24,000.

By the end of 1921, subscriptions in cash and pledges received, since the launching of the second campaign, totalled $47,000. Some friends, physicians, and patients had made contributions, but largely the subscriptions came from the nurses, mostly in amounts of less than $100. The returns from potential donors—those givers of gifts of $1,000 or more—had not satisfactorily

[8] Old Ben, whose full name was Benjamin Alexander Frisby, died in 1936.

materialized, although many of them had expressed interest and admiration of the cause and the intent to send a check at a later date.

Several months after the launching of the drive, it was clear that it would not be a whirlwind campaign. Unless potential donors appeared who would contribute appreciable sums, an endowment of $1,000,000 must remain a distant goal. It is true that the campaign was undertaken at a time of financial stress. It is also true that the number of graduates from the Johns Hopkins Hospital School of Nursing was much smaller than the number from great colleges and universities. The committee critically examined the year's work, lined up realistically those features that had been weak and those that had been strong, and then proceeded to move into the new year, firmly determined to use the experience of the past twelve months in a new attack on the problem.

Despite determination and hard work the next two years were periods of marking time. Some changes took place in committee personnel: Helen Crawford, as chairman of the Class Organization Committee, was compelled to resign because of ill health and was succeeded by Amy P. Miller; Mrs. Agnes C. Hartridge assumed the responsibilities of chairman of the Regional Committee. John C. Thomas, treasurer, requested that the endowment books and bank accounts be examined by a certified public accountant. Such examination was made by Haskins and Sells, submitted at the 1922 annual meeting of the Alumnae Association, and thereafter submitted yearly until the fund was transferred to the custody of the Board of Trustees of the Hospital. Also at the 1922 meeting, Yssabella Waters, the secretary, reported that of the approximate $10,000 voted for the conduct of the campaign about $192 remained. "To continue even in a small way the work for the coming year," said the secretary, "will require another vote of confidence of the Alumnae which will carry with it the ability to draw on the Treasury whatever may be needed throughout the following twelve months." The vote of confidence was promptly given in the form of a second appropriation of $10,000.

For the year 1922, the subscriptions in cash and pledges totalled $15,000; for the year 1923, $4,700. Not enough in 1922 and depressingly little in 1923. Still there was no wilting of spirit. Well did the committee know that it was exploring untravelled paths; that, added to the obstacles of pioneer work, were the "hard times" of the early Twenties. When, in the spring of 1922, the committee agreed to postpone active effort until the fall, Miss Nutting declared that this postponement was not to be interpreted as any slackening of purpose. Miss Nutting wrote:

"On the contrary, let it be seen as a period in which we are storing up energy and considering plans for a fresh and more vigorous effort. . . . And if we should find that there is a long, long trail ahead of us let us remember that no great reform has ever been reached without long, patient, and devoted struggle. . . . The endowment of Schools of Nursing will be their enfranchisement toward which it is our great privilege to lead the way."

The study, *Nursing and Nursing Education in the United States*, financed by the Rockefeller Foundation, was published in February 1923. As a result of the study the sponsoring committee concluded its report by urging: "That the development of nursing service adequate for the care of the sick and for the conduct of the modern public health campaign demands as an absolute prerequisite the securing of funds for the endowment of nursing education of all types. . . ." [9]

Dr. William H. Welch and Dr. Winford H. Smith were members of the sponsoring committee. Dr. Welch for many years had ardently supported the principle of endowment for schools of nursing as well as for other types of professional schools. Dr. Smith in his annual reports to the Hospital Board of Trustees during the Twenties had urged the need of endowment for the Hopkins School.

Miss Nutting was also a member of the sponsoring committee. One can well believe that she played a leading role in the drafting of both the report and the conclusions. Quick always to sense and grasp an occasion, three months before the report was in print, in November 1922, she approached the Rockefeller Foundation for the second time and asked George E. Vincent, then president

[9] *Nursing and Nursing Education in the United States*, p. 30

of the Foundation, whether an appeal was in order for the Johns Hopkins Hospital School of Nursing. Mr. Vincent's reply came through Edwin R. Embree, the secretary of the Foundation, who wrote:

"The trustees expressed themselves as still unwilling to enter the field of direct financial aid to specific schools of nursing. We are not unhopeful that the time may come when there is just the right combination of persons, institutions, and ideals, when the Foundation may feel that it is desirable to aid in developing some of the newer programs and proposals in nurse training."

A few months later a substantial gift to Yale University made possible the establishment of a school of nursing. Evidently the Foundation had found in Yale University "the right combination of persons, institutions, and ideals" and now felt it "desirable to aid in developing some of the newer programs and proposals in nurse training."

About this same time, another large sum was given to nursing education: Mrs. Chester Bolton's gift of $500,000 to Western Reserve University. Miss Nutting wrote:

"Nurses the world over will rejoice deeply in these two great gifts . . . but none more warmly, more fully than the members of our own Alumnae who have for nearly a decade been striving to secure similar gifts for the Johns Hopkins Hospital School of Nursing. Well do they know how imperative is the need of such gifts for the education of nurses."

And the rejoicing of the Alumnae was fruitful rejoicing. In the gift to Yale, the Endowment Committee discerned that an appeal to the Foundation might be effective, *given the right conditions*. The Endowment Executive Committee voted in May 1924, to make a special effort to obtain funds from the Rockefeller Foundation, providing a practicable plan, which might enlist the interest of the Foundation, could be developed for reorganizing the present system of training.

In the same year an event occurred which, while not directly attributable to the Endowment Fund Committee, was due in some measure to its insistence that changes in the School program and organization were in order. During the late fall of 1924, a study of the School was made by an outstanding leader in nursing education. One outcome of the study was the appointment of a new Training School Committee. The chairman of the Endowment Fund Committee was later to become a member of that committee; for the next ten years the Endowment Committee extended its activities to serve directly the School in other ways than the establishment of an endowment.

Other events occurred in the year 1924 which affected significantly the Endowment Committee. In May the committee lost its chairman. Since the twenty-fifth anniversary of the Hospital and School, a decade ago, Miss Nutting had constantly kept before the Alumnae Association its privilege and its obligation to work for the endowment with all of its strength, its energy, and its resources. She infused into the committee zeal and enthusiasm and, when the tide of giving ran low, sent cheering words of hope and encouragement. She was relentlessly unflagging in her efforts to accomplish the end for which the committee set out: the establishment of a million dollar endowment for her beloved School. It may be that what Miss Nutting achieved was more fundamental than the immediate attainment of that goal: the spreading of the doctrine of endowment for nursing education.

With deep regret Miss Nutting's resignation was accepted. She was asked to become honorary chairman. Mrs. Isabella Stevens Hunner, who was appointed to the original committee and who had served as vice chairman since the reorganization of the committee in 1921, was appointed chairman.

Early in 1924 the committee learned that a campaign was contemplated by the Hospital and the University for large endowments for both institutions and that funds for the School of Nursing would be included. By that time the receipts of the committee, including pledges and interest, totalled $87,000. Of that amount, $12,000 had been expended for the second drive. This left a fund of $75,000.

The question of cooperation in the University-Hospital campaign was brought before the Endowment Executive Committee; the Executive Committee voted "that we express our interest and approval of the plan and would like fuller information about the proposed uses of the fund for the School, and to know in what ways we can effectively cooperate."

The University-Hospital campaign for $50,000,000 was launched in the autumn of 1925. In the meantime the Endowment Committee had received the "fuller information" it desired. Daniel Willard, a Trustee of the University and chairman of the Johns Hopkins Half-Century Committee, prepared an article for the November 1925 *Alumnae Magazine*. Wrote Mr. Willard, ". . . the cooperation and support of the alumnae of your school will be most valuable." In outlining the general plan of the campaign, he said, "It has been decided that approximately $11,000,000 ought to be raised within the next two years, if possible, to take care of the more pressing needs." Evidently endowment of the School of Nursing was considered one of the "pressing needs," since the immediate program included an item of $500,000 for "general endowment" of the School. The Half-Century Committee's publicity material included an imposing pronouncement entitled *The Johns Hopkins Hospital.* In this publication it was declared that:

"The best of our schools, colleges, and universities are endowed institutions or receive their income directly from the State and not as an indefinite part of some other appropriation. The foremost authorities on nursing education are of the opinion that this profession . . . will never be adequately provided for from the standpoint of education until its schools have independent endowment. To safeguard the system of education of nurses is most important to the public, to physicians, and to the whole public health program." [10]

Among the committees organized by the Half-Century Committee was a permanent one called the Johns Hopkins Hospital Association. A subcommittee of the association was the Women's Board, consisting of a number of guilds working for the different departments of the Hospital. One of the guilds was the Nurses Guild of which Mrs. John S. Gibbs, Jr., was chairman—a fortunate circumstance for the School and the Alumnae Association. Mrs. Gibbs was the daughter of William T. Dixon, second president of the Board of Trustees of the Hospital, wife of a member of the Board of Trustees, and sister of Mrs. Mary B. Dixon Cullen, editor of the *Johns Hopkins Nurses Alumnae Magazine*. Mrs.

[10] The Johns Hopkins Half-Century Committee, *The Johns Hopkins Hospital.* Baltimore, 1925, p. 28

Gibbs invited Amy Miller and Mrs. Elizabeth Thomas Kent, two Alumnae representatives, to serve as members on the Nurses Guild.

To inform and interest important groups in Baltimore of the necessity of an endowment for a nursing school, a meeting was held on November 16, 1925 at the home of Mrs. Gibbs. The occasion was well attended. Mrs. William M. Manly, chairman of the Women's Board, presided. Among the speakers was Carolyn E. Gray, who had made a study of the School the previous year. "With an endowment," said Miss Gray, "the faculty of your school could take a long look ahead, could develop a definite program . . . your school is good—marvelously good—considering its handicaps. . . . But just to be good is not good enough for Hopkins. Everyone expects nothing short of the *best* from you." Mrs. Manly and Mrs. Gibbs assured the audience of their earnest desire to help secure the necessary endowment fund.

Early in 1926, it was announced that the Endowment Fund Committee had a new secretary and a new chairman. Yssabella Waters, who was elected secretary at the first meeting, had resigned. She it was who prepared from time to time the schedules and diagrams to keep before Alumnae members the status of the endowment fund and particularly the contributions of individual classes. Her reports were masterly summaries not only of work that had been accomplished but also of work still to be done. She faithfully and ably served as secretary of the committee for ten years; now she resigned because of continued absence from Baltimore. Margaret Hoyt was appointed her successor. Mrs. Hunner resigned as chairman in the spring, her resignation to take effect not later than the autumn. The committee accepted Mrs. Hunner's resignation with regret. Amy P. Miller, a member of the committee since its organization, was appointed chairman, November 25, 1925. Two months later, John C. Thomas, treasurer of the endowment fund since the opening of the second drive, sailed for a trip abroad. James D. Leeke, now treasurer of the Hospital, assumed Mr. Thomas' responsibilities for the fund during his absence and later became the endowment treasurer.

From the beginning an inherent purpose of the Alumnae Association in building an endowment was unmistakable—the creating of means that would enable the School to retain and maintain a leading position in nursing education. To this time the Endowment Fund Committee had largely focussed its efforts on the solicitation of contributions from Alumnae members and a public educational program with the hope, justly warranted, that the public would give substantially to the fund. This hope had not been realized. Now with the Half-Century Campaign on and with the assurance of the wholehearted cooperation and support of the Nurses Guild, the Endowment Committee decided that both the Guild and the committee should have direct and specific information concerning the type of school for which funds were sought. With the intent of planning definitely the reorganization of the School, it was agreed to request the Hospital Trustees through the Nurses Guild to enlarge the present Training School Committee; it was also agreed to suggest names to the Trustees for additional members.

As the Endowment Fund Committee moved into the year 1926, circumstances seemed propitious. No longer was the committee a voice "crying in the wilderness": its chairman and another alumna were members of the Nurses Guild; the Guild, a subdivision of the Half-Century Committee, was actively supporting both the endowment and the proposal that plans be developed for the reorganization of the School; the Hospital Trustees had acted favorably upon the request that the Training School Committee be enlarged and that the personnel be added as suggested by the Endowment Committee.[11]

The enlarged Training School Committee met in January. A subcommittee was appointed "to study the question of a program" for the School. The subcommittee outlined a program which dealt solely with the needs of the School as a good hospital school. A modified form of this program provided one of the documents upon which a third appeal to the Rockefeller Foundation was based.

In October 1926, the appeal which asked for a minimum of $500,000 was presented to the Rockefeller Foundation for the

[11] For membership of the enlarged Training School Committee, see pp. 203–4.

Hospital Board of Trustees by Judge Harlan, president of the Board, Dr. Smith, Dr. Welch, and Miss Lawler. The intent of this approach was to secure funds in support of a demonstration showing the educational possibilities in a school of nursing conducted by a hospital. Both the president of the Foundation, George E. Vincent, and the director of the Foundation Division of Studies, Edwin R. Embree, were sympathetic and expressed themselves as believing that such a demonstration could make a contribution but that the school selected for the project should not be identified with a university, as was the Johns Hopkins Hospital School of Nursing. For that reason the appeal did not have favorable consideration.

In 1925 the Rockefeller Foundation had given assistance to the Vanderbilt University School of Nursing. At that time the control of the Vanderbilt School changed from the Vanderbilt University Hospital to the Vanderbilt University. Within two years the Foundation had given to two schools—both university controlled institutions.

On May 13, 1926 Judge Harlan sent to Mrs. Cullen a copy of the minute adopted by the Board of Trustees and giving their action on the program outlined by the enlarged Training School Committee. Of the modifications made in the program, the one rejecting the appointment of a director of the School and substituting in her place an educational director was particularly disappointing to the Endowment Committee. Eight days later, fifty-five Hopkins nurses, attending the Health Congress in Atlantic City, gathered for a "Hopkins" breakfast. It was agreed by the group to recommend to the Alumnae Association that the Association request the Hospital Trustees to receive its representatives who would submit information that vitally concerned the welfare and progress of the School.

The following week the recommendation was presented by the Endowment Fund Committee at the annual meeting. No time was lost by either the committee or the Association. On May 31, 1926, the committee met and suggested the names of eleven Alumnae to send to the Association with the request that a committee of seven with two alternates be nominated from the eleven and that the names of the Alumnae so nominated be mailed to

Association members for their vote. Two months later, July 1926, the committee, thereafter referred to as the Special Committee of the Alumnae Association, was elected. It consisted of M. Adelaide Nutting, professor emeritus, Department of Nursing, Columbia University, New York, N.Y.; Elizabeth G. Fox, director, American Red Cross Public Health Nursing Service, Washington, D.C.; Anna C. Jammé, director, Bureau of Registration of Nurses, San Francisco, Calif.; Clara D. Noyes, director, American Red Cross Nursing Service, Washington, D.C.; Effie J. Taylor, professor of nursing, Yale University School of Nursing, New Haven, Conn.; Marion L. Vannier, director, School of Nursing and associate professor of nursing, University of Minnesota, Minn.; Anna D. Wolf, associate professor of nursing and superintendent of nurses, Albert Merritt Billings Hospital, the University of Chicago, Chicago, Ill.

With the Alumnae Special Committee elected, the next step was the appointment of a chairman. The committee was eager to have Miss Nutting steer it. Miss Nutting did not feel she could undertake the task. Every member of the Special Committee was keenly aware of the importance of the committee's work and the responsibility of its chairman. Wrote the chairman of the Endowment Fund Committee: "It seemed as if there had never been a group of women more distrustful of its ability to head a committee. Everyone thought some one else could do it better than she, but finally Miss Taylor, who held the same views with respect to herself, consented to undertake it provided each member of the committee would promise to aid her in every way possible." After sixteen months of painstaking effort the Special Committee submitted to the Board of Trustees of the Hospital its findings and recommendations. The recommendations proposed changes in the administrative and educational policies of the School and focussed upon the establishment of an affiliation with the Johns Hopkins University.[12]

While the work of the Special Committee was in progress the Endowment Committee suspended activities to add to the fund. Then, too, the great depression of the late Twenties and early

[12] See pp. 204–5.

Thirties contraindicated resumption of fund-raising effort. As the year 1929 began the committee reported a fund of $100,000, one-tenth of the set goal, after fifteen years of uncommon and persistent effort. Discouraged by the fact that the University, the School of Medicine, and the Hospital had been given considerable sums since the opening of the Half-Century Campaign, while the Nursing School endowment had increased less than $25,000, largely from income on investments and Alumnae contributions, the spirit of the committee must have been at low kindling point. But the spark was still there and ten years later the Alumnae Association began a third drive.

At the annual meeting, May 1929, the Endowment Fund Committee suggested that the endowment fund of $100,000 be dedicated to Miss Nutting and that it be named after her. "As she has done so much to lead modern thought and action toward . . . endowments for schools of nursing, it would seem fitting for her own school to honor her for what she has done. . . ." The Alumnae Association voted unanimously upon the suggestion, profoundly pleased to pay tribute to one who for many years had been its illustrious leader. The name of the fund was now the M. Adelaide Nutting Endowment Fund of the Johns Hopkins Hospital Nurses' Alumnae Association.

At the quarterly meeting of the Alumnae Association, February 1932, Miss Miller, chairman of the Endowment Fund Committee, reported the receipt of a letter from the Advisory Board of the School of Nursing. The Board requested of the Endowment Fund Committee an appropriation of $4,000 to finance a survey for the purpose of studying the facilities available for public health nursing in the basic curriculum and outlining a plan for a public health nursing course. The Endowment Committee, by a large majority, recommended the granting of the request.

An important outcome of the survey was the recommendation that an instructor in public health nursing be appointed on the School faculty. The Advisory Board again approached the Endowment Fund Committee and asked that the unexpended portion of the $4,000, appropriated for the survey, be used for the salary of a public health nursing instructor and that thereafter the salary of such instructor be paid by the endowment fund. The committee agreed to pay the salary for a two-year period. According to the report submitted at the annual meeting of the Alumnae Association in May 1933, "The majority did not feel it was advisable or in line with the spirit for which the fund was collected to bind ourselves to support this work for a longer time as it might interfere with our participation in a plan for more fundamental educational progress." Later, however, the committee underwrote the salary for a third year.

It is clear from the record that by 1934 the use of any part of the accumulated fund for purposes other than that originally intended—the building of a substantial endowment—raised questions in the minds of the committee members. In April 1934, the *Alumnae Magazine* published a concise history of the endowment with the title, "Twenty Years Later," by Amy P. Miller. Miss Miller squarely stated the issue, "what we as the legal custodians of this fund have the right to do." One month later at the annual meeting of the Association, Hester K. Frederick presented a carefully considered memorandum. Miss Frederick summarized in two questions the gist of the memorandum:

"Do we wish to incorporate this fund in such a way that not only the principal shall remain intact, but that the interest should also accumulate and be added to the principal until the fund can be increased to such a time when it can adequately endow the school of nursing?

"Or, do we wish to incorporate this fund in such a way that the principal shall remain intact, but that the interest may be used at times to further the educational advantages of the School of Nursing if such a cause presents itself and seems worthy of consideration by the endowment fund committee?"

At the same meeting the chairman of the Endowment Fund Committee reported that the committee was considering "some rather important steps" which, when formulated more definitely, would be presented to the Alumnae Association. The "steps" referred to consultations with a lawyer for a legal interpretation of the purposes to which the income from the fund might be applied.

In August 1935 the committee sent a questionnaire to the Alumnae membership. In essence the questionnaire asked whether the members were in favor of the Alumnae Association retaining the administration of the endowment fund, provided it could be done legally, or in favor of transferring the fund to the Hospital Board of Trustees. Only about 15 per cent of the members returned the form, a large majority of whom were in favor of the Association retaining the administration.

A second communication was sent to the membership in May 1936, stating one of the problems which confronted the Alumnae Association. In the 1921 drive the subscription blank had specified, "I agree to give to the Trustees of the Johns Hopkins Hospital for an Endowment Fund of the School of Nursing. . . ." According to the legal advice received, the wording of the blank indicated the intention of the Association and the subscribers to transfer eventually the fund to the Board of Trustees. Of the 286 members returning the May communication, 98 per cent were in favor of transferring the greater part of the fund to the Trustees of the Hospital.

At the quarterly meeting in November 1936, the Endowment Fund Committee presented the following recommendation to the voting body of the Association:

"That the amount of $130,000 be turned over to the Trustees of The Johns Hopkins Hospital as a fund to be known as The M. Adelaide Nutting Endowment Fund for the School for Nurses; the income from the Fund to be administered for the further advancement of educational work in the School for Nurses, for such projects as shall be recommended or approved by the Advisory Board of the School for Nurses; the remaining amount, $7,533.52, to be used as a working fund by the committee which will continue toward a larger fund for the Endowment."

The recommendation was favorably acted upon and promptly forwarded to the Hospital Board of Trustees. On December 8, 1936, the Board adopted the following resolution:

"Resolved, That the Trustees of the Johns Hopkins Hospital are willing to accept as an Endowment Fund for the Nurses Training School to be known as the 'M. Adelaide Nutting Endowment

Fund for the School of Nursing,' the amount of $130,000 to be turned over to them in cash or securities having a market value of $130,000 with power to the Trustees to hold and invest and reinvest the said fund from time to time in other securities in their discretion, and to use the income from the fund for the 'further advancement of educational work in the School of Nursing, for such projects as shall be recommended or approved by the Advisory Board of the School of Nursing.' Provided, however, that the income from this fund may be used for educational work heretofore paid for through funds provided by the Nurses Alumnae Association, but shall not be used for educational work now paid for out of funds of the Hospital until the 'M. Adelaide Nutting Fund' shall produce income sufficient to carry the entire educational program.

"AND BE IT FURTHER RESOLVED, That the Board of Trustees gives its approval to the use of $7,533.32 remaining in the fund collected by the Endowment Fund Committee as a working fund towards a larger fund for the endowment of the School of Nursing."

On January 30, 1937 the Alumnae Association transferred $130,000 of the endowment fund to the Trustees of the Johns Hopkins Hospital. The money remaining in the fund then amounted to $16,000. Upon the recommendation of the Endowment Fund Committee, the $16,000 was transferred from the care of that committee to the care of the Alumnae Association, to be known in the records of the Association as "The M. Adelaide Nutting Endowment Fund" and to be used "as a nucleus for a future drive to enlarge the Endowment for the School of Nursing."

The period from 1925 to 1939 was a crucial one in the life of the Endowment Fund Committee. Other than administering the business of the fund, the committee participated in and stimulated educational changes in the program of the School. During most of that period, Amy Phillips Miller, who had been voted a member of the committee at its first meeting in 1915, was chairman. Elected to office November 1925, she served in that capacity for ten years, giving all of her time without compensation to the activities of the committee. Bred in the Nutting tradition, Miss Miller passionately believed in its ideals and doctrines, the rock bottom of which was financial independence for schools of nursing. It was in the order of things that she should use her training and her talents, of talents she had many, to carry on courageously and vigorously the work toward the ultimate security of her own School.

Upon Miss Miller's resignation in November 1935, the vice chairman, Elma J. Hussey, directed temporarily the affairs of the committee. Mrs. Mary B. Dixon Cullen accepted the chairmanship in May 1936 with the stipulation that she would serve only until the autumn.

Although contributions to the endowment had practically ceased by the end of 1929, the Alumnae Association never gave up the idea of ultimately achieving a substantial endowment for the School. In the early Thirties, it was not the time to renew activities; the country was in the grip of an economic spasm. But by May 1936 the committee declared itself as "anxious that the Alumnae shall continue to enlarge the Fund with the possibility of an intensive effort in 1939, the 50th anniversary of the School."

As already stated, a fund of $16,000 remained after the transfer of $130,000 to the Trustees. The purpose of this fund, as specifically stated in the resolution of the Alumnae Association, was for continuing the work toward a larger endowment. The Board of Trustees concurred with that purpose. This concurrence was expressed in letters received from the president of the Hospital Trustees, Judge Henry D. Harlan; from the president of the University, Dr. Isaiah Bowman, then a member of the Advisory Board of the School of Nursing; and from Dr. Winford H. Smith, director of the Hospital. Judge Harlan wrote, "They [the Trustees] are in hearty accord with the desire that the School shall be adequately endowed to make and keep it one of the, if not the leading Nursing School in the United States. . . ." Dr. Bowman said in his letter, "Should an enlargement of the Fund be brought about, it would greatly aid in the combined effort that must now be made to safeguard our educational ideal that only the best possible training is good enough for a school of such influence and prestige." Dr. Smith said he was "glad to learn that the Alumnae are to continue their efforts to add to this fund."

Encouraged and hopeful, the Alumnae Association once more tackled a drive for increasing the endowment. Moreover the fiftieth anniversary of the Hospital and School seemed a propitious time to bring the endowment again into focus. Four months after the transfer of the fund to the Trustees, the Association voted to appoint a new Endowment Fund Committee. Caroline E. Falls, 1925, accepted the chairmanship of the new committee and Elizabeth A. Phillips (Mrs. R. R. Squier), 1925, the office of secretary-treasurer. Other Alumnae members who served on the committee were: Mrs. Helen Wilmer Athey, Christina M. Dick, Alta E. Dines, Elma J. Hussey, Elsie M. Lawler, Mrs. Dorothy Filler McBride (ex officio, as president of the Alumnae Association), Mary S. Purcell, Effie J. Taylor, Marion E. Thuma, 1926, and Ernestine Wiedenbach, 1925. The Trustees of the Hospital later adopted a resolution giving approval to the campaign and designated "the unrestricted gift of $4,231.87 in the will of Emil B. Vey to be added to the Endowment of the School of Nursing. . . ." The Advisory Board of the School also adopted a resolution supporting and commending the campaign.

By May 1938, the committee reported a plan for the campaign. The plan proposed "three fronts": approach to the individual, group activities in local centers, and a public information program. The plan further proposed that the Alumnae membership be organized geographically and that the geographic divisions launch the drive in their respective areas. The publicity material included "Within the Gates," an attractive pictorial book showing exterior and interior views of the Hospital, the School program in action, and episodes in the life of the School. The reaction of graduates in all parts of the country was wholeheartedly in favor of the campaign. The Gate House Shop again concentrated on earning money for the endowment, and early in 1940 turned over $4,500 to the committee, making a total of $28,500 earned by the Shop for the endowment fund. Contributions varying in amount from one to eight hundred dollars were received from thirty-two states and the District of Columbia, Europe, Canada, and such distant lands as China, India, and Africa.

The anniversary year came to an end, and with the end of the year the Endowment Fund Committee concluded its anniversary campaign. At the annual meeting in May 1940, the chairman recommended that "the amount of $13,666.62 be turned over to the Trustees of the Johns Hopkins Hospital to be added to the M. Adelaide Nutting Endowment Fund." With the unrestricted Hospital gift contributed by the Trustees, the fund was thus increased by approximately $18,000. The committee further recommended that "A chairman of the Endowment Fund Committee be appointed annually to keep alive the need for an Endowment Fund for the School of Nursing."

In terms of dollars, the net result of the 1939 campaign did not fulfill expectations and hopes, notwithstanding the enthusiasm and hard work of the committee and the Alumnae all over the country. Nevertheless, the drive did serve an important purpose. It demonstrated again the readiness of Hopkins nurses to organize and to work for their School, and it revived the endowment as a living, growing fund and brought the fund one step, even though a very small step, nearer the million-dollar goal.

In May 1941, Miss Falls resigned as chairman of the Endowment Fund Committee; the following November, Mrs. Mary B. Dixon Cullen accepted the chairmanship with Mrs. Helen Wilmer Athey, Alta E. Dines, and Anna D. Wolf as committee members. Mrs. Cullen had served the committee in various capacities; she knew the history of the endowment. Before accepting the chairmanship she made sure that the Board of Directors of the Alumnae Association should know her present point of view: she believed that the Association should cooperate with the Hospital Trustees in securing money from a national educational foundation. Also, before accepting the chairmanship, she told the Association she had asked Abraham Flexner, formerly associated with the General Education Board, if funds from such a source were available. Mr. Flexner replied that they were available but difficult to obtain. He said he was familiar with the long efforts of the Alumnae Association to secure an endowment.

The Endowment Fund Committee decided that Mrs. Cullen and Miss Wolf should confer with John S. Gibbs, Jr., president of the Hospital Trustees, with reference to Mr. Flexner's reply.

Mr. Gibbs expressed willingness to go to New York to see Mr. Flexner. When an appointment was sought Mr. Flexner wrote that "as yet his efforts in our behalf had yielded nothing, that he expected to come to Baltimore in the spring and would talk with us at that time." That was in November 1941; in December Pearl Harbor was attacked and this country was at war. Mr. Flexner did not come to Baltimore in the spring, but he did write to Mrs. Cullen that during a "global war" the time is "unpropitious" to solicit funds for an endowment. Two years later Mrs. Cullen received from Mr. Flexner another message. The message read: "The Johns Hopkins School of Nursing has revolutionized nursing, precisely as the University effected a revolution in higher education, and the Medical School in medical education and practice." One cannot doubt that Mr. Flexner had confidence in the School.

Mrs. Cullen held the chairmanship of the committee until the fall of 1944. In her final report she said, ". . . we must, with all our strength, secure that adequate endowment." Mrs. Cullen had served on the Endowment Fund Committee in various capacities over a period of twenty-nine years. At the first meeting in 1915 she was appointed treasurer and held that office for six years. When the committee was reorganized in 1921, John C. Thomas, treasurer of the Hospital, consented to serve as treasurer and Mrs. Cullen became assistant treasurer. At that time she was also appointed a member of the Executive Committee, chairman of the Publicity Committee, and chairman of the Finance Committee; she remained chairman of the Finance Committee for fifteen years. In May 1936, after the resignation of Amy P. Miller, Mrs. Cullen accepted the chairmanship of the Endowment Fund Committee "until autumn." But in 1941 she was again prevailed upon to take office as chairman.

Not only did Mrs. Cullen serve the endowment fund in so many important ways, but, as editor of the *Alumnae Magazine*, she wrote one editorial after the other, setting forth vigorously every circumstance that affected favorably or unfavorably the progress of the endowment. She must have been an astute financier; as treasurer and chairman of the Finance Committee, she shared much responsibility for endowment fund investments which, according to the record in 1936, "felt only slightly the effects of the recent financial upheaval." With her heart and her mind she strove over many years of disappointments and hopes to bring to fruition the endowment goal. She was indeed the unfaltering crusader.

There were others, too, who believed in the importance of financial independence for the School—nurses, hospital trustees, physicians, and friends. Many Alumnae members worked untiringly for the fund. John C. Thomas, treasurer of the Hospital, and his successor, James D. Leeke, both acted as treasurer of the endowment fund. For many years they ably served the committee and with Mrs. Cullen, the chairman of the Finance Committee, vigilantly guarded the investment of funds.

Of that company of men and women, whose counsel and help were freely and generously given, the names especially stand out of Mrs. John S. Gibbs, Jr., Dr. Henry M. Hurd, Dr. William H. Welch, Judge Henry D. Harlan, Dr. Winford H. Smith, Dr. Frank J. Goodnow, Dr. Joseph S. Ames, and Dr. Isaiah Bowman.

From 1915 to 1946 the Endowment Fund Committee had functioned as a special committee of the Alumnae Association. In 1946 the constitution and bylaws of the Association were revised and the Endowment Fund Committee made a standing committee. The membership and duties of the committee are given as follows: "The Endowment Fund Committee shall consist of five members who shall stimulate interest in and promote effort to increase the M. Adelaide Nutting Endowment Fund of the School of Nursing."

Even though the endowment activities had practically ceased by 1946, it is significant that the Alumnae Association should write into the bylaws a standing committee, "who shall stimulate interest in and promote effort to increase" the endowment fund. In so doing the Association, in considered and deliberate action, committed itself and Alumnae who would follow to carry through to realization the suggestion made by M. Adelaide Nutting long, long ago. The bylaw is there on the printed page, and as this history ends October 1949, it stands as a mandate to the Alumnae Association. If the past is an index of the future, the Association will again mobilize its forces to work for and to enlarge the endowment. It can render no greater service to the School.

The Johns Hopkins Hospital

Nurses' Alumnae Association

IT IS NO historical accident that the two women who shaped and gave substance to the School should have played conspicuous parts in the formation and growth of the Alumnae Association. There was no confusion in their goals—one led to the other: a professionally-conducted school of nursing, well-qualified graduate nurses, and a strong alumnae association. Isabel Hampton and Adelaide Nutting were not alone in their desire to create a group that could officially stand together, not only on professional, but also on public issues; the interest and zeal of many of the graduates, particularly those in the early classes, extended beyond the perimeter of nursing to the wider horizons of health, social, and civic affairs. As nurses and as public spirited citizens, the Alumnae Association provided them with an instrument for voicing their convictions and their aspirations for the common good.

On June 3, 1892, less than three years after the inauguration of the School, twenty-five members of the classes of 1891 and 1892 met in the classroom of the Nurses' Home "for the purpose of organizing an Alumnae Association." [1] A temporary chairman

[1] The Alumnae Association of the Johns Hopkins Hospital Training

was appointed; then followed the nomination and election of officers for the ensuing year. Helena Barnard, 1892, was elected president; M. Adelaide Nutting, 1891, vice president; Georgia M. Nevins, 1891, secretary and treasurer; and Susan C. Read (later Mrs. W. S. Thayer), 1891, corresponding secretary. Six days later Isabel A. Hampton and Lavinia L. Dock were elected honorary members of the new association.

The infant organization lost no time in drafting a constitution and bylaws and incorporating under the General Laws of the State of Maryland. It was fortunate in having the advice of Skipwith Wilmer, later a Trustee of the Hospital. At the first annual meeting a resolution was passed "that a vote of thanks be tendered to Mr. Wilmer, Attorney, on behalf of the Association for his generous aid in securing the Charter." The Certificate of Incorporation specifies the name of the new corporation as "The Alumnae Association of the Johns Hopkins Hospital Training School for Nurses of Baltimore City." In 1933, a less cumbersome title was adopted. Thereafter the official name of the Association was "The Johns Hopkins Hospital Nurses' Alumnae Association, Incorporated."

The object of the Association is stated in Article 1 of the 1892 Constitution as, "the promotion of unity and good feeling among the Alumnae, and the advancement of the interest of the profession of Nursing, and also of providing a home for its members, and of making provision for them if ill or disabled." Actually the organization was soon engaged in activities not strictly encompassed in the declared objectives, although they too received punctilious attention.

The first year must have been a busy one for the Association. At the first annual meeting in 1893, the officers could report that a charter had been obtained, bylaws drafted, a building fund and a sick benefit fund established, and a badge and motto adopted. In her presidential address Miss Barnard said:

"We have before us the possibility of becoming either a known

---

School was the third nursing school alumnae organized in the United States. The first was the Bellevue, 1889; the second, the Illinois Training School, 1891.

and felt power in the nursing world, or an inactive body, accomplishing nothing, merely existing. . . .

"To achieve anything worthy, we shall find it necessary to work as a whole, as one. . . .

"This is *your* Association, and it will be just what you make it. . . ."

It soon became apparent that the pioneer members chose to become "a known and felt power in the nursing world." The Association sent M. Grace O'Bryan, 1897, as a delegate to the 1904 annual convention of the Associated Alumnae of Trained Nurses of the United States. In her report Miss O'Bryan spoke of "the general feeling expressed at the Convention that the Johns Hopkins Hospital nurses stood for progress. . . ." Indeed during the first ten years of its existence the Association set in motion a vigorous program and engaged in some of its most far-reaching activities.

The organization promptly acted on the pledge given in the constitution, "of providing a home for its members, and of making provision for them if ill or disabled." The "home" was made possible in 1895 through the generosity of George W. Grafflin. Mr. Grafflin became interested in the Association's efforts to establish a home for its members through Charlotte Ewell, 1893, who nursed his daughter. He offered the Association the use of the house, 219½ East North Avenue, then vacant, with no obligation other than payment of ground rent and taxes and keeping the house in good repair. The offer was appreciatively accepted and the "Club House" officially opened July 4, 1895. On the evening of August 31, 1940, its hospitable doors quietly closed. In an editorial on "The Passing of Our Club" in the October 1940 issue of the *Alumnae Magazine*, "H.S.W.A." wrote, ". . . we shall not forget that for forty-five years those old walls housed many splendid women, nor the work that they have done for illness and the honour of their profession."

The Sick Benefit Fund at once became the concern of the Association. The fund was built over the years from a "tax" on the membership, from moneys set aside from the regular dues, from gifts, and from contributions of the Gate House Shop. Two bequests, $5,000 each, came from early graduates of the School:

one from Gertrude Hemming (Mrs. C. H. Frost), 1892, in memory of her sister, Evelyn M. Hemming (Mrs. R. S. Allen), 1897; and the other from Edith Carson (Mrs. S. H. Wilder), 1902. It would appear that the Benefit Fund was originally intended as a loan fund. The "loan" ruling, however, was not rigidly adhered to, and in instances where the circumstances warranted, the debt was cancelled. The requests for loans were never large in relation to the total Alumnae membership. When the question of interest on a loan came up at the 1908 annual meeting, Mary Cloud Bean, 1895, then president, replied, "There is absolutely no interest attached. On the contrary, a great deal of affection goes with it." The Sick Benefit Fund has a special historical interest in that it was one of the first activities undertaken by the Association and the only one of the projects, begun during the early Nineties, still functioning as this History came to a close at the end of 1949.

The origin of the motto and badge is also found in the first constitution and also goes back to the early Nineties. Article XIV of the original constitution states:

"The motto of the Association shall be 'Vigilando.' . . .

"The badge of the Association shall be in the form of a Maltese Cross, and bearing the colors of the Johns Hopkins University in blue and black enamel on a background of gold, the centre bearing the letters J.H.H., and on the back the year of graduating and the motto."

The story goes that from the several suggestions for a motto submitted by members of the Association, Miss Hampton favored "Vigilando," the motto adopted. Whether legend or fact, certain it is that Miss Hampton had a strong sense of the nurse's moral responsibility for vigilant watchfulness. At the third annual meeting she suggested that the Association have a "Code of Ethics," whereupon the assembled company "resolved that a Committee be appointed with Mrs. Robb as Chairman, on 'Code of Ethics.' . . ." The following year, 1896, the committee submitted a code which was adopted. It was signed by Isabel Hampton Robb, Katherine C. de Long, 1894, Alice B. P. Conover, 1894, and Mary W. Heriot, 1894, and developed under seven headings.

1. The duty of the nurse to the physician.
2. The duty of the nurse to the patient.
3. The duty of the nurse to her school.
4. The duty of nurses to each other.
5. The duty of the nurse to the public.
6. The duty of the physician to the nurse.
7. The duty of the public to the nurse.

In 1942 a committee [2] was appointed to consider the revision of the code. The original code, then having endured for forty-six years, must have influenced the thinking and the lives of many Hopkins nurses.

Before the nineteenth century ended the Association launched two other professional projects, one of which was to carry on for the next fifty years.

At the annual meeting in June 1896 the Registry Committee was appointed. Members of the committee were: Ethel B. Barwick, 1893, housekeeper at the Club, Lucy P. Welch, 1892, resident of the Club, Lucy S. Gilpin, 1895, a non-resident, Mary E. Gross (Mrs. J. M. T. Finney), 1891, "a doctor's wife," and M. Adelaide Nutting, chairman. One year later it was possible to report "that a registry is now formally opened at the Club House."

In the meantime registry rules governing membership, fees, and so on had been compiled. Private nursing in 1896 was an affair of the individual. Each private duty nurse set her own terms for service. Consequently it is not surprising that one of the registry rules read thus, "Nurses are required to provide the Registrar with their schedule of prices. . . ." Apparently the private duty nurses did not adhere rigidly to their specified fees, for the final rule stated, "They should also keep her informed as to whether they are willing to give up any of their time to patients unable to pay the full prices."

For many years two of the questions that confronted the registry were: whether trained nurses who were not graduated from

[2] Members of the Committee for the Revision of the Code of Ethics: Alta E. Dines, Virginia M. Dunbar, Ruth L. Greenfield, Harriet K. Mitchell, Mary G. Sanders (Mrs. H. A. Price), 1934, Anne A. Stevens, 1914, Dora E. Twentier, 1929, Ethel Rainey (Mrs. D. M. Ward), 1946, Ernestine Wiedenbach, and Anna D. Wolf, chairman. The revision was published in the December 1951 issue of the *Alumnae Magazine*.

Hopkins should be permitted to use the registry; whether the Hopkins registry should be given up and all registry service in the city provided by a central directory. It appears from the record that nurses graduated from other schools were permitted to use the Hopkins registry because of the revenue their registration yielded and because they were needed to answer calls. But the question of the Hopkins registry merging with a central directory was a more controversial issue. Miss Nutting, at the annual meeting in 1907, bespoke "broad mindedness and progress" in considering a central directory, and there were other members who urged an open spirit toward registry centralization. In 1910 the Baltimore Central Directory was opened. But the majority of the private duty nurses wanted the Johns Hopkins registry for Johns Hopkins nurses, and it was not until 1946 that the Alumnae Association closed the registry which it had sponsored for half a century.

At the 1898 annual meeting, the Association announced it had embarked on a pioneer venture: it had introduced "Trained Nursing for People of Moderate Incomes" in the city of Baltimore. The rich could buy the nursing it needed; the poor could secure nursing through public and private charities. The Association now sought to meet the needs of people of moderate means by making moderately-priced nursing available to them in their homes.

Twelve months earlier a special meeting of the Association had been called to outline plans for the hourly nursing project. A memorial fund, contributed to by the public, was proposed as a means to support the activity until it was sufficiently known and accepted to support itself. It was also agreed that the organization and management of the new service be the responsibility of the Registry Committee. Miss Nutting was then chairman of that committee.

Interesting documents are extant on the beginning of the enterprise. Two leaflets were promptly printed describing the service. In one it is stated:

"The plan as at present outlined provides that a nurse will be sent by the Association to families, schools, or to sick persons in lodging or boarding houses, by the hour, and a moderate fixed price by the hour be charged for her services. The nurse will endeavor to instruct some member of the family, so that the work may be carried on successfully during her absence."

Rates were given in the same leaflet:

One hour or less	$ .50
Each subsequent hour or part of an hour	.50
Obstetrical case—all night	3.00
Obstetrical case—all day	3.00

The Hourly Nursing Service must have met with considerable success during the early years of its existence. Later it encountered financial difficulties and in 1924 was regretfully discontinued. The Hourly Nursing episode in the history of the Association will always be associated with the name of Helena Barnard. Ada M. Carr has recorded:

"The establishment of Hourly Nursing in Baltimore was one of Miss Barnard's notable efforts and was in the beginning entirely her idea. . . . To start the work she gave her services for six months. . . . At her suggestion this plan of hourly nursing was put into the hands of the Alumnae Association. . . ."

One of the most notable achievements of the Alumnae Association is the *Johns Hopkins Nurses Alumnae Magazine*. At the eighth annual meeting of the Association in 1900, Miss Nutting moved and it was so voted "that we as an alumnae association publish a magazine quarterly." The first issue appeared December 1901. Members of the Publications Committee responsible for this epochal event were: Ada M. Carr, chairman, Helen C. Bartlett, Emily J. McDonnell, 1892, Amy P. Miller, M. Adelaide Nutting, M. Grace O'Bryan, Georgina C. Ross, and Virginia Rice, 1899. The Association now could bring information and news to its members, wherever they were, through an official channel, not only on the activities of the organization and individual members but on all the great and stirring questions of the times. Ada M. Carr was the first editor.

The first number of the *Magazine* speaks eloquently of the Publications Committee's aspirations for the new venture. The committee boldly produced a journal of twenty-six pages, bound in blue and black (the colors of the badge), with the badge and

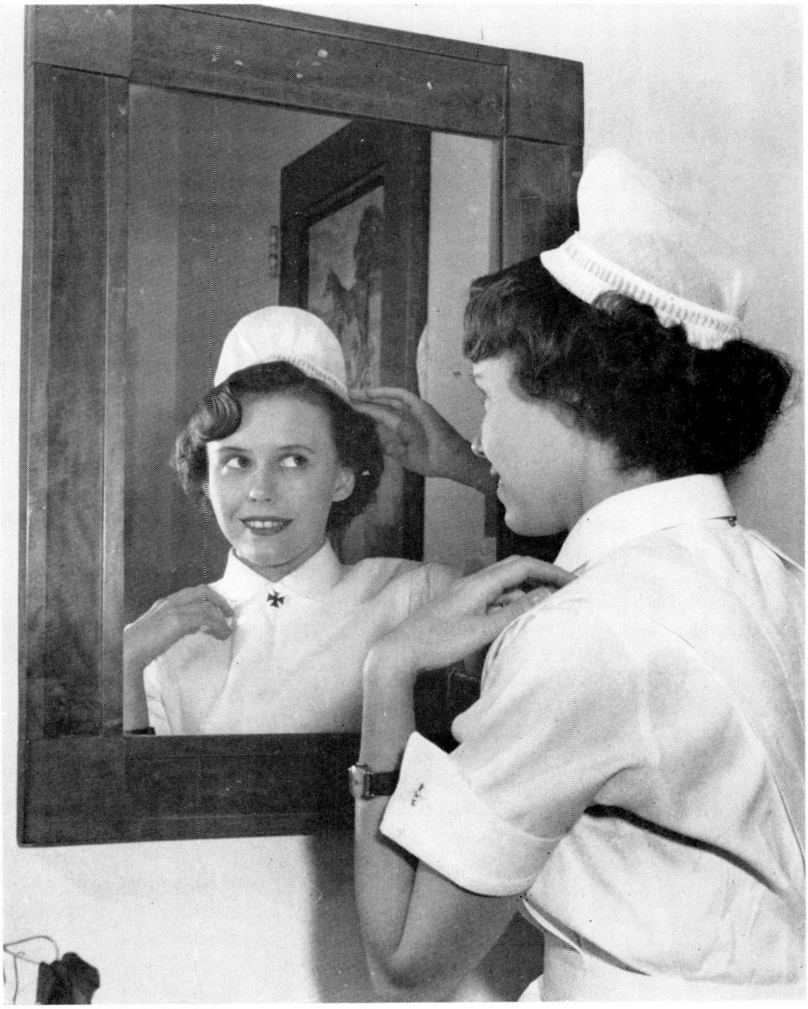

Vigilando

motto reproduced on the cover and also on the first page of the *Magazine*. Later the cover was changed to blue and white for reasons of economy. The annual subscription price was fifty cents. To help finance the project advertisements were sought, but the only concern risking a display in the initial issue was Meinecke and Company of New York City. When the second number appeared, three months later, five Baltimore firms, as well as the New York one, bought space, and financial prospects were brighter. Indeed Miss Carr was "pleased" to announce in May 1902 "that the Committee would now be able to repay the Association the loan necessary to defray expense of getting out the first number of the Alumnae Magazine."

Nevertheless subscriptions lagged and the patronage of advertisers was uncertain. It soon became apparent that a more stable way had to be found to finance the *Magazine*. At the annual meeting in 1903 the yearly dues were increased to three dollars, this sum to include subscription to the *Magazine*. Now the Association was financially responsible for the publication. Mary Bartlett Dixon, as chairman of the Publications Committee, gave "a most gratifying report" in January 1905, and again four months later. The number of advertisers had increased and altogether the outlook for the *Magazine* was encouraging.

Not only was the first number impressive in format, it was equally so in content. The content included "Report of Quarterly Meeting," "Delegates' Reports" on the convention of the Associated Alumnae of Trained Nurses, a brief article on "The Tuberculosis Question," a delightfully refreshing account of "An Outing in Idaho," a description of the new "Preliminary Course" at the Johns Hopkins School of Nursing, and a notice of an exhibition of the Maryland State Federation of Women's Clubs. The first issue was an indication of the varied interests that were to stamp the *Magazine*. Regularly the official reports of the Association were printed in the publication, as were also matters of professional nursing significance in the city, the state, and the nation, and discussions of vital social and public questions. Any voice on any good public cause could be assured a hearing, even though the Publications Committee maintained on it an official neutral attitude. Woman suffrage evidently gave much concern to an early graduate. This graduate wrote a letter to the Publications Committee which the committee published with the editorial note, "The Publications Committee endorses neither side of the Woman Suffrage Movement: but is willing to hear briefly, from members of the Alumnae Association their sentiments for or against the movement."

Of the authors whose writings appeared in the *Magazine*, there were many who wrote with grace and distinction; only a few can be mentioned. These few include M. Adelaide Nutting, Lavinia L. Dock, Dr. Henry M. Hurd, Dr. William Osler, Dr. William H. Welch, and Frank R. Kent.

Among the editors of the *Magazine* were some of the most distinguished members of the Alumnae Association: Ada M. Carr who possessed a sensitive and facile pen; Mary Bartlett Dixon, editor for sixteen years, who had convictions and the courage to express them; Clara D. Noyes, long a figure in the national and international scene, who brought to the *Magazine* a national flavor and an unerring sense of news.

About the time the *Alumnae Magazine* was begun, the library activity was initiated. Helena Barnard, at a meeting of the Alumnae Association in October 1901, urged the establishment of a library in the Johns Hopkins Nurses' Club. Speaking as chairman of the Library Committee Miss Barnard said, ". . . it has been felt by some of our members that the time has arrived when the dignity of our Club House should be augmented by the addition of a suitable collection of books. . . ." Miss Barnard then outlined the kinds of materials that should be assembled: reference books, books of general cultural value, and materials of historical as well as current interest. A handsome bookcase, that originally belonged to the Club, is now in the Historical Library of the School. This bookcase provides silent testimony to the earnest interest with which the Library Committee's report must have been received and the promptness of the Association in carrying out the committee's suggestions. It bears a plate with the inscription:

Library Established
January—1902
Section 1. Professional and Technical

The Library Committee gave its report in October 1901; the Alumnae library was established three months later, in January 1902.

In an article, "Alumnae Library, 1902–1945," by Ruth Brewster Sherman in the *Johns Hopkins Nurses Alumnae Magazine*, January 1949, Miss Sherman records that the William H. Welch Medical Library gave the Association the loan of two rooms at the time it was opened and that thereafter the Association deposited about half of its books in the Welch Library and kept the other half at the Club House.

The Club House was closed in 1940 and the books housed there were moved to the library of the School of Nursing as a loan. Two years later in the autumn of 1942, when the School was enjoying its newly remodeled library and the services of a full-time librarian, the books belonging to the Association on deposit in the Welch Library were transferred to the School, also as a loan. In 1945 the Library Committee recommended "that the Association give the Alumnae Library to the Training School, to be added outright to the School Library." The recommendation was approved by the Alumnae Association.

An enterprise of the Library, due to Miss Sherman's diligence, was "the building up of the system of libraries" that have either complete or partial files of the *Johns Hopkins Nurses Alumnae Magazine*. The "system" included historical, public, medical, university, and organization libraries, twenty-seven in number, located in cities from the east to the west coast. All had permanent, complimentary subscriptions.

Miss Sherman served as a member of the Library Committee for thirty-five years; for thirty-one she was chairman of the committee. At the annual meeting of the Association in May 1949, Mrs. Helen Wilmer Athey proposed that a bookplate be placed in the Alumnae collection as a tribute to Miss Sherman for her interest and efforts in gathering and preserving irreplaceable documents, finally deposited with the School. The Alumnae Association unanimously approved Mrs. Athey's proposal.

The idea of one other activity was projected before the Association reached its tenth birthday. In April 1902 the endowing of a bed in the Hospital for Alumnae members was discussed, "but owing to the large amount required . . . the question was dropped." From time to time the discussion was revived. A considerable amount was contributed by the Alumnae membership and a generous sum from the earnings of the Gate House Shop. Finally the Association was able to turn over $35,000 to the Trustees of the Johns Hopkins Hospital, and the idea of an endowed bed, born in 1902, became a reality in 1936.[3]

The history of the Endowment Fund Committee is given in detail in the study of the work of that committee. While the fund which the Association was able to build by the end of 1949 was far short of the goal, the work of the committee stands as a monument to the zeal of a tireless group of women.

Out of the work of the Committee on the Endowment Fund came the Gate House Shop. Since 1921 the Shop earned money, first for one Alumnae enterprise, then for another. Its wares included magazines, notepaper, postcards, candy, and many other useful little commodities. It dispensed Hopkins caps to any place on the globe. Mrs. Helen Wilmer Athey packed the caps, addressed them, and deposited them in the post office of the Hospital. Day after day, in the humid heat of Baltimore summers and the snow and sleet of Baltimore winters, Mrs. Athey could be seen in the Shop and the corridors of the Hospital. "Neither snow, nor rain, nor heat, nor darkness" stayed her rounds. She had her rewards—in the Shop's savings and the uses made of them. By the end of 1949, the little Shop could report total earnings of $60,600. Of that total, approximately the sum of $29,000 was given to the Endowment Fund, $7,700 to complete the necessary amount for the Endowed Bed, $3,500 to the Sick Benefit Fund; $1,900 for a station wagon to transport students to and from Sherwood Forest; and varying sums to other causes that affected the welfare of either the graduates or students. To Mrs. Helen Wilmer Athey, the guiding genius of the Shop, who steered its course for many years, to Mabel V. Bent (Mrs. W. W. Cator), 1902, and to a host of others who gave faithful service, the Alumnae Association members are deeply indebted.

[3] Mrs. Edith Carson Wilder, who died in 1941 and who bequeathed in her will $5,000 to the Sick Benefit Fund, also bequeathed $5,000 to the Hospital "for additional hospital care for sick Alumnae members."

Four years after the founding of the Alumnae Association of the Johns Hopkins Hospital Training School, the Associated Alumnae of Trained Nurses of the United States and Canada was organized. Mrs. Isabel Hampton Robb was elected the first president of the new organization and Helena Barnard, the first secretary. With Mrs. Robb at the helm, it is small wonder that the Hopkins Alumnae Association promptly voted to "become a member of the national association" and proceeded to take a lively interest in its activities. This interest in the infant national organization was indicative of the role that Alumnae members were to play in the rapidly expanding nursing scene. Throughout the years the graduates of the School have engaged in and wielded a considerable influence in national and international nursing affairs. Their names may be found on the rosters of important organization boards and committees, and in important positions in the service of their government.

As the twentieth century began, matters of state organization and state registration were agitating nursing groups. Early in 1901 Miss Dock spoke to the Alumnae Association on the "advantages" of registration. Anna E. Rutherford (Mrs. R. S. Dickey), 1891, then president of the Association, gave a report "at the annual meeting of the State Federation of Women's Clubs" in which she spoke on state registration, especially stressing the protection it gave the public from the incompetent "nurse" and bespeaking the support and cooperation of the Federation membership. M. Adelaide Nutting, a member of the board of directors of the Alumnae Association, took a leading part in the Maryland state registration movement and in the organization of the Maryland State Nurses' Association, of which she was the first president. Other Hopkins graduates on the first board of directors of the State Association were Georgina C. Ross and Susan Shrive, 1897.

Reading through the minutes of the Alumnae Association impresses one with the wide scope of interests and the intense sense of social and civic responsibility that characterized the organization, especially in the first two decades of its existence. Literally during that period, it took for its domain the whole field of public welfare. In 1900 the Association was accepted as a member of the Maryland State Federation of Women's Clubs and for many years sent delegates to the conventions of the Federation and received from its delegates full reports. It appointed a committee in 1901 to aid the medical profession and the municipal authorities in their fight against tuberculosis and another in 1908 to investigate almshouses. Among the nonnursing activities in which the Association interested itself were those of the Consumers' League, improvement of sanitary conditions in the Lexington Market of Baltimore, civil service reform, and child labor legislation.

For almost twenty-five years the work of the officers had been on a volunteer basis. In 1916 provision was made for a paid corresponding secretary-treasurer. Then in 1936, the positions of secretary-treasurer and editor of the *Alumnae Magazine* were combined. Claire R. P. Craigen, 1912, was appointed to the dual position. Miss Craigen reorganized the Alumnae Association office and instituted important administrative changes in the Association activities. She resigned early in 1946. Later in the same year the office of executive secretary was created. L. Judith Richardson, 1929, was the first appointee to the position.

The affection, the pride, and the hopes of the Alumnae Association for its parent School have manifested themselves in manifold ways. Of activities in behalf of the School, the work of the Endowment Fund Committee has been the most outstanding. Second only to that committee's work was the survey of the School made by the Alumnae Special Committee in 1927. Out of that survey came the Advisory Board of the School of Nursing which provided for two Alumnae representatives. By this representation a direct channel of communication was established between the School and the Alumnae Association.

In 1949 the Johns Hopkins Hospital Nurses' Alumnae Association had reached the ripe age of fifty-seven years. In this bird's-eye sketch many important events and activities of the Association necessarily have been omitted to be filled in at a later day when a life-size history is written. Many fine and able women have been members of the Association. From their ranks have come nurses who have served with distinction at home and in all parts of the globe and who have won honors for themselves, their School, and their Alumnae Association.

Appendix

UNDER the organization shown in Diagram 1, recommendations for changes in policy, revisions of the curriculum, and major modifications in administrative procedures in the School of Nursing might originate either in the School or in McCoy College. To consider such recommendations a special sub-committee with representatives from the School and the College was set up, and when agreement was reached the recommendations were forwarded to the Sub-Committee on Nursing Education. If the recommendations were not approved by that committee, they were returned to the Special Sub-Committee for further consideration; if approved by the Sub-Committee on Nursing Education and if action of higher authority was required, the recommendations were forwarded to the Medical Planning and Development Committee. If approved by the Medical Planning and Development Committee, that committee transmitted the recommendations to the Joint Committee of Boards of Trustees. Upon approval of the Joint Committee they were then forwarded to the separate Boards of Trustees of the Hospital and the University for action and/or information as appropriate. The Sub-Committee on Nursing Education was responsible in seeing to it that recommendations authorized by both Boards of Trustees were properly put into effect. On the operating level it was expected that a number of joint permanent sub-committees of the School of Nursing and of McCoy College would be functioning regularly and that joint special sub-committees would be appointed as indicated.

The organization as shown in Diagram 1 was operating in April 1953, at the time the History was completed.

DIAGRAM I

LINES OF COMMUNICATION OF THE SCHOOL OF NURSING WITH THE BOARDS OF TRUSTEES OF THE JOHNS HOPKINS HOSPITAL AND THE JOHNS HOPKINS UNIVERSITY

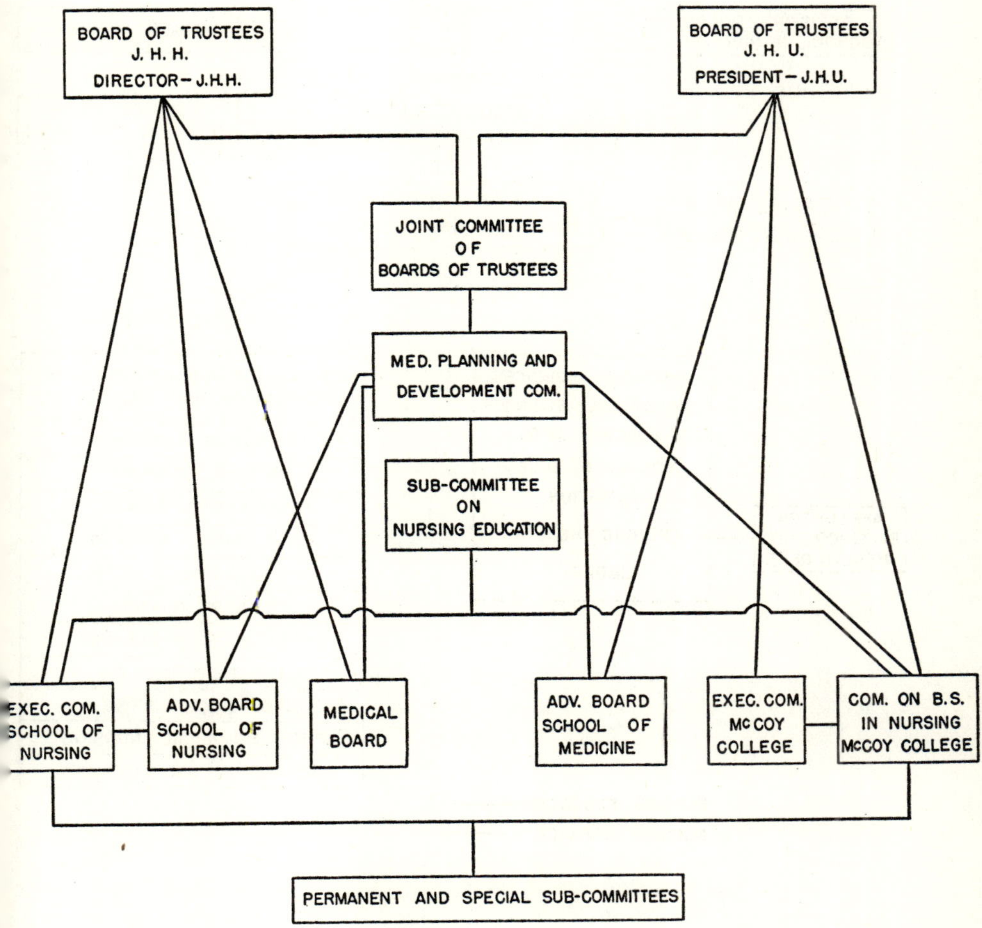

NOTE: THE LOOPS IN THE HORIZONTAL LINE DENOTE THERE IS NO INTERCEPTION OF CROSSING LINES.

…Y, 1948

DIAGRAM 2

THE JOHNS HOPKINS HOSPITAL
ORGANIZATION AND ADMINISTRATION OF THE SCHOOL OF NURSING AND NURSING SERVICE

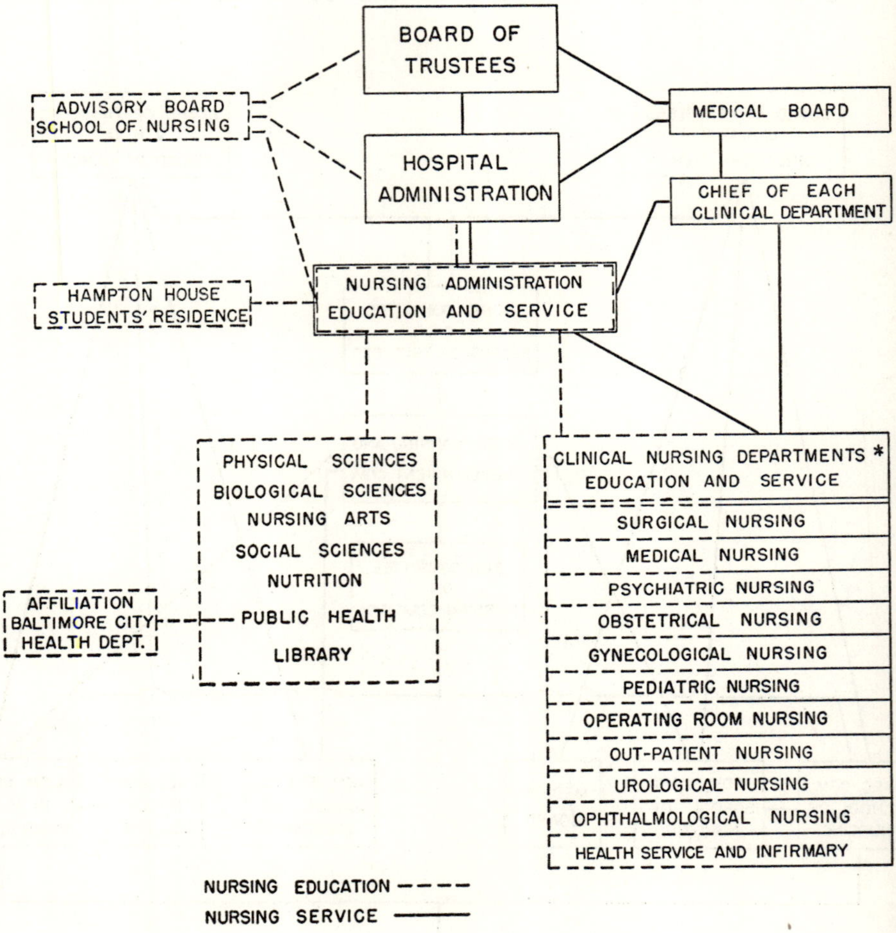

* IN THE CLINICAL NURSING DEPARTMENTS EDUCATION AND SERVICE CANNOT BE SHARPLY DIFFERENTIATED SINCE STUDENTS GIVE VARYING AMOUNTS OF SERVICE IN THE PROCESS OF LEARNING NURSING.

MAY, 1948

DIAGRAM 3

THE JOHNS HOPKINS HOSPITAL
ORGANIZATION AND ADMINISTRATION OF CLINICAL NURSING DEPARTMENTS

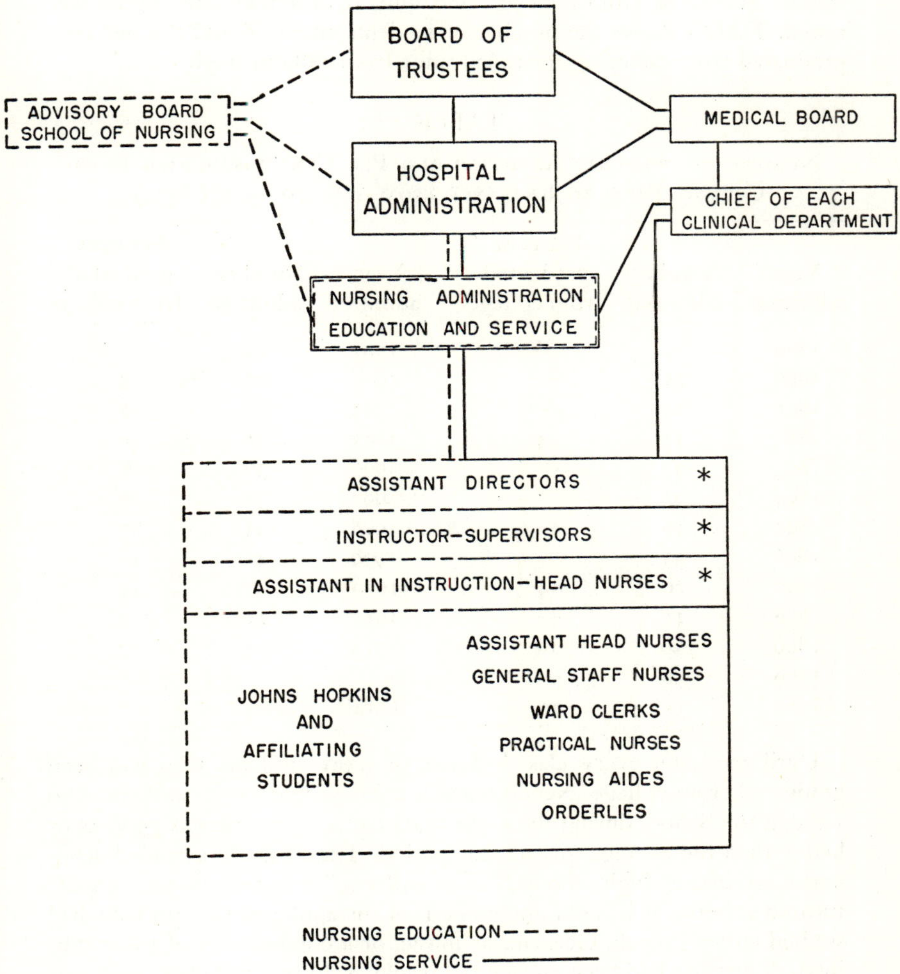

* RESPONSIBLE FOR BOTH EDUCATION AND SERVICE

MAY, 1948

STATISTICS

Students Admitted and Per Cent Graduated from College Prior to Entrance, 1889 to 1912 (incl.)

Before 1913, if a student had been graduated from college before admission to the Johns Hopkins Hospital School of Nursing, her record stated "graduated from college," and only occasionally the degree was noted. Table 1 shows the number of students admitted and the per cent graduated from college prior to entrance from 1889 through 1912.

TABLE 1

NUMBER OF STUDENTS ADMITTED AND PER CENT GRADUATED FROM COLLEGE PRIOR TO ENTRANCE FROM 1889 TO 1912 (INCL.)

Year admitted	Number admitted	Per cent graduated from college	Year admitted	Number admitted	Per cent graduated from college
1889	17	6%	1902	45	2%
1890	25	—	1903	37	5
1891	23	—	1904	39	8
1892	25	4	1905	38	8
1893	25	—	1906	36	8
1894	41	7	1907	48	8
1895	35	—	1908	45	7
1896	35	—	1909	45	11
1897	29	14	1910	47	19
1898	22	—	1911	43	5
1899	30	10	1912	54	17
1900	36	—			
1901	31	10	Total	851	7

Until 1901, not every class had one or more students who had been graduated from college. Nevertheless it is likely that many students who were in the School during the early years had an education as good as or better than the average girl of that period. They usually attended academies, seminaries, high schools, "ladies colleges," convent schools, or were tutored at home. It was not uncommon for the applicant to report she had studied either French, German, or music, or a combination of those subjects. A number had been engaged in teaching. In the first class, 1889, one student had the degree of master of arts; otherwise the degrees noted were baccalaureate degrees. Eight hundred and fifty-one students were admitted from 1889 through 1912; of this number fifty-nine, or 7 per cent, were graduated from college.

Students Admitted and Per Cent Having Degrees Prior to Entrance, 1913 to 1949 (incl.)

From 1913 through 1949 the degree earned by a student before admission to the School was specified. The per cent of students holding degrees varied widely, from 13 to 100 per cent.

TABLE 2

NUMBER OF STUDENTS ADMITTED AND PER CENT HAVING DEGREES PRIOR TO ENTRANCE FROM 1913 TO 1949 (INCL.)

Year admitted	Number admitted	Per cent with degrees	Year admitted	Number admitted	Per cent with degrees
1913	62	13%	1932	94	30%
1914	65	22	1933	92	45
1915	80	23	1934	89	42
1916	69	30	1935	89	43
1917	80	23	1936	86	48
1918	95	38	1937	97	38
1919	83	22	1938	84	37
1920	73	15	1939	83	34
1921	71	23	1940	82	34
1922	78	13	1941	101	36
1923	85	22	1942	195	40
1924	82	17	1943	202	20
1925	61	25	1944	214	38
1926	97	21	1945	108	79
1927	116	23	1946	30	100
1928	125	17	1947	27	100
1929	94	27	1948	69	35
1930	98	16	1949	66	26
1931	75	23	Total	3,399	32

The first peak in the curve occurred in 1918 during World War I. In that year the largest per cent of college women and the largest class up to that time were admitted to the Johns Hopkins Hospital School of Nursing. These increases were doubtless due to the work of the Committee on Nursing of the General Medical Board of the Council of National Defense. The committee carried on a national campaign to increase enrolment and to stimulate the entrance of college women in schools of nursing in order to meet immediate and postwar needs.

The years between 1933 and 1941 are marked by a larger proportion of college graduates than any previous year except 1918. Then in 1941 America entered World War II and another nation-wide campaign was waged by the National Nursing Council for War Service, again to expand enrolment and to interest college women in nursing. The Johns Hopkins School itself carried on an intensive recruitment program and despite the large number of entrants in 1942 and 1944 maintained its previous educational record. Late in 1944 a baccalaureate degree was made the educational requirement for admission to the School. All students admitted during 1945 had degrees except about one-fifth with two or three years of college from the Bryn Mawr College Summer School of Nursing. During 1946 and 1947 all entrants had baccalaureate degrees. In 1948 the minimum educational requirement reverted to high school graduation and the per cent of students with degrees dropped sharply, although the largest proportion still had either a degree or two or three years of college; in 1948, 91 per cent and in 1949, 85 per cent.

DIAGRAM 4

PER CENT OF STUDENTS HAVING DEGREES PRIOR TO ENTRANCE FROM 1913 TO 1949 (INCL.)

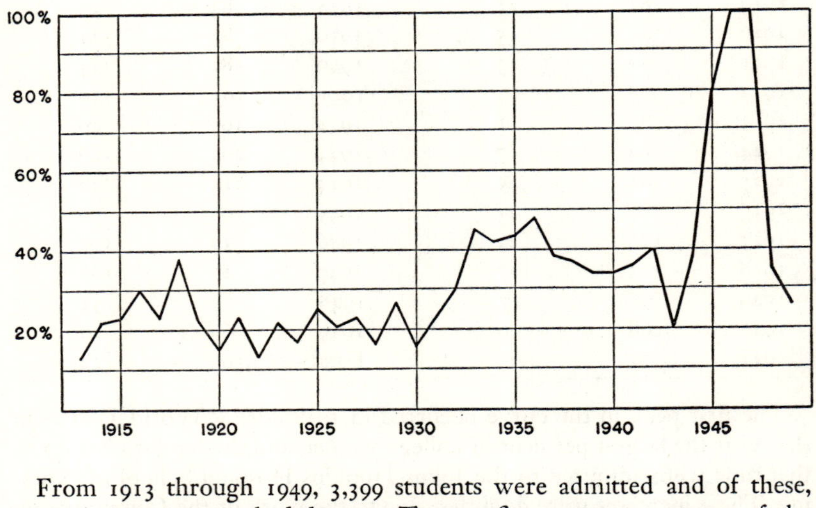

From 1913 through 1949, 3,399 students were admitted and of these, 1,071, or 32 per cent, had degrees. Twenty-five, or two per cent, of the degree-holding students had the degree of master of arts.

Total Students Admitted, 1889 to 1949 (incl.)

The total number of students admitted from 1889 through 1949 was 4,250.

Total Students Graduated, 1891 to 1949 (incl.)

In 1896 the program was changed from two to three years. Five students admitted in 1896 elected to complete their program in two years; all other students in three years.

TABLE 3

NUMBER OF STUDENTS GRADUATED FROM 1891 TO 1949 (INCL.)

Year graduated	Number graduated	Year graduated	Number graduated	Year graduated	Number graduated
1891	17	1911	35	1931	76
1892	19	1912	36	1932	67
1893	17	1913	39	1933	55
1894	21	1914	36	1934	57
1895	24	1915	45	1935	57
1896	33	1916	55	1936	56
1897	28	1917	43	1937	59
1898	5	1918	68	1938	47
1899	27	1919	50	1939	50
1900	24	1920	64	1940	73
1901	18	1921	83	1941	64
1902	28	1922	69	1942	69
1903	28	1923	58	1943	58
1904	25	1924	60	1944	84
1905	38	1925	64	1945	132
1906	32	1926	69	1946	149
1907	32	1927	68	1947	176
1908	31	1928	71	1948	59
1909	38	1929	84	1949	23
1910	40	1930	64	Total	3,097

During the sixty years of the School's existence, 3,097 students were graduated.

BYLAWS
of
THE FACULTY
of
THE JOHNS HOPKINS HOSPITAL SCHOOL OF NURSING

Article I

Name

The name of this organization shall be the Faculty of the Johns Hopkins Hospital School of Nursing.

Article II

Objects

The objects of the Faculty of the Johns Hopkins Hospital School of Nursing shall be:

(a) To formulate all policies which will further the aims of the School and the Nursing Service and to present these to the Advisory Board of the School of Nursing or to appropriate committees of the Hospital and the Johns Hopkins University.

(b) To promote all policies approved by the Board of Trustees of the Hospital.

(c) To foster interdepartmental relationships and general interest in the welfare of patients, students, and graduate staff.

(d) To promote professional growth and to stimulate research in nursing education.

Article III

Membership

The active members of the Faculty shall consist of:

(a) The director, associate and assistant directors, instructors, assistant instructors, assistants in instruction, supervisors, assistant supervisors, and head nurses who are full or part time appointees.

(b) Special members upon election by the Faculty at any one of its regular meetings.

Article IV

Officers

Section 1. The officers shall be chairman, vice chairman, secretary-treasurer.

Section 2. The chairman shall be the director of the School of Nursing. The vice chairman and the secretary-treasurer shall be appointed annually by the Executive Committee.

Article V

Duties of Officers

Section 1. The duties of the officers shall be such as are implied by their respective titles and as herein set forth in the bylaws.

Section 2. The chairman shall preside at all meetings; shall have the power to call meetings; shall appoint all committees not otherwise provided for; shall be an ex officio member of each committee and shall, in case of tie, cast the deciding vote.

Section 3. The vice chairman shall carry all responsibilities of the chairman in her absence.

Section 4. The secretary-treasurer shall conduct, in general, the correspondence of the Faculty; shall keep the minutes of the meetings of the Faculty and submit them to the Faculty for correction and approval. She shall have custody of all records and papers belonging to the Faculty not otherwise provided for. She shall receive all moneys belonging to the Faculty and shall pay bills incurred by the Faculty as authorized by the chairman.

Article VI

Meetings

Section 1. The Faculty shall hold regular meetings, the time and place to be determined by the Executive Committee.

Section 2. Special meetings may be called at the discretion of the chairman.

Article VII

Dues

Section 1. The dues of each member of the Faculty shall be one dollar yearly, payable in October.

Section 2. New members appointed between October 1 and March 31 shall pay one dollar; new members appointed between April 1 and September 30 shall pay fifty cents.

Article VIII

Standing Committees

Section 1. There shall be thirteen standing committees.

Section 2. The standing committees shall be:

(a) Executive Committee.
(b) Committee on the Basic Curriculum.
(c) Committee on Graduate Studies.
(d) Committee on Admissions to the Basic Professional Program.

(e) Committee on Admissions to Programs for Graduate Nurses.
(f) Committee on Nursing Arts.
(g) Committee on Library, Publications, and Illustrative Material.
(h) Committee on Staff Education.
(i) Committee on Records and Grading.
(j) Committee on Residences.
(k) Committee on Student and Staff Health.
(l) Committee on Student and Staff Relationships.
(m) Committee on Revisions and Resolutions.

Section 3. Membership.

(a) The Executive Committee shall consist of the director of the School of Nursing, the associate and assistant directors and the director of residences.
(b) The other standing committees shall consist of not less than three members to be nominated and elected by the Executive Committee each year after the first fall meeting.

Section 4. Chairmen.

(a) The chairman of the Executive Committee shall be the director of the School of Nursing.
(b) The chairman of the Committee on the Basic Curriculum shall be the associate director of the School of Nursing.
(c) The chairman of the Committee on Nursing Arts shall be the assistant director in charge of instruction in nursing arts.
(d) All other chairmen of committees shall be nominated and elected by the Executive Committee each year after the first fall meeting.

Section. 5. Reports.

(a) The secretary of the Executive Committee shall present a written report of the activities of that committee at each monthly meeting.
(b) The chairmen of all other committees shall present a written annual report at the May meeting.
(c) A report may be called for from any committee by the chairman of the Faculty if she deems it timely or advisable.
(d) In the absence of the chairman of a committee another member of that committee shall give the report.

Article IX

Duties of Committees

Section 1. Executive Committee. The functions of this committee shall be to consider the policies and activities of the School and of the Nursing Service; to recommend to the Advisory Board of the School of Nursing or to appropriate committees of the Hospital and the Johns Hopkins University educational policies and such other matters as may be deemed desirable for the development of the School; to transact the general business within the approved and established policies; and to appoint standing and special committees as designated.

This committee shall have five subcommittees as follows:

(a) Subcommittee on Faculty Selection. This committee shall consist of the director of the School of Nursing, the associate directors, and the assistant director of the department for which the applicant is being considered for appointment. It shall review functions of and necessary qualifications for faculty members and recommend individuals for appointment.

(b) Subcommittees to Give Consideration to the Progress of Johns Hopkins Students.

(1) Subcommittee on the Progress of Students in the Preclinical Period.

(2) Subcommittee on the Progress of Students in the Clinical Period, Unit I.

(3) Subcommittee on the Progress of Students in the Clinical Period, Unit II.

The functions of these subcommittees shall be to consider the status of students within their respective groups, and to make necessary recommendations to the Executive Committee regarding their acceptability for the profession of nursing, for their promotion, and for their graduation.

(c) Subcommittee on Affiliations. The functions of this committee shall be to recommend the acceptability of agencies with which the School of Nursing may wish to affiliate and to study the performance of affiliating students.

Section 2. Committee on the Basic Curriculum. The functions of this committee shall be to study the basic curriculum and to plan and recommend a program of study in keeping with modern professional and educational policies.

Section 3. Committee on Graduate Studies. The functions of this committee shall be to consider matters relative to courses offered graduate students; to cooperate with the Johns Hopkins University in the promotion of programs of study for graduate nurses; and to make recommendations accordingly.

Section 4. Committees on Admissions.

(a) Committee on Admissions to the Basic Professional Program.

(b) Committee on Admissions to Programs for Graduate Nurses.

The functions of these committees shall be to study matriculation requirements for the basic professional course and for programs for graduate nurses, respectively, and to recommend policies in relation to these requirements to the Executive Committee; to examine qualifications of applicants; and to recommend them for admission or rejection to the director of the School.

Section 5. Committee on Nursing Arts. The functions of this committee shall be to review nursing principles and practices and to recommend changes to the Executive Committee. A Medical Advisory Committee appointed by the Medical Board shall confer with the committee and approve all major changes.

Section 6. Committee on Library, Publications, and Illustrative Material. The functions of this committee shall be to regulate activities of the library; to determine all accessions and subscriptions to current literature; and to arrange for the use of teaching aids.

Section 7. Committee on Staff Education. The functions of this committee shall be to plan such activities as may encourage individual professional development; to foster support of professional organizations through active participation; and to stimulate interest in original contributions to nursing.

Section 8. Committee on Records and Grading. The functions of this committee shall be to review current records and grading and to make recommendations for necessary changes; to set up new forms as the need arises; and to give guidance in the interpretation of the grading system and the use of records.

Section 9. Committee on Residences. The functions of this committee shall be to promote agreeable living arrangements and to recommend policies for the administration of the nurses' residences.

Section 10. Committee on Student and Staff Health. The functions of this committee shall be to consider policies and special problems relating to the health service for students and graduates and to assist in the interpretation of the policies of the health service and in the stimulation of interest in the promotion of health of the various groups.

Section 11. Committee on Student-Staff Relationships. The functions of this committee shall be to formulate and promote plans for student-staff relationships.

Section 12. Committee on Revisions and Resolutions. The functions of this committee shall be to consider and recommend to the Faculty any revision of these bylaws and to propose any resolutions deemed necessary.

Article X

Voting Body and Quorum

Section 1. The voting body shall consist of all active members of the Faculty.

Section 2. Two-thirds of the total number of active members shall constitute a quorum at any regular meeting of the Faculty.

Section 3. Two officers and ten active members shall constitute a quorum at any special meeting.

Article XI

Duties of Voting Body

Section 1. It shall be the duty of all members to be present at all Faculty meetings.

Section 2. It shall be the duty of a member, when it is impossible to be present at a meeting, to notify the secretary prior to the meeting.

Article XII

Roll Call

There shall be roll call at each regular meeting of the Faculty.

Article XIII

Amendments

The bylaws may be amended or repealed or new bylaws adopted at any meeting by a two-third vote of the active members present.

Article XIV

Order of Business

The order of business shall be:

(a) Call to order.
(b) Approval of the minutes.
(c) Reports of standing committees.
(d) Reports of special committees.
(e) Unfinished business.
(f) New business.
(g) Announcements and communications.
(h) Adjournment.

Original—June 1941

Revised—June 1942, April 1943, November 1944, November 1946, May 1948.

MEMBERSHIP OF THE CAMPAIGN ORGANIZATION IN 1921 FOR THE ENDOWMENT FUND OF THE SCHOOL OF NURSING

Executive Committee. M. Adelaide Nutting, chairman, Mrs. Isabella Stevens Hunner, vice chairman, Yssabella G. Waters, Mrs. Mary B. Dixon Cullen, Elsie M. Lawler, Effie J. Taylor

Advisory Council. Dr. Frank J. Goodnow, Judge Henry D. Harlan, Dr. William H. Welch, Dr. Winford H. Smith, Dr. Joseph S. Ames, Dr. Lewellys F. Barker, Dr. Hermann M. Biggs, Dr. Thomas S. Cullen, Dr. Livingston Farrand, Dr. John M. T. Finney, John M. Glenn, Dr. William S. Halsted, Dr. John Howland, Dr. Henry M. Hurd, Dr. William G. MacCallum, Dr. Adolf Meyer, Dr. William S. Thayer, Dr. J. Whitridge Williams

Secretary. Yssabella G. Waters

Treasurer. John C. Thomas, assistant treasurer, Mrs. Mary B. Dixon Cullen

Finance Committee. Mrs. Mary B. Dixon Cullen, chairman, Mrs. Helen Wilmer Athey, Elsie M. Lawler

Class Organization Committee. Helen H. Crawford, 1901, chairman, Mrs. Helen Wilmer Athey, Virginia L. McMaster (Mrs. J. R. Foard), 1896, Amy P. Miller, M. Hilda Miller, 1919, Mildred H. Bentley (Mrs. K. M. Wilson), 1912

Regional Committee. Elizabeth G. Fox, chairman

Publicity Committee. Mrs. Mary B. Dixon Cullen, chairman, Effie J. Taylor, secretary, Ada M. Carr, Mary E. Lent

Potential Donors Committee. Mary E. Lent, chairman

Alumnae General Committee. Mrs. Helen Wilmer Athey, Mary Carey (Mrs. F. H. Baetjer), 1902, Helen C. Bartlett, Mary C. Bean, Helen F. Boyd (later Mrs. A. Powell), 1915, Margaret S. Brogden, 1902, Mrs. Helen Hutchinson Caples, Emma E. Carter, 1907, Helen H. Crawford, Nancy P. Ellicott, Mrs. Dorothy Filler McBride, Alice Fitzgerald, 1906, Louisa Riggs (Mrs. R. H. Follis), 1902, Hester K. Frederick, Anna M. French, 1896, Mary A. Goldthwaite, 1916, Mrs. Agnes C. Hartridge, Alice M. Hillman (Mrs. W. L. Sanders), 1921, Helen T. Holliday (Mrs. J. R. Lehman), 1909, Anna C. Jammé, Mary E. Lent, Amy P. Miller, Angela R. Mitchell (Mrs. G. S. Shipley), 1918, Martha C. Perkins (Mrs. J. D. Norris), 1897, Clara D. Noyes, Evelyn Oliver, 1903, Katherine M. Olmsted, 1912, Florence M. Patterson, Mary E. Shearn, 1895, Annah Winn, 1897, Anna D. Wolf.

Women's Committee. Mrs. William Bauernschmidt, Mrs. Edward F. Buchner, Mrs. Benjamin W. Cochran, Dr. Claribel Cone, Mrs. Charles E. Ellicott, Mrs. Thomas B. Futcher, Elizabeth Gilman, Mrs. Frank J. Goodnow, Mrs. William W. Guth, Mrs. Frank S. Hambleton, Mrs. Louis P. Hamburger, Mrs. Henry D. Harlan, Mrs. Donald R. Hooker, Lady Arthur Newsholm, Lady William Osler, Dr. Florence Sabin, Dr. Mary Sherwood, Mrs. Edward Shoemaker, Mrs. Winford H. Smith, Mrs. Knox Taylor

A Note on Sources

At Johns Hopkins the credo from the first days was, "Observe, record, tabulate, communicate." Daniel C. Gilman, president of the University, who administered the Hospital a few months before the arrival of Dr. Hurd, established the precedent of writing explicit annual reports of the University and publishing in the *Circular of Information* full details of the programs offered and other pertinent University matter. The Hospital Trustees authorized the publication of the *Johns Hopkins Bulletin* in September 1889 and the following month, the *Johns Hopkins Hospital Reports.*

The School of Nursing was thus begun in an atmosphere where recording and communicating were established as inherent to well-ordered administration and public relations. Miss Parsons, who directed the Nursing Department prior to Miss Hampton's arrival, rendered a report for each month between May and October 1889. Needless to say Miss Hampton at once began using her "own pen." Monthly reports were continued and each year a comprehensive account of the Nursing Department, describing fully the developments both in the School and the nursing service, was submitted to the superintendent of the Hospital. The School reports were meticulously written in longhand until January 1906 and are fine examples of a period when writing by hand was an art.

The earliest reports of the head of the School and of the administrator of the Hospital include the outlines of all courses given in the Training School curriculum. The School reports also give course examination questions and the grade made in each course by each student. The *Day Book* records in chronological sequence the experience of each student from the day she entered the School until the day she completed her course. It is possible to compile for every student admitted to the School of Nursing a transcript of the courses she had and the grades she made in them. Not only reports and records but the applications of all candidates for admission and the correspondence between them and the School have been preserved.

The first *Circular of Information* was published in the first number of the *Johns Hopkins Hospital Bulletin*, December 1889, less than three months after the School of Nursing was inaugurated. One copy of the first *Circular* in four-page pamphlet form is fortunately on file in the School office. Historically this bulletin is priceless. It describes the requirements for admission when the School was established, gives the length of the program, and discusses the conditions under which the School then operated.

Other documents in the School files are reports of studies of the School made by a member of the nursing staff or an outside agency; committee reports; minutes; correspondence; and newspaper clippings, which often provide dramatic accounts of some episode in the School's history. There are bulletins and leaflets dating back to the Nineties on public health and other movements related to nursing. The library accession books make it possible to reconstruct the library content from the early days of the School. The old oak bookcase in the Main Residence Hall, given to the School by the Teresians at the beginning of the century, ceases to be a mute piece of furniture and becomes historically eloquent as a symbol of interest and concern in the proper facilities for the housing of the growing library. Many people, who have lived through significant periods in the history of the School, are rich reservoirs of information. They have generously helped when interviewed by the authors to fill in and interpret events. To these men and women and to all whose foresight and wisdom made possible the wealth of material on the founding and the growth of the School of Nursing, the authors are deeply indebted. History cannot be written without records in some form—the spoken word, the written word, an old chair or a bookcase, a picture or a photograph; these are the bricks out of which the past is rebuilt and made to live again.

Following are the main sources which have contributed to this historical narrative.

Accession Books, Library, 1900–12; 1922–49

No accession records on file for period between 1912–21.

American Journal of Nursing, 1–49, 1900–49

Chesney, Alan M. *The Johns Hopkins Hospital and the Johns Hopkins University School of Medicine.* Vol. 1, 1867–1893. Baltimore, Johns Hopkins Press, 1943

Circulars of Information, Johns Hopkins Hospital Training School for Nurses,[1] *1889, 1896, 1901 to 1949–50*

No *Circular* was published for the school year 1945–46. Other periods for which *Circulars* are not on file: 1923, 1933–34, 1934–35.

Constitution and Bylaws of the Alumnae Association of the Johns Hopkins Hospital Training School for Nurses of Baltimore City.

Original Certificate of Incorporation dated December 6, 1892. In 1933 the legal name of the Association was changed to "The Johns Hopkins Hospital Nurses' Alumnae Association, Incorporated."

Dome, The

Student Handbook prepared by the Student Association of the Johns Hopkins Hospital School of Nursing.

French, John C. *A History of the University Founded by Johns Hopkins.* Baltimore, Johns Hopkins Press, 1946

Interviews by Authors

With graduates of the School of Nursing, ex-director of Hospital, and others.

Johns Hopkins Hospital, 1889–1939: A Brief Account of Its Founding and of Its Achievements during the First Fifty Years of Its Existence. Baltimore, Press of Schneidereith and Sons, n.d.

Johns Hopkins Nurses Alumnae Magazine, 1–48, 1901–49

Letters in School Archives

These relate to transactions and special episodes in the life of the School.

Minutes of Advisory Board of School of Nursing, 1930–49

The first meeting was held October 1930, four meetings held in 1931, and from six to eight during each of the next four years. After 1935 four regular meetings were held annually.

Minutes of Executive Committee of Faculty, School of Nursing, 1941–49

Regular meetings held weekly, September through June.

Minutes of Faculty, School of Nursing, 1941–49

Regular meetings held monthly, September through May.

Minutes of the Society of the Teresians, 1905–25

Pamphlets, Bulletins, and Newspaper Clippings

These materials date back to the Nineties.

Reports of the American Society of Superintendents of Training Schools for Nurses, Annual, 1894–1949

First and second convention reports not published until 1897. Name of organization changed at the 1912 convention to "National League of Nursing Education."

Reports of Committees of Advisory Board of School of Nursing, 1931–49

Reports of Committees of the Alumnae Association of the Johns Hopkins Hospital Training School for Nurses, 1895–1949

[1] First officially referred to as "Johns Hopkins Hospital School of Nursing" in 1935.

While the first committee report found is in the report of the third annual meeting in 1895, reference is made to the report of a "Publishing Committee" at the first annual meeting in 1893. The reports of the Endowment Fund Committee provided the bulk of the information on the work of that committee.

Reports of Committees of Johns Hopkins Hospital Training School for Nurses

The appointment of administrative committees and committees for educational projects began during the first half of the life of the School. Many of these reports contain valuable historical information. After the faculty was organized in 1941, standing committees of the faculty were designated.

Reports of Department of Instruction, Annual, 1923–24 to 1941–42

No report for 1924–25 on file.

Reports of Superintendent of the Hospital,[2] *Annual, 1890–1949*

The first report is for eight and one-half months, from May 15, 1889, date of opening of Hospital, to January 31, 1890.

Reports of Superintendent of Nurses and Principal of the Training School[3] *to Advisory Board of the School, 1930–49*

These reports were submitted irregularly until 1941; thereafter the director of the School of Nursing and nursing service submitted a report at all regular meetings.

Reports of Superintendent of Nurses and Principal of the Training School, Annual, to the Superintendent of the Hospital, 1890–1949

First report for eight and one-half months, May 15, 1889 to January 31, 1890.

Reports of Superintendent of Nurses and Principal of the Training School, Monthly, to the Superintendent of Hospital, 1889–1949

The first report is dated May 1889. There are few months for which reports are not on file during the sixty years of the School's existence. In 1908 the practice began of including the reports for the summer months in either the September or October report.

Reports and Minutes of Regular and Special Meetings of the Alumnae Association of the Johns Hopkins Hospital Training School for Nurses, 1892–1949

Student Applications and Correspondence with School, 1889–1949

Student Assignment Records, 1889–1949

Sunpapers of Baltimore

[2] Title changed to "Director of Hospital," Dec. 1920.

[3] Title changed to "Director of School of Nursing and Nursing Service," Nov. 1940.

Index

Frances Butler
Ruth Brewster Sherman.